Handbook of
Targeted Cancer Therapy and Immunotherapy

THIRD EDITION

Handbook of
Targeted Cancer Therapy and Immunotherapy

THIRD EDITION

Editors

Daniel D. Karp, MD

Professor of Medicine
Department of Investigational
  Cancer Therapeutics
Principal Investigator of the
  MD Anderson Clinical &
  Translational Science
  Award (CTSA)
The University of Texas MD
  Anderson Cancer Center
Houston, Texas

Gerald S. Falchook, MD, MS

Director
Drug Development Unit
Sarah Cannon Research Institute
  at HealthONE
Presbyterian/St. Luke's Medical
  Center
Denver, Colorado

JoAnn D. Lim, PharmD, BCOP

Clinical Pharmacy Specialist,
  Phase I
Division of Pharmacy
Department of Investigational
  Cancer Therapeutics
The University of Texas MD
  Anderson Cancer Center
Houston, Texas

Managing Editor

Jackie Bronicki, MLIS, CCRA

Grant Program Manager
Investigat onal Cancer
  Therapeutics
The University of Texas MD
  Anderson Cancer Center
Houston, Texas

Wolters Kluwer

Philadelphia • Baltimore • New York • London
Buenos Aires • Hong Kong • Sydney • Tokyo

Acquisitions Editor: Nicole Dernoski
Development Editor: Thomas Celona
Editorial Coordinator: Priyanka Alagar
Marketing Manager: Kirsten Watrud
Production Project Manager: Catherine Ott
Manager of Graphic Arts and Design: Steve Druding
Manufacturing Coordinator: Beth Welsh
Prepress Vendor: S4Carlisle Publishing Services

Third edition

9 8 7 6 5 4 3 2 1

Printed in Singapore

Library of Congress Cataloging-in-Publication Data

ISBN-13: 978-1-975179-24-3

Cataloging in Publication data available on request from publisher.

MKO322

Contributors

Ahmed Abdelhakeem, MD
The University of Texas MD Anderson Cancer Center

Kavitha Balaji, PhD
AstraZeneca

Sarah Baldwin, RN, ANP-BC, BSN, MSN
The University of Texas MD Anderson Cancer Center

Tamara G. Barnes, RN, MSN, CNS, AOCNS
The University of Texas MD Anderson Cancer Center

Laura Beatty, PA-C
The University of Texas MD Anderson Cancer Center

Prajwal C. Boddu, MD
Yale School of Medicine

Lindsay Gaido Bramwell, MSN, RN, ACNS-BC
Flatiron Health

Sara Eresser, MPAS, PA-C
The University of Texas MD Anderson Cancer Center

Amanda Brink, DNP, APRN, FNP-BC, AOCNP
The University of Texas MD Anderson Cancer Center

Manojkumar Bupathi, MD, MS
Rocky Mountain Cancer Centers
Sarah Cannon Research Institute at HealthONE

Maria E. Cabanillas, MD
The University of Texas MD Anderson Cancer Center

Isabel Cepeda, MSN, RN, AGN-P
The University of Texas MD Anderson Cancer Center

Niamh Coleman, MBBCH, BAO, PhD
The University of Texas MD Anderson Cancer Center

Anthony Conley, MD
The University of Texas MD Anderson Cancer Center

Senthil Damodaran, MD, PhD
The University of Texas MD Anderson Cancer Center

Ecaterina Dumbrava, MD
The University of Texas MD Anderson Cancer Center

Gerald S. Falchook, MD, MS
Sarah Cannon Research Institute at HealthONE

Renata Ferrarotto, MD
The University of Texas MD Anderson Cancer Center

Siqing Fu, MD, PhD
The University of Texas MD Anderson Cancer Center

Goldy C. George, PhD
The University of Texas MD Anderson Cancer Center

Sangeeta Goswami, MD, PhD
The University of Texas MD Anderson Cancer Center

Roman Groisberg, MD
Rutgers Cancer Institute of New Jersey

Mouhammed A. Habra, MD
The University of Texas MD Anderson Cancer Center

Laura L. Holman, MD, MS
The University of Oklahoma College of Medicine

David S. Hong, MD
The University of Texas MD Anderson Cancer Center

Filip Janku, MD, PhD
The University of Texas MD Anderson Cancer Center

Milind Javle, MD
The University of Texas MD Anderson Cancer Center

Tapan M. Kadia, MD
The University of Texas MD Anderson Cancer Center

Radhika Kainthla, MD
The University of Texas MD Anderson Cancer Center

Daniel D. Karp, MD
The University of Texas MD Anderson Cancer Center

Ahmed O. Kaseb, MD
The University of Texas MD Anderson Cancer Center

Gregory Kaufman, MD
The University of Texas MD Anderson Cancer Center

Maliha Khan, MD
The University of Texas MD Anderson Cancer Center

Ed Kheder, MD
The University of Texas MD Anderson Cancer Center

Holly Kinahan, RN, MSN, NP-C, AOCNP
The University of Texas MD Anderson Cancer Center

E. Scott Kopetz, MD, PhD
The University of Texas MD Anderson Cancer Center

JoAnn D. Lim, PharmD, BCOP
The University of Texas MD Anderson Cancer Center

Xiaochun Liu, MD, PhD
Bristol-Myers Squibb

Kathrina Marcelo-Lewis, PhD
The University of Texas MD Anderson Cancer Center

Erminia Massarelli, MD, PhD, MS
City of Hope

Hossein Maymani, MD
Rocky Mountain Cancer Centers

Meredith A. McKean, MD, MPH
Sarah Cannon Research Institute at HealthONE

Sandra Montez, RN
The University of Texas MD Anderson Cancer Center

Shyamm Moorthy, PhD
The University of Texas MD Anderson Cancer Center

Justin Moyers, MD
The University of Texas MD Anderson Cancer Center
University of California, Irvine College of Medicine

Mariela B. Murphy, MD
The University of Texas MD Anderson Cancer Center

Aung Naing, MD
The University of Texas MD Anderson Cancer Center

Robert Orlowski, MD, PhD
The University of Texas MD Anderson Cancer Center

Lance C. Pagliaro, MD
Mayo Clinic

Shubham Pant, MD
The University of Texas MD Anderson Cancer Center

Amy B. Patel, MPAS, PA-C
The University of Texas MD Anderson Cancer Center

Michael Pearlman, MD, PhD
Blue Sky Neurology
Sarah Cannon Research Institute at HealthONE

Naveen Pemmaraju, MD
The University of Texas MD Anderson Cancer Center

Allan A. L. Pereira, MD, PhD
Instituto Hospital de Base

Sarina A. Piha-Paul, MD, MS
The University of Texas MD Anderson Cancer Center

Patrick Pilie, MD
The University of Texas MD Anderson
Cancer Center

Matthew J. Reilley, MD
University of Virginia

Jordi Rodon-Ahnert, MD, PhD
The University of Texas MD Anderson Cancer Center

Jason Roszik, MBA, PhD
The University of Texas MD Anderson Cancer Center

Shiraj Sen, MD, PhD

Arlene O. Siefker-Radtke, MD
The University of Texas MD Anderson Cancer Center

Raphael Steiner, MD
The University of Texas MD Anderson Cancer Center

Ana Stuckett, PhD
The University of Texas MD Anderson Cancer Center

Vivek Subbiah, MD
The University of Texas MD Anderson Cancer Center

Nizar M. Tannir, MD, FACP
The University of Texas MD Anderson Cancer Center

Debu Tripathy, MD
The University of Texas MD Anderson Cancer Center

Gabriele Urschel, DNP, RN, FNP-C, AOCNP
The University of Texas MD Anderson Cancer Center

viii

Jason R. Westin, MD, MS, FACP
The University of Texas MD Anderson
Cancer Center

Shannon N. Westin, MD, MPH
The University of Texas MD Anderson Cancer Center

Michael K. K. Wong, MD, PhD
The University of Texas MD Anderson Cancer Center

Scott E. Woodman, MD, PhD
The University of Texas MD Anderson Cancer Center

Ralph G. Zinner, MD
University of Kentucky College of Medicine

Preface

The exponential growth of oncology drug development and personalized/targeted therapy in recent years has presented a challenge to even the most experienced cancer researchers. Many of us struggle to keep up with the hundreds of clinical trials conducted each year. To help with this challenge, we have made major updates in this third edition of our concise handbook. Our goal is to make the results of clinical trials of targeted cancer treatments and immunotherapy more easily accessible to cancer researchers and clinicians. We are very proud of the reception the first and second editions have received from oncologists, medical staff, students, and even patients, and we are excited about the updated and widely expanded content included in this third edition.

As medical oncologists conducting clinical trials in large phase I cancer center departments, we have had the privilege of observing oncology drug development from a unique perspective. We work at the intersection between exciting preclinical discoveries and the clinical realities of first-in-human clinical trials. This book was conceived with a broad audience in mind. It is our hope that this book will find use among academic oncologists, community oncologists, lab scientists, pharmacists, nurses, residents, clinical fellows, midlevel providers, postdoctoral fellows, and the numerous other staff who are essential for clinical and translational cancer research. Indeed, some motivated patients or family members may even find this book helpful in their quest to identify the most promising cancer treatments available.

We approach this book primarily from the viewpoint of clinician investigators. We have focused on agents for which clinical data are available, either published or publicly presented at a national meeting. We did not have the space in this work to mention the many clinical trials for which results were not yet available at the time these pages were sent to press, and we apologize in advance to anyone who is surprised or offended to discover that their favorite agent was not included. Furthermore, we expect that by the time this work is available for purchase, results of ongoing clinical trials will have become available and could significantly alter various aspects of the therapeutic landscape.

Importantly, this collection is a handbook, not a textbook. Our goal was to create a publication that was small enough to fit comfortably into a lab coat pocket so that it may be easily accessible for reference in the clinic. To our knowledge, there is not another book available with the scope of this work in such a concise format.

The book is divided into four core sections. Please note that throughout the book we have used color-coding to produce an intuitive organizational framework. For example, in Section 1, Food and Drug Administration (FDA)-approved agents are highlighted in green; in Section 3, we have categorized and color-coded what we call the signaling "families" (mTOR, MAP Kinase, SRC, JAK-STAT, etc.). In Section 4, FDA-approved drugs are still in green, whereas those in early phase are in orange and late-phase development are in blue. To conserve pages, the references have been abbreviated in the print book but appear in full form in the companion ebook.

The first section, Targets by Organ Site, contains the "secret sauce" of our publication. Organized by tumor type and molecular target, this section provides a concise description of clinical experience with various targeted agents and immunotherapies in an easy-to-read table format. Each organ site includes tabular information on common molecular alterations observed and targeted therapies that have shown efficacy. Although our book does not have a traditional textbook format, we include the second section, Carcinogenesis from the Perspective of Targeted Therapy and Immunotherapy, as a primer for cancer researchers. We have built on Hanahan and Weinberg's Hallmarks of Cancer, which we consider to be a seminal work. As clinicians, we have added our own clinical flavor to their observations.

If the medication section describes the many different vehicles on the cancer treatment highway, then the third section, Molecular Targets and Pathways, is a roadmap each vehicle is designed to travel. The numerous cellular pathways involved in cancer survival and proliferation are arranged functionally, with emphasis on actionable molecular targets. Understanding each of these pathways gives context and rationale for modern cancer drug development. In the fourth section, Targeted and Immunotherapy Agents, the more than 270 drugs reflect the rapid acceleration of drug development in "precision oncology." For the sake of conciseness, we have chosen the most immediately relevant information that most clinicians and researchers would want to know. Mechanism of action, dosing schedule, FDA approval and/or clinical trial investigations, and common toxicities are listed for each agent.

For historical context, we are mindful that effective systemic treatments for cancer were first introduced less than 80 years ago. In spite of the gains in recent years, there is still much need for improvement. Success in drug development is still typically measured in months, not years, of life extended. It is our hope that, in addition to its use in the clinic, this book will facilitate new discoveries that result in better treatments for our patients.

Daniel D. Karp
Gerald S. Falchook
JoAnn D. Lim

Acknowledgments

We would like to acknowledge and thank the many people who made the third edition of this book possible. In particular, we would like to express our appreciation to the dedicated coauthors of each individual subsection. We are truly grateful for their willingness to share their knowledge and insights within the pages of this compilation. We would also like to thank the many individuals who have inspired and supported us in so many ways, including the senior leadership at MD Anderson and Sarah Cannon, as well as our colleagues at Wolters Kluwer Health, Thomas Celona and Nicole Dernoski. We are extremely appreciative of our spouses and families, who have always been so supportive but who have been especially understanding and encouraging during this project. We also would like to express our sincere gratitude to Leonard and Norma Forey, whose ongoing support and encouragement has been instrumental to the success of our third edition. Even though we lost Norma in 2019, we feel her spirit and support continue to improve our efforts. Finally, we want to recognize Jackie Bronicki for the enormous amount of work she performed in making the third edition a reality.

Above all, we would like to thank our brave patients and their supportive families, to whom this book is dedicated.

Contents

SECTION 1 Targets by Organ Site 1
Gerald S. Falchook, Editor

SECTION 2 Carcinogenesis from the Perspective of Targeted Therapy and Immunotherapy 160

Daniel D. Karp

SECTION 3 Molecular Targets and Pathways 229

Ecaterina Dumbrava and Jordi Rodon-Ahnert, Editors
Kavitha Balaji, Ecaterina Dumbrava, Roman Groisberg,
Filip Janku, Daniel D. Karp, Ed Kheder, Kathrina Marcelo-Lewis,
Hossein Maymani, Sandra Montez, Shyamm Moorthy, Patrick Pilie,
Matthew J. Reilley, Jordi Rodon-Ahnert, Shiraj Sen, Ana Stuckett,
Contributors

SECTION 4 Targeted and Immunotherapy Agents 336

JoAnn D. Lim and Justin Moyers, Editors

*Sarah Baldwin, Tamara G. Barnes, Laura Beatty, Sara Bresser,
Amanda Brink, Isabel Cepeda, Lindsay Gaido Bramwell,
Holly Kinahan, JoAnn D. Lim, Justin Moyers, Amy B. Patel,
Gabriele Urschel, Contributors*

Targets by Organ Site

Color Key

 Green FDA-approved agents for tumor type

 Black agents not yet approved by the FDA

- CBR: clinical benefit rate (CR + PR + SD)
- CR: complete response
- d: days
- DOR: duration of response
- HR: heart rate
- mo: month
- mTOR: mechanistic target of rapamycin
- N/A: not applicable
- ND: newly diagnosed
- ORR: overall response rate
- OS: overall survival
- PFS: progression-free survival
- PR: partial response
- Pts, pt: patients, patient
- RFS: relapse-free survival
- RR: response rate (PR + CR)
- RT: radiation treatment
- SD: stable disease
- TTP: time to progression
- wk, wks: week, weeks
- WT: wild-type
- yr: year

Adrenocortical Carcinoma (ACC)

Actionable Target	Abnormality	Prevalence (%)	Clinical Experience with Targeted Agent
BRAF	Mutation	3	**Sorafenib** (VEGFR/RAF inhibitor): • Phase 2, with **paclitaxel**: RR 0% (1)
EGFR	Mutation/overexpression	4	**Erlotinib** (EGFR inhibitor): • Phase 2, with **gemcitabine**: RR 10% (2)
IGF-2	Overexpression	60–90	**Cixutumumab** (IGF-1R inhibitor): • Phase 1, with **temsirolimus**: Durable SD 40% (3) **Linsitinib** (IGF-1R inhibitor): • Phase 3: no effect on survival compared to placebo (4)
MET	Overexpression	Unknown	**Cabozantinib**: Retrospective cohort. RR 19% (5,6)
PD-1/PD-L1	Expression	PD-L1: 11% (7)	**Pembrolizumab**: RR 14%–23% (7–9)

Actionable Target	Abnormality	Prevalence (%)	Clinical Experience with Targeted Agent
NTRK	Fusion		**Entrectinib** (FDA approved 2019) (TRK inhibitor): • Phase 1/2 (STARTRK-2, STARTRK-1, ALKA-372-001): ORR 57% across all tumor types (95% CI 43–71), including a 7% complete response rate (1) **Larotrectinib** (FDA approved 2018) (TRK inhibitor): • Phase 1/2: ORR 79%, CR 24 pts, PR 97 pts, SD 19 pts (2)
PD-1/PD-L1	MSI-H or dMMR pts		**Dostarlimab-gxly** (PD-1 inhibitor) (FDA approved 2021): • Phase 1: ORR 41.6%, CR 9.17%, 32.5% PR, DOR 34.7 mo (95.4% with duration ≥6 mo) (3) **Pembrolizumab** (PD-1 inhibitor) (FDA approved 2018): • Phase 2 (KEYNOTE-158): ORR 34.3% pts, DOR ≥24 mo 77.6%, PFS 4.1 mo, OS 23.5 mo (4)

Biliary Tract Adenocarcinoma (Gallbladder, Bile Duct, Cholangiocarcinoma)

Actionable Target	Abnormality	Prevalence	Clinical Experience with Targeted Agent
BRAF	Mutation	5%	**Selumetinib** (MEK 1/2 inhibitor): • Phase 2: RR 12% (3 pts had confirmed PRs, including 1 pt with unconfirmed CR) (1) **Dabrafenib + Trametinib** (BRAF inh + MEK inh): • Phase 2: ORR 47% (independent reviewer assessed) in patients with BRAF V600E-mutated biliary tract cancer (2)
FGFR2 fusions	FGFR2-BICC1 and several other fusions	10%–15% of IHCCA	**Infigratinib** (FGFR inhibitor): • Phase 2: RR 15%, disease control rate (ORR + SD) 75%, PFS 25 wk. Among 61 pts, most had *FGFR2* alterations, including translocation (n = 48), mutation (n = 8), and amplification (n = 3) (3). **Pemigatinib**: • Phase 2: ORR of 35.5% in patients with FGFR2 fusions or rearrangements (4) **Futibatinib** (**TAS-120**) (FGFR1-4 inhibitor): • Phase 2 FOENIX CCA2: ORR of 25% in cholangiocarcinoma patients with FGFR2 fusions (5) **Derazantinib**: • Phase 1/2: ORR 20.7%; PFS 5.7 OS in patients with unresectable intrahepatic cholangiocarcinoma with FGFR2 fusion (6)

Actionable Target	Abnormality	Prevalence	Clinical Experience with Targeted Agent
HER2/neu	Amplification	4%	**Trastuzumab** (anti-HER2 antibody): • Phase 2, with **pertuzumab** (anti-HER2 dimerization inhibitor): 4 PRs, 3 SD >4 mo, out of 11 pts with HER2+ biliary cancer (HER2-amplified/overexpressed, n = 8; HER2-mutated, n = 3 [D277Y, S310F, and A775-G776insYVMA]) (7) **Zanidatamab (ZW25)** (bispecific HER2-antibody): • Phase 1: 47% ORR; mDOR 6.6 mo in HER2-overexpressing biliary tract carcinoma patients (8) **Neratinib** (mutations): • Phase 2 SUMMIT trial: ORR 10.5%; CBR 31.6%; PFS 1.8 mo in HER2-mutant biliary tract cancer patients (9)
IDH1	R132 mutation	20% of IHCCA	**Ivosidenib** (IDH1 inhibitor): • Phase 1 trial, for IDH1R132 mutant pts: OS 10.8 mo (vs. 9.7 OS with placebo); PFS 2.7 OS (placebo at 1.4 OS) (10)

(*continued*)

Actionable Target	Abnormality	Prevalence	Clinical Experience with Targeted Agent
NTRK	Fusion		**Entrectinib** (TRK inhibitor): • Phase 1/2 (STARTRK-2, STARTRK-1, ALKA-372-001): ORR 57% across all tumor types (95% CI 43–71), including a 7% complete response rate (11) **Larotrectinib** (TRK inhibitor): • Phase 1/2: ORR 79% in all tumor types, CR 24 pts, PR 97 pts, SD 19 pts. RR 50% in cholangiocarcinoma cancer pts (12)
PD-1			**Nivolumab** (anti-PD-1): • Phase 2: ORR of 22%; PFS 3.7 mo, OS 14.2 mo (13) **Ipilimumab + Nivolumab**: • Phase 2 subgroup analysis: ORR 23% in patients with advanced biliary tract cancers (14) **Bintrafusp alfa (M7824)** (bifunctional fusion protein of anti-PD-L1 +TGF-beta RII): • Phase 1: ORR 20%; PFS 2.5 OS; OS 12.7 mo in patients with pretreated biliary tract cancer (15)
PD-L1/CTLA4			**Durvalumab monotherapy or in combination with Tremelimumab (+Cisplatin/Gemcitabine)**: • Phase 2: ORRs 73.4% for Durvalumab alone; 73.3% for Durvalumab + Tremelimumab (16)

Actionable Target	Abnormality	Prevalence (%)	Clinical Experience with Targeted Agent
CTLA-4	Expression	Present	**Ipilimumab + Nivolumab:** • Phase 2: RR 38%, OS 15.3 mo (1)
FGFR3	Mutation	20	**For second-line, selected FGFR3 and FGFR2 alterations and fusions:** Erdafitinib (FGFR3 inhibitor): • Phase 2: RR 40%; OS 13.8 mo (2)
Her-2	Expression	~30	**RC48-ADC** (antibody–drug conjugate): • Phase 2: RR 60% (3)
IL-2/CD122	Expression, present on immune cells to stimulate clonal expansion of tumor-infiltrating immune cells	Present	**Bempegaldesleukin** (cytokine signaling): • Phase 2: RR 48% (4)
Nectin-4	Expression	94	**For third-line treatment:** Enfortumab Vedotin (antibody–drug conjugate): • Phase 2: RR 41%, OS 12.8 mo (5)

(continued)

Actionable Target	Abnormality	Prevalence (%)	Clinical Experience with Targeted Agent
PD-1/PD-L1	PD-L1 expression only needed for front-line therapy	Variable	**For front-line, maintenance, platinum eligible:** **Avelumab** (PD-L1 inhibitor): • Phase 3, pts in CR, PD, or SD, OS 21.4 mo (6) **For front-line, cisplatin-ineligible and PD-L1 high, or platinum ineligible:** **Pembrolizumab** (PD-1 inhibitor): • Phase 2: RR 28.6%, OS 11.3 mo (7) **Atezolizumab** (PD-L1 inhibitor): • Phase 2: RR 23%, OS 15.9 mo (8) **For second-line, platinum failures:** **Pembrolizumab** (PD-1 inhibitor): • Phase 3: RR 21.1%, OS 10.3 mo (9) **Nivolumab** (PD-1 inhibitor): • Phase 2: RR 19.6%, OS 8.7 mo (10)
Trop-2	Expression	83	**Sacituzumab Govitecan** (antibody–drug conjugate): • Phase 2: RR 27%, 77% had decrease in measurable disease. DoR 7.2 mo, PFS 5.4 mo, OS 10.9 mo (11)

Actionable Target	Abnormality	Prevalence (%)	Clinical Experience with Targeted Agent
Biallelic mismatch repair deficiency (bMMRD)	Mutation	Unknown	**Nivolumab** (PD-1 inhibitor): • bMMRD is caused by homozygous germline mutations in 1 of the 4 MMR genes (*PMS2*, *MLH1*, *MSH2*, and *MSH6*) and is arguably the most penetrant cancer predisposition syndrome with 100% of biallelic mutation carriers developing cancers in the first 2 decades of life (1). • Durable responses of recurrent GBM to immune checkpoint inhibition (1)
BRAF V600	Mutation	N/A	**Dabrafenib** (BRAF inhibitor) + **Trametinib** (MEK inhibitor): • Phase 2, high-grade glioma (HGG): ORR 33% (3 CR, 12 PR); median DOR 36.9 mo (95% CI, 7.4–44.2). PFS and OS 3.8 mo (95% CI, 1.8–9.2) and 17.6 mo (95% CI, 9.5–45.2), respectively (2) • Phase 2, low-grade glioma (LGG): ORR 69% (1 CR, 6 PR, 2 MR); DOR, PFS, and OS not reached (2) **Vemurafenib** (BRAF inhibitor): • Open-label/multicohort: ORR 25% (95% CI, 10%–47%), PFS 5.5 mo (95% CI, 3.7–9.6 mo) (3)

(continued)

Actionable Target	Abnormality	Prevalence (%)	Clinical Experience with Targeted Agent
Cytosine deaminase	N/A	N/A	**Vocimagene Amiretrorepvec (Toca511)** (retroviral replicating vector): • Phase 1, with **5-fluorocytosine**: OS 13.6 mo, statistically improved relative to external control (HR 0.45, $p = 0.003$) (4)
EGFR	Amplification and/or mutation	57.4	**ABT-414** (EGFR antibody–drug conjugate with anti-microtubule agent monomethyl auristatin F): • Phase 1: PFS 6.1 mo (5) **Erlotinib** (EGFR inhibitor): • Phase 2, with temozolomide and RT (ND): PFS 8 mo, OS 19.3 mo (6) **Gefitinib** (EGFR inhibitor): • Phase 2, combination with RT (ND pediatric): PFS at 1 yr 21%, OS at 1 yr 57% (7) **Vandetanib** (VEGFR/EGFR/RET inhibitor): • Phase 1, with RT (ND): SD 90%, PFS 8 mo, OS 11 mo (8) • Phase 1/2, with RT (recurrent disease): PFS 3 mo, OS 6 mo (9)
	Amplification/ overexpression	40	
	Mutation	6	
FGFR	Mutation	N/A	**Debio1347** (FGFR inhibitor): • Phase 1 expanded access in 4 pediatric pts: 2 PR, 2 SD (10)

Actionable Target	Abnormality	Prevalence (%)	Clinical Experience with Targeted Agent
IDH1	Mutation	Unknown	**AG-120** (IDH1 inhibitor): • Phase 1: 10 out of 20 pts with IDH1 mutant–positive glioma had SD, with 4 maintained beyond 5 mo (11) **IDH1 Peptide Vaccine:** • Phase 1 in IDH1R132H mutant Grade 3 and 4 gliomas: Vaccine-induced immune responses were observed in 93.3% of pts across multiple MHC alleles. 3 yr PFR and DFR 63% and 84%, respectively (12) **Ivosidenib** (IDH1 inhibitor): 35 pts w/ nonenhancing glioma: ORR 2.9%, PFS 13.6 mo, 1 PR, 30 SD; 31 pts w/ enhancing glioma: PFS 1.4 mo, 14 SD (13)
IL13Rα2	Expression	Unknown	**Chimeric antigen receptor (CAR)–engineered T cells targeting the tumor-associated antigen interleukin-13 receptor alpha 2 (IL13Rα2):** • Case report: After CAR T-cell treatment, regression of all intracranial and spinal tumors was observed, along with corresponding increases in levels of cytokines and immune cells in the cerebrospinal fluid. This clinical response continued for 7.5 mo after the initiation of CAR T-cell therapy (14).

(*continued*)

Actionable Target	Abnormality	Prevalence (%)	Clinical Experience with Targeted Agent
MGMT	Methylation	45	• Methylation of promoter region of gene in tumors associated with superior responses to temozolomide, OS 21.7 vs. 15.3 mo (15)
NTRK	Fusion		**Entrectinib** (FDA approved 2019) (TRK inhibitor): • Phase 1/2 (STARTRK-2, STARTRK-1, ALKA-372-001): ORR 57% across all tumor types (95% CI 43–71), including a 7% complete response rate (16) **Larotrectinib** (FDA approved 2018) (TRK inhibitor): • Phase 1/2: ORR 79%, CR 24 pts, PR 97 pts, SD 19 pts (17)
PDGFR	Overexpression	Unknown	**Imatinib** (BCR-Abl/cKIT/PDGFR inhibitor): • Phase 2 (advanced disease): RR 3.4%, SD 19%, OS 26 wk (with hydroxyurea) (18) **Sunitinib** (VEGFR/PDGFR/RET/KIT/FLT3 inhibitor): • Phase 2 (recurrent disease): No objective responses (19)

(*continued*)

Actionable Target	Abnormality	Prevalence (%)	Clinical Experience with Targeted Agent
PIK3CA	Mutation	5	**Temsirolimus** (mTOR inhibitor): • Phase 1, with **temozolomide and RT** (ND): ORR 4%, SD 96% (median follow-up of 10 mo) (20)
PIK3R1	Mutation	4	
PTEN	Mutation/deletions	17	**Everolimus** (mTOR inhibitor): • Phase 1, with **temozolomide and RT** (ND): ORR 6%, SD 83% (after 6 mo) (21)
POLE	Mutation	Unknown	**Pembrolizumab** (PD-1 inhibitor): • Case report: Germline DNA mismatch repair deficiency and tested positive for a *POLE* mutation encoding L424V substitution. Patient had evidence of a clinical and immunologic response (22)
TGF-β	Overexpression	Unknown	**LY2157299** (TGF-β inhibitor): • Phase 1: ORR 18% (23) **Trabedersen** (AP12009, TGF-β inhibitor): • Phase 1/2: RR 38% (24)
VEGFR	Expression	100	**Bevacizumab** (VEGF inhibitor): • Phase 2 (single agent) (recurrent disease): RR 28%, PFS at 6 mo 43% (25) • Phase 2, with irinotecan, RT: RR 38%, PFS at 6 mo 50% (25) • Phase 2: RR 35%, PFS at 6 mo 29% (single agent and RT) (26) **Sorafenib** (VEGFR/PDGFR/RAS/RET inhibitor): • Phase 1, with RT: OS 18 mo (ND), 24 mo (recurrent disease) (27)

Actionable Target	Abnormality	Prevalence (%)	Clinical Experience with Targeted Agent
EGFR (28)	Overexpression	40	**Lapatinib** (EGFR/HER2 inhibitor): • Phase 2, NF2: ORR 24% (time to response: 4.5 mo), PFS at 12 mo 64% (29) **Erlotinib** (EGFR inhibitor): • Phase 2, NF1: SD 5% (30)
NF1/NF2	Loss	100	**Everolimus** (mTOR inhibitor): • Phase 2: RR 0% (31)
PDGFR	Overexpression	Unknown	**Imatinib** (BCR-Abl/cKIT/PDGFR): • Phase 2, NF1: ORR 17% (26% in those treated for >6 mo) (32)
VEGFR	Expression	100	**Bevacizumab** (VEGF inhibitor): • Retrospective review, NF2: ORR 55% (33) • Case study: 2 pts treated with single-agent SD of 9+ and 10+ mo, 2 pts treated with combination with **temsirolimus** (mTOR inhibitor) SD 4+ and 9+ mo (with 33% volumetric reduction) (34)

Actionable Target	Abnormality	Prevalence (%)	Clinical Experience with Targeted Agent
PTCH1	Mutation (hedgehog pathway activation)	7	**Vismodegib** (SMO/hedgehog inhibitor): • Phase 1, pediatric pts: ORR 33% (activated hedgehog pathway), 0% (without activation) (35) • Phase 1, advanced disease: 1/1 PR **Erismodegib** (SMO/hedgehog inhibitor): • Phase 1, advanced disease: ORR 8% (CR) (36) • Phase 1: 1 PR and 1 metabolic PR (activated hedgehog pathway) (37)
VEGFR	Expression	100	**Bevacizumab** (VEGF inhibitor): • Phase 1, with irinotecan and temozolomide, pediatric pts: ORR 67% at 3 mo and 55% at 6 mo, PFS 11 mo, OS 13 mo (38)

Actionable Target	Abnormality	Prevalence (%)	Clinical Experience with Targeted Agent
EGFR	Overexpression	40	**Erlotinib** or **gefitinib** (EGFR inhibitors): • Phase 2: PFS at 6 mo 29% (irrespective of drug) (39)
PDGFR	Overexpression	Unknown	**Imatinib** (BCR-Abl/cKIT/PDGFR inhibitor): • Phase 2, with **hydroxyurea**: SD at 6 mo 67% (40)
VEGFR	Expression	100	**Bevacizumab** (VEGF inhibitor): • Retrospective analysis: RR 29% of tumors (duration 3.7 mo), PFS at 6 mo 93%, PFS at 12 mo 62% (41)

Actionable Target	Abnormality	Prevalence (%)	Clinical Experience with Targeted Agent
AKT1	Mutation	3–8	**AZD5363/Capivasertib** (AKT inhibitor): • Phase 2, basket study: ORR 30%, 4 confirmed PR, PFS 5.5 mo, in pts with AKT1 mutations (1) • Phase 1; ORR 20%, in combination with fulvestrant, ORR 36% in fulvestrant pretreated and 20% in fulvestrant naïve (2)
ESR1	Mutation	20–30*	• Predicts resistance to aromatase inhibitors and associated with shorter survival (3) • Specific variants predict for lack of response to fulvestrant or everolimus (e.g., Y537S) (4,5) **Fulvestrant** (estrogen receptor downregulator): • In ESR1 mutants, PFS 5.7 vs. 2.6 mo for exemestane (6) • PlasmaMATCH—Extended-dose **fulvestrant**: 8% RR, 12% CBR, DOR 7 mo (7)
FGFR1	Amplification	10–15	• Associated with endocrine resistance and poor prognosis (8) • Predicts for response to FGFR inhibitors (9,10)

(continued)

Actionable Target	Abnormality	Prevalence (%)	Clinical Experience with Targeted Agent
HER2 (ERBB2)	Mutation	2[†]	• Typically, exclusive with HER2 amplifications (11) • Kinase domain mutations predict response to TKIs (e.g., neratinib) (12) • Extracellular domain mutations predict for response/resistance to trastuzumab/pertuzumab (13) **Neratinib (dual HER2/EGFR inhibitor):** • Phase 2: CBR (CR/PR/SD ≥6 mo) 31% (14) • Phase 2 SUMMIT basket trial: RR 30% (15). SUMMIT breast trial: RR 17%, PFS 3.6 mo, DOR 6.5 mo. In combination with fulvestrant, RR 30%, PFS 5.4 mo, DOR 9.2 mo (16). In combination with trastuzumab and fulvestrant, RR 39% (17) • Phase 2, PlasmaMATCH: with Neratinib and fulvestrant: 25% RR (1 CR, 4 PR), CBR 45%, DOR 5.7 mo, PFS 5.4 mo (7)

Actionable Target	Abnormality	Prevalence (%)	Clinical Experience with Targeted Agent
PIK3CA	Mutation	30–35	• Predicts response to PI3K/AKT/mTOR inhibitors **Alpelisib** (alpha-selective PI3K inhibitor): • Phase 3: SOLAR-1, with fulvestrant: PFS 11 vs. 5.7 mo, RR 36% vs. 16% for fulvestrant alone (9) • Phase 1b, with letrozole: CBR 44% in PIK3CA mutants vs. 20% in WT (18,19) **Everolimus** (mTOR inhibitor): • Phase 3: PFS 10.6 vs. 4.1 mo for placebo (20). Pts with no or one genetic alteration in CCND1, PI3K, or FGFR pathways had greater treatment effect. • Phase 2, with tamoxifen: CBR 61% vs. 42% for placebo (21) • Phase 1b, with anastrozole: CBR 27% with PI3K pathway alterations vs. 8% without alterations (22) **Buparlisib** (alpha-selective PI3K inhibitor): • Phase 3, with fulvestrant: In pts with PIK3CA mutations, PFS 4.7 vs. 1.6 mo for placebo (23)

(*continued*)

Actionable Target	Abnormality	Prevalence (%)	Clinical Experience with Targeted Agent
PTEN	Mutation/loss	3/29	• May predict response to PI3K/AKT/mTOR inhibitors **Alpelisib** (alpha-selective PI3K inhibitor): • Phase 3: SOLAR-1 (post hoc analyses) with fulvestrant: PFS 6.2 vs. 1.9 mo for fulvestrant alone (9) in PTEN loss (without PIK3CA mutation), PFS 7.7 vs. 3.6 mo in PTEN loss (with PIK3CA mutation) (22,24)

*Variable, based on prior AI exposure. Uncommon in primary breast cancer.
†Higher prevalence in invasive lobular carcinoma (10%).

Actionable Target	Abnormality	Prevalence (%)	Clinical Experience with Targeted Agent
HER2 (ERBB2)	Amplification	20	**Trastuzumab** (HER2 inhibitor): • Phase 3: Single agent, first line, RR 26% (25) • Phase 3, with **chemotherapy**: RR 50% vs. 32% for chemo alone, PFS 7.4 vs. 4.6 mo (26) • Phase 3, with **lapatinib**, neoadjuvant: RR 51% vs. 30% with trastuzumab alone vs. 24% with lapatinib alone (27) **Lapatinib** (dual HER2/EGFR inhibitor): • Phase 2: Single agent, after trastuzumab, RR 12.6% (28) • Phase 3, with **trastuzumab**: PFS 11.1 vs. 8.1 mo for lapatinib (29) • Phase 3, with **capecitabine**: PFS 8.4 vs. 4.1 mo for capecitabine (30) **Pertuzumab** (HER2 dimerization inhibitor): • Phase 3, with **trastuzumab** and **docetaxel**: PFS 18.5 vs. 12.4 mo with trastuzumab and docetaxel, RR 80% vs. 69% (31) • Single agent, RR 3.4% (32). With **trastuzumab**, RR 17.6% (33) • Phase 3, with adjuvant trastuzumab: invasive disease events 7.1% vs. 8.7% for trastuzumab alone (33)

(continued)

Actionable Target	Abnormality	Prevalence (%)	Clinical Experience with Targeted Agent
			Neratinib (dual HER2/EGFR inhibitor): • Phase 3, after adjuvant trastuzumab: IDFS 94.2% vs. 91.9% with placebo (34) • Phase 3, for metastatic BC: with capecitabine, PFS 8.8 vs. 6.6 mo (lapatinib and capecitabine), ORR 33% vs. 27% (35)
HER2 (ERBB2)	Amplification	20	**T-DM1 (Ado-Trastuzumab Emtansine)** (antibody–drug conjugate to HER2; trastuzumab linked with emtansine): • Phase 3: PFS 9.6 vs. 6.4 mo for lapatinib and capecitabine, RR 44% vs. 31% (36) • Phase 3: PFS 6.2 vs. 3.3 mo for treatment of physician's choice, third line or greater (37) **Trastuzumab Deruxtecan (DS-8201)** (topoisomerase inhibitor–drug conjugate to HER2): • Phase 2: ORR 61%, CR 6%, DOR 14.8 mo (38) **Tucatinib** (selective HER2 inhibitor): • Phase 2: in combination with trastuzumab and capecitabine, PFS 7.8 vs. 5.6 mo (trastuzumab and capecitabine alone), OS 21.9 vs. 17.4 mo, ORR 41% vs. 23% (39). Median CNS-PFS 9.9 vs. 4.2 mo (40)

Actionable Target	Abnormality	Prevalence (%)	Clinical Experience with Targeted Agent
			Margetuximab (Fc-modified trastuzumab analog): • Phase 2: with chemotherapy (capecitabine, eribulin, gemcitabine, or vinorelbine), PFS 5.8 vs. 4.9 mo, RR 25% vs. 14% (trastuzumab with chemotherapy) (41)
PIK3CA	Mutation	25–30	• PIK3CA mutations or PTEN loss associated with decreased response with trastuzumab (42,43) • Decreased PFS with pertuzumab, 12.5 vs. 21.8 mo for WT (44). No difference in outcomes with T-DM1 based on PIK3CA mutations (45) • Decreased pCR with trastuzumab and lapatinib, 28.6% vs. 53.1% for WT (46) • PIK3CA mutations or PTEN loss associated with decreased response with trastuzumab (32,33) • Decreased PFS with pertuzumab, 12.5 vs. 21.8 mo for WT (34). No difference in outcomes with T-DM1 based on PIK3CA mutations (35) • Decreased pCR with trastuzumab and lapatinib, 28.6% vs. 53.1% for WT (36)

(continued)

Actionable Target	Abnormality	Prevalence (%)	Clinical Experience with Targeted Agent
			Everolimus (mTOR inhibitor): • Phase 3, with **trastuzumab** and **paclitaxel**, in pts with hyperactive PI3K pathway*, PFS 13.9 vs. 10.9 mo for placebo (47,48) • Phase 3, with **trastuzumab** and **vinorelbine**, in pts with hyperactive PI3K pathway*, PFS 8.1 vs. 5.6 mo for placebo (48,49)

*PIK3CA mutations and/or PTEN loss and/or AKT1 mutation.

Actionable Target	Abnormality	Prevalence (%)	Clinical Experience with Targeted Agent
AR	Expression	12	**Bicalutamide** (androgen receptor inhibitor): • Phase 2: CBR 19%, PFS 12 wk (50) **Enzalutamide** (androgen receptor inhibitor): • CBR at 16 wk 25%, PFS 2.9 mo (51)
BRCA1/2	Mutation (germline)	5	**Talazoparib** (PARP inhibitor): • Phase 3: PFS 8.6 vs. 5.6 mo for standard therapy in gBRCA1/2. RR 63% vs. 27% (52) Olaparib (PARP inhibitor): • Phase 3: PFS 7.0 vs. 4.2 mo for standard therapy in germline BRCA1/2. RR 59.9% vs. 28.8% (53) • Phase 2: RR 20% vs. 9.5% with prior platinum (54) **Veliparib** (PARP inhibitor): • Phase 2: with carboplatin and paclitaxel, PFS 14.5 vs. 12.6 mo (carboplatin and paclitaxel alone) (55) **Carboplatin**: • Phase 3: RR 68% vs. 33 % in BRCA mutants (56) • Phase 2 (carboplatin/cisplatin): RR 54.5% vs. 25.6% in non-BRCA carriers (57) *(continued)*

Actionable Target	Abnormality	Prevalence (%)	Clinical Experience with Targeted Agent
NTRK	Translocation	<1	**Common in secretory breast cancers:** Entrectinib (NTRK inhibitor) tissue-agnostic FDA approval: • Phase 1/2 (ALKA, STARTRK-1, STARTRK-2) basket trial, ORR 57% across all tumors. RR 83% in breast cancer (58) Larotrectinib (NTRK inhibitor) tissue-agnostic FDA approval: ORR 75%, median DOR and PFS not reached (59)
PD-1/PD-L1	Overexpression	Variable	Atezolizumab (PD-L1 inhibitor): • Phase 3: with nab-paclitaxel, PFS 7.5 vs. 5 mo (nab-paclitaxel alone), OS 25 vs. 18 mo, RR 59% vs. 43%, CR 10% vs. 1.1%, in PD-L1 positive (>1% in IC, SP142 assay) (60,61) Pembrolizumab (PD-1 inhibitor): • Phase 3: with chemotherapy (nab-paclitaxel, paclitaxel, carboplatin, and gemcitabine), PFS 9.7 vs. 5.6 mo (chemotherapy alone) for CPS ≥10 (22C3 assay) (62) • Phase 1: RR 18.5%, median duration of response not reached (15 to ≥47.3 wk), CBR (CR/PR/SD ≥ 6 mo) 25.9%. PD-L1 positivity (expression in stroma or >1% of tumor cells by IHC) (63)

Actionable Target	Abnormality	Prevalence (%)	Clinical Experience with Targeted Agent
			• FDA approved for MSI-H or dMMR cancers (1%–2% of breast cancers) (64) **Avelumab** (PD-L1 inhibitor): • Phase 1: ORR 5.2% in TNBC (22% ORR in PD-L1 positive) (65)
PIK3CA	Mutation	8	• Higher prevalence in metaplastic cancers ~40% (66,67) **Temsirolimus** (mTOR inhibitor): • Phase 1, with **bevacizumab** anc **liposomal doxorubicin**: RR 32% in metaplastic (66) **Ipatasertib** (AKT inhibitor) • Phase 2: with paclitaxel, PFS 9 vs. 4.9 mo (paclitaxel) for PIK3CA/AKT1/PTEN alterations (68) **Capivasertib** (AKT inhibitor): • Phase 2: with paclitaxel, PFS 9.3 vs. 3.7 mo (paclitaxel) for PIK3CA/AKT1/PTEN alterations (69)
PTEN	Mutation/loss	35	**Ipatasertib** (AKT inhibitor): • Phase 2: with paclitaxel, PFS 6.2 vs. 3.6 mo (paclitaxel), RR 48% vs. 26% for PTEN low (68)

(continued)

Actionable Target	Abnormality	Prevalence (%)	Clinical Experience with Targeted Agent
TMB	≥10 mutations/MB	Variable	**Pembrolizumab** (PD-1 inhibitor): tissue-agnostic FDA approval for TMB-high (≥10 mutations per MB) (70) • Phase 2: KEYNOTE-158, ORR 29%, CR 4%
Trop-2	Expression		**Sacituzumab Govitecan (Trodelvy™)** (Trop-2-directed antibody and topoisomerase inhibitor): • Phase 3: PFS 5.6 vs. 1.7 mo for chemotherapy alone, OS 12.1 vs. 6.7 mo, ORR 35% vs. 5% (71)

Actionable Target	Abnormality	Prevalence (%) (1,2)	Clinical Experience with Targeted Agent
AKT	Mutation		**Temsirolimus** (mTOR inhibitor): • Phase 2: RR 3%, SD 58% (3) **Trametinib** (MEK inhibitor): • Phase 2 (with AKT inhibitor GSK2141795): 0 confirmed responses (4)
KRAS	Mutation		
PIK3CA	Mutation	37.5 (squamous cell) 14%–25% (adenocarcinoma)	
PTEN	Protein loss	13 (squamous cell) 3.6% (adenocarcinoma)	
EGFR	Overexpression	54–71 (all histologies)	**Cetuximab** (EGFR inhibitor): • Phase 2, with topotecan and cisplatin: Trial terminated due to toxicity (5) • Phase 2 frontline with chemoradiation vs. chemoradiation alone: 2-yr OS 83% vs. 87% favoring chemoradiation alone (6) • Phase 2, with carboplatin and paclitaxel vs. carboplatin/paclitaxel alone: RR 43% chemo alone vs. 38% for cetuximab arm (7) • Phase 2 (with carboplatin/paclitaxel vs. chemo alone): PFS 7.6 vs. 5.2 mo (chemo alone), OS 17 vs. 17.7 mo (chemo alone) (8)

(continued)

Actionable Target	Abnormality	Prevalence (%) (1,2)	Clinical Experience with Targeted Agent
			Erlotinib (EGFR inhibitor): • Phase 2: RR 0%, SD 16% (9) • Phase 2 (frontline with chemoradiation): CR 94.4%, 3-yr OS 80% (10) **Gefitinib** (EGFR inhibitor): • Phase 2: RR 0%, SD 20% (11) **Matuzumab** (EGFR inhibitor): • Phase 2: RR 5%, SD 24% (12) **Lapatinib** (HER2 inhibitor): • Phase 2: RR 5%, SD 44% (13) • Phase 1 (with cisplatin and hyperthermia): Deemed not feasible due to toxicity (14)
Microsatellite instability (15)		6	**Pembrolizumab** (PD-1 inhibitor): • Phase 1b: ORR 12.5%, 6-mo OS 66.7% (16) • Phase 2 (with GX-188E vaccine): CR 15%, PR 27% (17)
PD-1/PD-L1	Expression	80 PD-1 (squamous cell) 17 PD-L1 (squamous cell) 38 PD-1 (adenocarcinoma) 0 PD-L1 (adenocarcinoma)	• Phase 2: ORR 12.2%—all in PD-L1 positive tumors (18) **Nivolumab** (PD-1 inhibitor): • Phase 2: PR 4%, SD 36% (19) • Phase 1/2: ORR 26.3%, OS 21.9 mo (20) **Camrelizumab** (PD-1 antibody): • Phase 2 (with apatinib): ORR 59.5%, PFS 7.6 mo (21)

Actionable Target	Abnormality	Prevalence (%) (1,2)	Clinical Experience with Targeted Agent
PDGFR	Expression	Not determined	**Imatinib** (PDGFR/BCR-Abl/KIT inhibitor): • Phase 1: RR 0%, SD 8% (22)
Tissue Factor (TF)	Expression		Tisotumab Vedotin-tftv (ADC) (FDA approved 2021): • Phase 2: ORR 24%, CR 7%, PR 17% (23)
VEGF	Expression	Associated with poorer prognosis (4)	Bevacizumab (VEGF inhibitor): • Phase 2: RR 11%, SD 24% (24) • Retrospective analysis, with 5-FU or capecitabine: RR 34%, SD 33% (25) • Phase 3, with cisplatin/paclitaxel or topotecan/paclitaxel: RR 48% (26) **Apatinib** (VEGFR-2 inhibitor): • Phase 2 (with chemo or chemoXRT vs. chemo or chemoXRT alone): PFS 10.1 vs. 6.4 mo (chemo/chemoXRT alone); ORR 64.3% vs. 33.3% (chemo/chemoXRT alone) (27) • Phase 2 (with camrelizumab): ORR 59.5%, PFS 7.6 mo (28) **Sunitinib** (VEGFR/PDGFR/RET/KIT/FLT3 inhibitor): • Phase 2: RR 0%, SD 84% (29) **Anlotinib** (VEGFR inhibitor): • Phase 2: ORR 32.1%, PFS 3.9 mo (30) **Pazopanib** (VEGFR inhibitor): • Phase 2: RR 9%, SD 24% (31)

Actionable Target	Abnormality	Prevalence (%)	Clinical Experience with Targeted Agent
BRAF	Mutation	5–8	**Vemurafenib** (BRAF inhibitor): • Phase 2, with cetuximab (EGFR inhibitor) and irinotecan: PFS 4.3 vs. 2.0 mo (HR 0.48), PR 17% vs. 4%, DCR (PR + SD) 65% vs. 21% favoring the arm with vemurafenib (1) **Dabrafenib** (BRAF inhibitor): • Phase 1/2, with trametinib and panitumumab: RR and SD of 10% and 90% for dabrafenib + panitumumab, 0% and 55% for trametinib + panitumumab, and 21% and 68% for dabrafenib + trametinib + panitumumab (2) **Encorafenib** (BRAF V600E) (BRAF inhibition) (FDA approved): • Phase 3, with cetuximab (EGFR inhibitor) ± binimetinib (MEK inhibitor) vs. chemotherapy: RR 26% vs. 2%, OS 9.0 vs. 5.4 mo (HR 0.52; $p < 0.001$) in BRAF V600E-mutated CRC pts who had progressed on 1 or 2 prior regimens (3) • Phase 2, with cetuximab (EGFR inhibitor) + binimetinib (MEK inhibitor) vs. chemotherapy: RR 50%, PFS 4.9 mo in first line (4)

Actionable Target	Abnormality	Prevalence (%)	Clinical Experience with Targeted Agent
HER2 (ERBB2)	Amplification	2–11	**Trastuzumab** (HER2 inhibitor) + **Lapatinib** (HER2 inhibitor/EGFR inhibitor): • Phase 2: RR 30%, PR 26%, including 1 (4%) CR, SD 44%, in pts with refractory KRAS WT and HER2-amplified/overexpressed (5) **Pertuzumab** (HER2 inhibitor) + **Trastuzumab** (HER2 inhibitor): • Phase 2a: RR 32%, PR 30%, including 1 (2%) CR in pts with refractory KRAS WT and HER2-amplified/overexpressed (6) **Trastuzumab Deruxtecan** (HER2 inhibitor): • Phase 2: RR 45.3%, including 1 CR and 23 PRs; median duration of response was not reached (7)
KRAS G12C		1–3	**Sotorasib** (KRAS^{G12C} inhibitor): • Phase 1: RR 7.1%, DCR 73.8% and PFS 4.0 mo in the subgroup of mCRC harboring the *KRAS* p.G12C mutation in third-line or later setting (8) • Phase 1b/2, + panitumumab (EGFR inhibitor): RR 27%, DCR 81% in previously treated mCRC (9) *(continued)*

Actionable Target	Abnormality	Prevalence (%)	Clinical Experience with Targeted Agent
			Adagrasib (KRAS^{G12C} inhibitor): • Phase 1/2, monotherapy: RR 22%, DCR 87% in second line and later (10) • Phase 1/2 + cetuximab (EGFR inhibitor): RR 43%, DCR 100% in second line and later (10)
MSI-H, dMMR	Loss of at least one mismatch repair protein by IHC (MSH2, MLH1, MSH6, PMS2), or microsatellite instability high by PCR or NGS assay	15 (5 of stage IV)	**Pembrolizumab** (PD-1 inhibitor) (FDA approved for pts with MSI-H or dMMR including mCRC in first line): • Phase 3, monotherapy in first line: 16.5 vs. 8.2 mo, RR 43.8% vs. 33.1% compared with chemotherapy (11) **Nivolumab** (PD-1 inhibitor) (FDA approved for pts with MSI-H or dMMR including mCRC in second line): • Phase 2, monotherapy: RR 31%, DCR 69% in MSI-H tumors in pretreated patients with dMMR/MSI-H (12) • Phase 2 + ipilimumab (CTLA4 inhibitor) PR and SD of 52.4% and 31% in MSI-H tumors • Phase 2 + ipilimumab (CTLA4 inhibitor) in first line: RR 69%, PFS and OS not reached (13) **Atezolizumab** (PD-L1 inhibitor): • Phase 1b, with bevacizumab: RR 30% and SD 60% in MSI-H pts (14)

Actionable Target	Abnormality	Prevalence (%)	Clinical Experience with Targeted Agent
POLE	Abnormality	1	• PD-1/PD-L1 inhibitors: In a retrospective cohort, RR 27% to PD-1/PD-L1 inhibition (15)
NTRK	Fusion		**Entrectinib** (FDA approved 2019) (TRK inhibitor): • Phase 1/2 (STARTRK-2, STARTRK-1, ALKA-372-001): ORR 57% across all tumor types (95% CI 43–71), including a 7% complete response rate. RR 25% in colorectal cancer pts (16) **Larotrectinib** (FDA approved 2018) (TRK inhibitor): • Phase 1/2: ORR 79% across all tumor types, CR 24 pts, PR 97 pts, SD 19 pts. RR 50% in colorectal cancer pts (17)
RAS (KRAS/NRAS)	Mutation (resistance)	30–50	**Cetuximab** (EGFR inhibitor) (FDA approved): • Phase 3, monotherapy: RR 13% in WT KRAS vs. 1% in mutant KRAS (codons 12/13). PFS (3.7 vs. 1.9 mo) and OS (9.5 vs. 4.8 mo) favored cetuximab compared with BSC in WT KRAS. No difference in mutant KRAS pts (18).

(*continued*)

Actionable Target	Abnormality	Prevalence (%)	Clinical Experience with Targeted Agent
			• Phase 3: RR 72%, PFS 10.3 mo, OS 33.1 mo in first-line setting associated with chemotherapy in WT KRAS and NRAS (19) **Panitumumab** (EGFR inhibitor) (FDA approved): • Phase 3, monotherapy: RR 16% in WT KRAS vs. 1% in mutant KRAS. In pts with WT KRS, NRAS, and BRAF, RR 18%. In pts with WT KRAS and mutations in NRAS or BRAF, RR 0% (20) • Phase 3: PFS 10.0 vs. 8.6 mo, OS 23.9 vs. 19.7 mo with chemotherapy in KRAS WT pts on first-line setting (21)
VEGF/VEGFR			**Regorafenib** (VEGFR inhibitor) (FDA approved): • Phase 3, monotherapy: OS 6.4 vs. 5.0 mo, PFS 1.9 vs. 1.7 mo. RR 1% vs. 0.4% compared with placebo (22). **Ramucirumab** (VEGFR2 inhibitor): • Phase 3: OS 13.3 vs. 11.7 mo, PFS 5.7 vs. 4.5 mo, RR 13.4% vs. 12.5% in association with chemotherapy compared with placebo + chemotherapy (23)

Actionable Target	Abnormality	Prevalence (%)	Clinical Experience with Targeted Agent
			Bevacizumab (VEGF inhibitor) (FDA approved): • Phase 3: RR 45% vs. 35%, OS 20 vs. 16 mo; TTP 11 vs. 6.0 mo with chemotherapy in first line (24) **Aflibercept** (VEGF inhibitor) (FDA approved): • Phase 3: RR 19.8% vs. 11.1% placebo, OS 13.5 vs. 12.1 mo placebo; PFS 6.9 vs. 4.7 mo placebo with chemo in second line (16) **Anlotinib** (VEGFR inhibitor) (FDA approved): • Phase 3, monotherapy: OS 8.6 vs. 7.2, PFS 4.1 vs. 1.5 mo, RR 4.3% vs. 0.7%, DCR 75.9% vs. 30.7%, compared to placebo in refractory mCRC (17)

Actionable Target	Abnormality	Prevalence	Clinical Experience with Targeted Agent
EGFR	Mutation	19% (1)	**Gefitinib** (EGFR TKI): • Phase 2: OS 3.7 vs. 3.6 mo with placebo (2) **Afatinib** (EGFR TKI): • Phase 2: ORR 14.3%, DCR 73.3%, OS 6.6 mo (3) **Icotinib** (EGFR TKI): • Phase 2: Median OS 24 mo in the RT plus icotinib group vs. 16.3 mo in the RT group (4)
	Overexpression	30%–90%	**Panitumumab** (EGFR inhibitor): • Phase 3: Trial was stopped at interim futility analysis (5)
MSI-H, dMMR	Mutation/ expression	N/A	**Dostarlimab-gxly** (PD-1 inhibitor) (FDA approved 2021): • Phase 1: ORR 41.6%, CR 9.17%, 32.5% PR, DOR 34.7 mo (95.4% with duration ≥6 mo) (6) **Pembrolizumab** (PD-1 inhibitor) (FDA approved for pts with MSI-H or dMMR 2018): • PR in 1 pt, DOR range 18.2+ mo (7) • Phase 2 (KEYNOTE-158): ORR 34.3% pts, DOR ≥24 mo 77.6%, PFS 4.1 mo, OS 23.5 mo (8)

Actionable Target	Abnormality	Prevalence	Clinical Experience with Targeted Agent
PI3K	Mutation	PI3KCA 13%	**BKM120** (PI3K inhibitor): • Phase 2: DCR 51.2%, OS 9.0 mo (9)
PD-1	Overexpression	PD-L1/PD-L2 43.9% (6)	Nivolumab (PD-1 inhibitor)*: • Phase 2: ORR 17%, DCR 42%, OS 10.8 mo (10) Pembrolizumab (PD-1 inhibitor): • Phase 1b: ORR 30% (11) **Sintilimab** (PD-1 inhibitor): • Phase 2: Median OS 7.2 mo in Sintilimab group vs. 6.2 mo in chemotherapy group (12) **Avelumab** (PD-L1 inhibitor): • Phase 3: Median OS 4.6 vs. 5 mo in chemotherapy alone group (13)

*Asian pts.

Gastric/Gastroesophageal Junction Adenocarcinoma

Actionable Target	Abnormality	Prevalence	Clinical Experience with Targeted Agent
AKT	Overexpression	22% (1)	**Ipatasertib** (AKT inhibitor): • Phase 2: PFS 6.6 mo in ipatasertib + mFOLFOX6 vs. 7.5 with mFOLFOX6 only (2)
Claudin-18.2	N/A	48%	**Zolbetuximab (IMAB362)** (anti-claudin-18.2 antibody): • Phase 2: IMAB362 + EOX OS 13.2 vs. 8.4 mo with EOX (3)
CTLA-4	Overexpression		**Tremelimumab** (CTLA-4 inhibitor): • Phase 2: ORR 5%, TTP 2.83 mo, OS 4.83 mo (4) **Ipilimumab** (CTLA-4 inhibitor): • Phase 2: OS 12.7 vs. 12.1 mo with BSC (5) **Nivolumab + Ipilimumab** (CTLA-4 inhibitor): • Phase 1/2: ORR and OSNivo 3 mg/kg Q2W: 12% and 6.2 mo • Nivo 1+Ipi 3 mg/kg Q3W: 24% and 6.9 mo • Nivo 3+Ipi 13 mg/kg Q3W: 8% and 4.8 mo (6)

Actionable Target	Abnormality	Prevalence	Clinical Experience with Targeted Agent
EGFR	Overexpression	30%–90%	**Cetuximab** (EGFR inhibitor): • Phase 3, with cisplatin/capecitabine: RR with cetuximab 51% (HER2+), 27% (HER2−), OS 10.7 vs. 9.4 mo (without cetuximab) (7) **Panitumumab** (EGFR inhibitor): • Phase 3, with epirubicin/oxaliplatin/capecitabine: OS 8.8 vs. 11.3 mo (without panitumumab) (8)
FGFR2b	Amplification	9% (9)	**Bemarituzumab (FPA144)** (anti-FGFR2B antibody): • Phase 1: ORR of 22%, DCR 55.6%, DOR 15.4 wk (10) **AZD4547** (FGFR1/2/3 inhibitor): • PFS 1.8 vs. 3.5 mo with paclitaxel (11)
HER2	Overexpression/amplification	20%–30%	**Trastuzumab** (HER2 inhibitor): • Phase 3, with cisplatin/5-FU/capecitabine: RR 47% (with trastuzumab), OS 13.8 vs. 11.1 mo (without trastuzumab) (12) **Lapatinib** (HER2/EGFR inhibitor): • Phase 3, with capecitabine/oxaliplatin: RR 53% (with lapatinib), OS 12.2 vs. 10.5 mo (without lapatinib) (13)

(*continued*)

Actionable Target	Abnormality	Prevalence	Clinical Experience with Targeted Agent
			Pertuzumab (HER2 inhibitor): • Phase 3 (with trastuzumab and chemotherapy): OS 17.5 vs. 14.2 mo in trastuzumab and chemotherapy only group HR 0.84; $p = 0.057$ (14) **Margetuximab** (HER2 inhibitor) plus **Pembrolizumab**: • Phase 1b/2: median follow-up was 19.9 mo (single-arm study) (15).
HGF/c-MET	Overexpression	21%	**Tivantinib** (MET inhibitor)*: • Phase 2: RR 0% (unselected pts), SD 37%, PFS 43 d (16) **Foretinib** (MET inhibitor): • Phase 2: RR 0% (unselected pts), SD 23% (17) **Rilotumumab** (HGF inhibitor): • Phase 3: plus epirubicin, cisplatin, and capecitabine, OS 8.8 mo in rilotumumab vs. 10.7 mo in placebo group (18) **Onartuzumab** (MET inhibitor): • Phase 3: plus mFOLFOX, OS 11.0 mo for onartuzumab vs. 11.3 mo for placebo (19)

Actionable Target	Abnormality	Prevalence	Clinical Experience with Targeted Agent
Matrix metalloproteinase 9 (MMP9)	Overexpression	N/A	**Andecaliximab (GS-5745)** (MMP9 inhibitor): • Phase 1: GS-5745 + FOLFOX, ORR 50%, DOR 9.4 mo (20)
mTOR	Overexpression	20%	**Everolimus** (mTOR inhibitor): • Phase 3, with best supportive care: 5.4 vs. 4.3 mo (best supportive care only) (22)
PIK3CA	Mutation	24% (21)	
PARP	Amplification	N/A	**Olaparib** (PARP inhibitor): • Phase 2: plus paclitaxel, OS 13.1 vs. 8.3 mo with placebo (23)
PD-1/PD-L1	Overexpression	PD-L1 40% (24)	**Nivolumab** (PD-1 inhibitor): • Phase 3: OS 5.3 vs. 4.1 mo with placebo* (25) **Pembrolizumab** (PD-1 inhibitor) (FDA approved after 2 lines of therapy in PD-L1-positive pts): • Phase 2: ORR 13.3%, OS 11.4 mo **Avelumab** (PD-L1 inhibitor): • Phase 1b: ORR 9.7% (2L), 9% (1L, maintenance); DCR 29% (2L), 57.3% (1L, maintenance) (26)

(*continued*)

Actionable Target	Abnormality	Prevalence	Clinical Experience with Targeted Agent
Stat3	Amplification	N/A	**Napabucasin (BBI608)** (Stat3 inhibitor): • Phase 1b/2: BBI608 + paclitaxel wkly, ORR 31%, DCR 75%, OS 39.3 wk (27)
VEGFR	Overexpression	30%–60%	**Bevacizumab** (VEGF inhibitor): • Phase 3, with cisplatin/capecitabine: RR 38% (with bevacizumab), OS 12.1 vs. 10.1 mo (without bevacizumab) (28) Ramucirumab (VEGFR2 inhibitor): • Phase 3: OS 5.2 vs. 3.8 mo (supportive care) (29)
VEGFR-2	Overexpression	30%–60%	**Apatinib** (VEGFR2 inhibitor): • Phase 3: OS 6.5 vs. 4.7 mo with placebo* (9) **Regorafenib** (VEGFR/multikinase inhibitor): • Phase 2: OS 5.8 vs. 4.5 mo with placebo (30)

*Apatinib is approved only in China.

Actionable Target	Abnormality	Prevalence	Clinical Experience with Targeted Agent
AR	AR positivity *86% SDC, 26% Ac NOS, 15% AcCC, 5% MEC, 5% ACC (1)*		**Androgen deprivation therapy (ADT):** • PFS 4 mo, OS 17 mo (2) • **Phase 2 bicalutamide** (antiandrogen) with **leuprorelin** (GnRH agonist): ORR 42%, PFS 8.8 mo, OS 30.5 mo (3) • **Bicalutamide** (antiandrogen) alone or with **goserelin** (LHRH agonist) or **leuprolide** (LHRH agonist): ORR 25%–50% (4) • **Bicalutamide** (antiandrogen) with **triptorelin** (LHRH agonist): ORR 65%. PFS 12%, 5-yr OS 19% (5) • Adjuvant **Bicalutamide** (antiandrogen) alone, **LHRH analogue** alone, or combination: 3-yr disease-free survival 48.2% (6)
HER2	HER2 alteration/amplification *20% MEC, 30%–40% SDC (7)*		**Pertuzumab** with **Trastuzumab** (HER2 inhibitors): ORR 60%, PFS 8.6 mo, OS 20.4 mo (8) **Ado-Trastuzumab** (HER2 inhibitor): ORR 90% (9) **Docetaxel** (chemotherapy) and **Trastuzumab**: 57 SDC pts with ORR 70.2%, PFS 8.9 mo, OS 39.7 mo (10)

(continued)

Actionable Target	Abnormality	Prevalence	Clinical Experience with Targeted Agent
NTRK	ETV6-NTRK1/2/3 fusions *15% AcCC (11), 30% mammary analogue secretory carcinoma of salivary glands (MASC) (12)*		**Larotrectinib** (FDA approved 2019) (NTRK inhibitor): • **Integrated study of Ph1 adult, Ph1/2 pediatric, and Ph2 adult/adolescent**: 12 MASC pts with ETV6–NTRK gene fusions with ORR 80% (13) • Phase 1/2: ORR 79%, CR 24 pts, PR 97 pts, SD 19 pts for all tumor types, RR 90% in salivary cancer (14) • **Entrectinib** (FDA approved 2019) (NTRK inhibitor): • **Integrated study of 3 Ph1/2 trials**: 7 MASC pts with ETV6–NTRK fusions with ORR 86% (15)
PD-1/PD-L1	N/A		**Pembrolizumab** (anti-PD-1 antibody): • Phase 1b KEYNOTE-028 with ORR 28%, PFS 4 mo, OS 13 mo (16)

Actionable Target	Abnormality	Prevalence	Clinical Experience with Targeted Agent
PD-1/PD-L1	N/A	*90%* (all HNSCC)	**Nivolumab** (anti-PD-1 antibody): • Phase 3: ORR 13.3% with nivolumab vs. 5.8% with investigator's choice, OS 7.5 mo with nivolumab vs. 5.1 mo investigator's choice (17) **Pembrolizumab** (anti-PD-1 antibody): • Phase 3 KEYNOTE-048: OS 14.9 mo with pembrolizumab vs. 10.7 mo chemotherapy in CPS ≥20, OS 12.3 mo with pembrolizumab vs. 10.3 mo with chemotherapy in CPS ≥ 1, ORR 18% (18) **Pembrolizumab** (anti-PD-1 antibody) and chemotherapy (platinum and 5-fluorouracil): • Phase 3 KEYNOTE-048: OS 13.0 mo with pembrolizumab + chemotherapy vs. 10.7 mo chemotherapy regardless of CPS score (18)

CPS, combined proportion score.

Actionable Target	Abnormality	Prevalence	Clinical Experience with Targeted Agent
PD-1/PD-L1	N/A	N/A	**Pembrolizumab** (anti-PD-1 antibody): • Phase 2 KEYNOTE-028: ORR 26% (19) **Nivolumab** (anti-PD-1 antibody): • Phase 1/2 CheckMate 356: ORR 20.7%, PFS 2.4 mo, OS NR (20) • Phase 2 NCI-9742: ORR 20.5%, 1-yr PFS 19.3%, 1-yr OS 59% (21) **JS001/Toripalimab** (anti-PD-1 antibody): • Phase 2 trial: ORR 25.2%, disease control rate 54.8% (22)

NR, not reached.

Actionable Target	Mutation	Prevalence	Clinical Experience with Targeted Agent
MET	Mutation (increases transcription of angiogenesis and growth factor receptors)	In addition to *MET* mutations, copy number gain of chromosome 7 (containing loci of both the MET receptor gene, *MET*, and its ligand, *HGF*) is common, occurring in 45%–75% of sporadic PRCC cases, and copy number alterations of *MET* occur in 81% of type 1 and 46% of type 2 PRCCs.	**Savolitinib:** • Phase 2: RR 18% of papillary RCC pts with MET-driven disease vs. 0% with MET-independent disease, PFS 6.2 vs. 1.4 mo (1) Sunitinib: • Phase 2 (non-MET selective). ORR 4%, PFS 5.6 mo (95% CI 2.9–6.7), OS 6.4 mo (2)

(continued)

Actionable Target	Mutation	Prevalence	Clinical Experience with Targeted Agent
mTOR			**Everolimus** (mTOR inhibitor): • Phase 3: ORR 2%, PFS 4.9 vs. 1.9 mo with placebo (3) **Temsirolimus** (mTOR inhibitor): • Phase 3: ORR 9%, PFS 5.5 vs. 3.1 mo with IFN-α (4)
PD-1/PD-L1			**Nivolumab** (PD-1 inhibitor): • Phase 1: RR 27% (5) • Phase 3: OS 25.0 mo with nivolumab vs. 19.6 mo with everolimus (6) • With **ipilimumab** (CTLA4 inhibitor): RR 40.4%; ongoing responses in 42.1% and 36.8% of pts in the N3I1 and N1I3 arms, respectively; 2-yr OS 67.3% and 69.6% in the N3I1 and N1I3 arms, respectively (7) • Phase 3 (second or later lines): 60-mo OS 26% vs. 18% with everolimus alone; OS 25.8 vs. 19.7 mo with everolimus; 60-mo PFS 5% vs. 1% with everolimus; ORR 23% vs. 4% with everolimus; DOR 18.2 vs. 14.0 mo with everolimus (8) alone
			BMS-936559 (PD-L1 inhibitor): • Phase 1: Responses in 2/17 pts (9)

Actionable Target	Mutation	Prevalence	Clinical Experience with Targeted Agent
VEGF, VHL, and angiogenesis	Mutation	VHL mutations in 43% (90% in sporadic cancers)	**Bevacizumab** (VEGF inhibitor): • Phase 3: ORR 26%–31% with IFN-α vs. 10% IFN-α alone (10, 11) **Cabozantinib** (VEGFR/MET/AXL): • Phase 3 (first-line treatment) IMDC intermediate or poor risk: PFS 8.6 vs. 5.3 OS with sunitinib alone; ORR 20% vs. 9% with sunitinib; OS 26.6 vs. 21.2 mo with single-agent sunitinib (12, 13) • Phase 3 (as second-line treatment): ORR 17% vs. 3% with everolimus alone; OS 21.4 vs. 16.5 mo with everolimus (14,15) **Sunitinib** (VEGFR/PDGFR/RET/KIT/FLT3 inhibitor): • Phase 3: ORR 47% vs. 17% with IFN-α alone, OS 26.4 vs. 21.8 mo with IFN-α alone (16) **Sorafenib** (VEGFR/PDGFR/RAF/RET): • Phase 3: ORR 10%, PFS 5.5 vs. 2.8 mo with placebo (17) **Pazopanib** (VEGFR/PDGFR/c-KIT): • Phase 3: ORR 30%, PFS 9.2 vs. 4.2 mo with placebo (18)

(continued)

Actionable Target	Mutation	Prevalence	Clinical Experience with Targeted Agent
			Axitinib (VEGFR/PDGFR/c-KIT): • Phase 3: PFS 6.7 vs. 4.7 with single-agent sorafenib (19) **Trebananib** (TIE2 inhibitor): • Phase 1: ORR 29% (with **sorafenib**), 53% (with **sunitinib**) (20)
			PT2385 (HIF-2α antagonist): • Phase 1: CR 2%, PR 12%, SD 52% (21) **Cediranib** (VEGFR inhibitor): • Phase 2 (first-line treatment): ORR 38%, PFS 8.9 mo, OS 28.6 mo (22) • Phase 2 (in advanced disease): ORR 34%, PFS 12.1 vs. 2.8 mo (with placebo) (23)

Actionable Target	Abnormality	Clinical Experience with Targeted Agent
BCL-2	Overexpression	**Venetoclax** (BCL-2 inhibitor): • Phase 2: As monotherapy in R/R AML: ORR 19%, additional 19% with PR and incomplete hematologic recovery. 33% CR rates in IDH-mutated AML (1) • Phase 1b with azacitidine/decitabine in treatment-naïve AML >65 yr: ORR 75% (venetoclax 400 mg), 80% (venetoclax 800 mg) (2) • Phase 1, with low-dose cytarabine in treatment-naïve AML >65 yr: CR or CRi 54%, 60-d mortality 15% (3)
CD33	Expression	**SGN-33A** (anti-CD33 antibody): • Phase 1, single agent in treatment-naïve AML: CR/CRi rates 60% (4) • Phase 1/2, with azacitidine/decitabine in treatment-naïve AML: CR/CRi rates 65%; OS not reached for median of 13.5+ wk (5) • Phase 1, with cytarabine and daunorubicin in ND AML: CR/CRi 76%; OS in MRD negative CR/CRi pts, not reached (6)
Cytogenetics	Inv(16), t(8;21)	**Gemtuzumab Ozogamicin** (anti-CD33 antibody) + FLAG: • Phase 1: CR/CRp 96%, relapse-free survival at 34 mo 83% (7)

(continued)

Actionable Target	Abnormality	Clinical Experience with Targeted Agent
FLT3	Internal tandem duplication (ITD)	**Sorafenib** (VEGFR inhibitor): • Compassionate use, monotherapy: Median time from allo-SCT to relapse = 192 d (8) • Phase 2, with idarubicin + cytarabine: CR 92%, CR with incomplete platelet recovery (CRp) 8% (9) • Phase 2, with azacitidine: CR 16%, PR 3%, CR with incomplete count recovery (CRi) 27%; median duration of CR/CRi 2.3 mo (10) Midostaurin (PKC-α/VEGFR2/c-KIT/PDGFR/FLT3 inhibitor): • Phase 3, 7 + 3 ± midostaurin in pts with FLT3 mutated AML: CR rates similar (59% [mido] vs. 54%), but significant improvement in OS ($p = 0.007$) and EFS ($p = 0.004$) with midostaurin (11) **Quizartinib** (FLT3 inhibitor): • Phase 2: ≥18 yr: CR 46%, OS 22.9 wk (in FLT3-ITD positive) (12); ≥60 yr: CR 50% (in FLT3-ITD positive) (13) Gilteritinib (FLT3/AXL/ALK inhibitor): • Phase 1/2, monotherapy in R/R AML: ORR 49% in FLT3 mutated and 12% in WT FLT3 (14)
IDH1	Mutation	**Ivosidenib** (IDH1 inhibitor): • Phase 1/2 study as monotherapy in R/R AML: ORR 33%, CR 15.5%, CRi/CRp 15.5%, PR 2%; 60 d mortality 21%; mDOR 10.2 mo (15) **IDH305** (IDH1 inhibitor): • Phase 1, as monotherapy in R/R AML/MDS: ORR 33%, CR or CRi 14.3%, PR 19% (16)

Leukemia: Acute Myeloid Leukemia (AML) (continued)

Actionable Target	Abnormality	Clinical Experience with Targeted Agent
IDH2	Mutation	**Enasidenib (IDH2 inhibitor):** • Phase 1/2, as monotherapy in R/R AML: ORR 41%, CR 26%, PR 15% (17)
MEK	RAS activating mutation	**Trametinib (MEK inhibitor):** • Phase 1/2: CR or CRp 12%, PR 2%; hematologic improvement 7% (18)
MDM2	Overexpression	**RG7112 (MDM2 inhibitor):** • Phase 1, as single agent in R/R AML: ORR 23%, CR with or without complete count recovery 10%, PR 13% (19)
NPM RARα PLZFRARα PML-RARα	t(5;17) t(11;17) t(15;17)	**All-Trans Retinoic Acid (ATRA):** • Pilot study, with idarubicin: CR 90% (20) • Phase 3, with arsenic trioxide (ATO), in pts with low-intermediate risk APL: CR 100%, at 2 yr, disease free survival rate 97%; cumulative incidence of relapse 1%, EFS 97% (21)

.onable Target	Type	Prevalence (%)	Clinical Experience with Targeted Agent
CD19	Precursor B cell	80	**Blinatumomab** (CD3-CD19 bispecific monoclonal antibody): • Phase 2 in pts with R/R B-ALL: CR/CRh rate of 43%, median RFS 5.9 mo (22) • Phase 3, blinatumomab vs. chemotherapy in R/R ALL: Blinatumomab superior in complete remission rates (34% vs. 16%; $p < 0.001$) and OS (7.7 vs. 4.0 mo; $p = 0.01$) (23) • Phase 2 in MRD+: Conversion to MRD neg 81%; RFS in responders 23.6 mo; OS 36.5 mo (24)
CD19	Precursor B cell	80	**Tisagenlecleucel** (murine anti-CD19 CAR T-cell therapy): • Phase 2, single-arm ELIANA trial in pts with R/R B-ALL: Overall remission rates 82.5%; RFS 75% and 64% at 6 and 12 mo; OS 89% and 79% at 6 and 12 mo (pivotal Phase 2 global ELIANA trial) (25)

Leukemia: Acute Lymphoblastic Leukemia (ALL)
(*continued*)

Actionable Target	Type	Prevalence (%)	Clinical Experience with Targeted Agent
CD20	Precursor B cell	40–50	**Rituximab** (CD20 monoclonal antibody): • Phase 2, with hyper-CVAD: CR 96%, CR duration 70% at 3 yr, OS 75% at 3 yr (26) **Ofatumumab** (CD20 monoclonal antibody): • Phase 2, with hyper-CVAD: CR 94%, CR duration 100% at 1 yr, OS 95% at 1 yr (27)
CD22	Precursor B cell	>90	**Inotuzumab Ozogamicin** (toxin-conjugated CD22 monoclonal antibody): • Phase 3 InO vs. standard salvage in pts with R/R B-ALL: Significantly higher CR rate (81% vs. 29%, $p < 0.001$); MRD rate (78% vs. 28%, $p < 0.001$); PFS (5 vs. 1.8 mo, $p < 0.001$); and OS (7.7 vs. 6.7 mo; $p = 0.04$) (28) • Phase 2: ORR 58%, CR rate 19%, CR with no platelet recovery 30%, bone marrow CR with no recovery of counts 9%, OS 6.2 mo, median remission duration 7 mo (29)

CRh, complete response with partial hematologic recovery.

Leukemia: Chronic Myeloid Leukemia (CML)

Actionable Target	Abnormality	Clinical Experience with Targeted Agent

Tyrosine kinase	BCR-ABL	**Imatinib (BCR-ABL inhibitor):**
		• Phase 2: Complete cytogenetic responses (CCyRs) 41%, complete hematologic response 95%, PFS 89% at 18 mo (30)
		Dasatinib (BCR-ABL, SRC inhibitor):
		• Phase 3: CCyRs 86%, major molecular response (MMR) 64% at 24 mo, transformation to accelerated/blast phase 2.3% (31)
		Nilotinib (BCR-ABL inhibitor):
		• Phase 3:
		  • 300 mg BID: CCyRs 87%, MMR 71% at 24 mo, complete molecular response (reduction of BCR-ABL levels to ≤0.0032%) 26%, 24-mo OS (CML-related deaths) 98.9%
		  • 400 mg BID: CCyRs 85%, MMR 67% at 24 mo, complete molecular response (reduction of BCR-ABL levels to ≤0.0032%) 21%, 24-mo OS (CML-related deaths) 98.9% (32)

	BCR-ABL, Src-Abl	**Bosutinib (BCR-ABL, Src inhibitor):** • Phase 3: CCyRs 70%, MMR 41% at 12 mo, transformation to accelerated/blast phase 2% (33)
	BCR-ABL (including T315I mutation)	**Ponatinib (BCR-ABL inhibitor):** • Phase 2: CCyRs 46%, MMR 34%, major cytogenetic response 56% (34)

Leukemia: Chronic Lymphocytic Leukemia (CLL)

Actionable Target	Abnormality	Clinical Experience with Targeted Agent
BCL-2	Overexpressed	**Venetoclax** (Bcl-2 inhibitor): • Phase 1: RR 85% (CR/CRi 13%, PR 72%) (35) • Phase 1, combined with rituximab: ORR 86%, CR 51%. MRD in 80% of CR; 2-yr PFS probability 82% (36)
BTK	Pathway activated	**Ibrutinib** (BTK inhibitor): • Phase 1b/2: RR 71%, PFS 75% at 26 mo, OS 83% at 26 mo (37) **Acalabrutinib** (BTK inhibitor) • Phase 3 (first line): 2-yr PFS 87% (93% with obinutuzumab) (38) • Phase 3 (salvage): 1-yr PFS 88% (39) **Zanubrutinib** (BTK inhibitor): • Phase 2 (salvage): RR 84.6% (3.3% CR); 1-yr OS 96% (40)

CD20	Present	**Fludarabine** + **Cyclophosphamide** + **Rituximab** (anti-CD20 antibody) (FCR):
		• Phase 3: RR 90% (CR 44%), PFS 51.8 mo, OS 87% at 3 yr (41)
		Ofatumumab (anti-CD20 antibody):
		• Phase 2 (42)
		  • Rituxan treated: RR 43%, PFS 5.3 mo, OS 15.5 mo
		  • Rituxan refractory: RR 44%, mPFS 5.5 mo, OS 15.5 mo
		  • Rituxan naïve: RR 53%, PFS 5.6 mo, OS 20.2 mo
		Obinutuzumab (anti-CD20 antibody):
		• Phase 3, with chlorambucil: PFS 26.7 mo, RR 77.3% (CR 22.3%, PR 55%) at 3 mo, hazard ratio for death 0.41 (95% CI 0.23–0.74) compared with chlorambucil monotherapy (43)
		
		(continued)

Leukemia: Chronic Lymphocytic Leukemia (CLL)
(continued)

Actionable Target	Abnormality	Clinical Experience with Targeted Agent
PI3kinase	Delta (δ) isoform	**Idelalisib** (PI3K-δ inhibitor): • Phase 3, with rituximab: RR 81%, OS 92% at 12 mo, lymph node RR 93% (reduction of 50% or more in lymphadenopathy), PFS 93% at 24 wk (44)
	Delta (δ), gamma (γ) isoform	**Duvelisib** (PI3K-δ, γ inhibitor): • Phase 3 (salvage): ORR 74%, PFS 13.3 mo (45)

Leukemia: Myeloproliferative Neoplasm (MPN)

Actionable Target	Abnormality	Clinical Experience with Targeted Agent
Janus kinase 2 (JAK2)	Somatic, constitutively activated mutation, V617F	**Ruxolitinib** (JAK2 inhibitor): • Phase 3, COMFORT-I trial, for intermediate 2 or high-risk myelofibrosis: Spleen volume reduction of 35% or more at 24 wk: 41.9% (0.7% in placebo); ≥50% improvement in total symptom score at 24 wk: 45.9% (5.3% in placebo) (46) • Phase 3, COMFORT-II trial: Spleen volume reduction of 35% or more at 48 wk: 28% (vs. 0% in best available treatment) (47) **Sotatercept** (JAK2 inhibitor): • Phase 2, for myelofibrosis with anemia: 36% of pts had anemia response (48)

Actionable Target	Abnormality	Prevalence (%)	Clinical Experience with Targeted Agent
BRAF	Mutation	4	**Sorafenib** (VEGFR/RAF inhibitor): • Phase 3 vs. placebo: RR 2%, OS 10.7 vs. 7.9 mo with placebo (1) **Sorafenib** + **Erlotinib** (EGFR inhibitor): • Phase 3 vs. sorafenib + placebo: RR 6.6% vs. 3.9%, OS 9.5 vs. 8.5 mo, PFS 3.2 vs. 4.0 mo (2) **Sorafenib** + **Refametinib** (MEK inhibitor): • Phase 2: RR 6.2%, SD 42%, PFS 114 d, OS 290 d (3)
PD-L1	Overexpression	25	**Nivolumab** (anti-PD1 antibody): • Phase 1/2: 77% treated with prior sorafenib, RR 15%, PFS 4.1 mo, OS 15.0 mo (4) **Pembrolizumab** (anti-PD1 antibody): • Phase 2: 79.8% treated with prior sorafenib, RR 18.3%, PFS 4.9 mo, OS 13.2 mo (5) **Nivolumab** + **Ipilimumab** (anti-CTLA4 antibody): • Phase 1/2: RR 33%, DOR 4.6–30.5+ mo (6) **Durvalumab** (anti-PD-L1 antibody) + **Bevacizumab** (anti-VEGF antibody): • Phase 3 vs. sorafenib: RR 25.6% vs. 5.5%, PFS 6.8 vs. 4.3 mo, OS at 12 mo: 67.2% vs. 54.6% (7)

Liver Cancer (Hepatocellular) (continued)

Actionable Target	Abnormality	Prevalence (%)	Clinical Experience with Targeted Agent
PIK3CA	Mutation	6	**Sirolimus** (mTOR inhibitor): • Phase 2: RR 8%, SD 32%, PFS 15.3 wk (8) **Everolimus** (mTOR inhibitor): • Phase 1/2: RR 4%, PFS 3.8 mo (9) **Temsirolimus** (mTOR inhibitor): • Phase 1/2: RR 3%, SD 56%, PFS 2.8 mo, OS 8.9 mo (10)
PTEN	Mutation	4	
TSC2	Mutation	5	
TGF-β	Overexpression	84	**Galunisertib** (TGF-β inhibitor): • Phase 2: 85% treated with prior sorafenib, PFS 4.2 mo, OS 16.8 mo (11)
VEGF	Overexpression	76	**Linifanib** (VEGFR/PDGFR inhibitor): • Phase 3 vs. sorafenib: RR 13% vs. 7%, PFS 5.4 vs. 4.0 mo, OS 9.1 vs. 9.8 mo (12) **Brivanib** (VEGFR/FGFR inhibitor): • Phase 3 vs. sorafenib: RR 12% vs. 9%, PFS 4.2 vs. 4.1 mo, OS 9.5 vs. 9.9 mo (13) **Regorafenib** (VEGFR2/PDGFR inhibitor): • Phase 3 vs. best supportive care after progression on sorafenib: RR 11% vs. 4%, OS 10.6 vs. 7.8 mo, PFS 3.1 vs. 1.5 mo (14)

(continued)

Actionable Target	Abnormality	Prevalence (%)	Clinical Experience with Targeted Agent
			Lenvatinib (VEGFR1, 2, 3 inhibitor): • Phase 3 vs. sorafenib in 1L: RR 4·1% vs. 9·2%, PFS 7.4 vs. 3.7 mo, OS 13.6 vs. 12.3 mo (15) • Proof-of-concept study vs. TACE in intermediate-stage HCC beyond up-to-seven criteria and Child–Pugh A liver function: RR: 73.3% vs. 33.3%, PFS 16 vs. 3 mo, OS 37.9 vs. 21.3 mo (16) **Ramucirumab** (VEGFR2 inhibitor): • Phase 3 vs. placebo in AFP ≥400 ng/mL: RR 5% vs. 1%, PFS 2.8 vs. 1.6 mo, OS 8.5 vs. 7.3 mo (17) **Cabozantinib** (VEGFR 1, 2, and 3, MET, AXL, TIE-2, RET, c-Kit, and FLT-3 inhibitor): • Phase 3 vs. placebo: RR: 4% vs. <1%, PFS 5.2 vs. 1.9 mo, OS 10.2 vs. 8 mo (18)

Genetic Abnormality	Prevalence	Clinical Experience with Targeted Agent
ALK/EML4-ALK	*ALK* rearrangement is detected in approximately 5% (1) Similar frequencies of *ALK* gene rearrangements have been reported in Asian and Western populations (2,3)	Second-generation inhibitors are now preferred to crizotinib in the first line (e.g., *alectinib*, given the benefit of longer-term follow-up of clinical trials with this agent compared with others). **Alectinib** (ALK inhibitor): • Phase 3: PFS not estimable vs. 10.2 mo with crizotinib. ORR 92% vs. 79% with crizotinib (4) • Phase 3: PFS (12-mo event-free survival rate) 68.4% vs. 48.7% with crizotinib. PFS was not reached with alectinib. RR 82.9% vs. 75.5% with crizotinib (5) **Brigatinib** (ALK inhibitor): • Phase 3: PFS 67% vs. 43% mo with crizotinib. ORR 71% vs. 60% with crizotinib (6) **Lorlatinib** (ALK inhibitor): • Phase 3: PFS at 12 mo 78% vs. 39% with crizotinib. ORR 76% vs. 58% with crizotinib (7) **Ceritinib** (ALK inhibitor) (less preferred than alectinib or brigatinib): • Phase 3: PFS 16.6 vs. 8.1 mo with chemotherapy. ORR 72.5% vs. 26.7% with chemotherapy (8) **Crizotinib** (ALK inhibitor) (crizotinib is more effective than chemotherapy for ALK-positive NSCLC, it should only be used if a next-generation ALK inhibitor is not available): • Phase 3: PFS 10.9 vs. 7.0 mo with chemotherapy. ORR 74% vs. 45% with chemotherapy (9) • Phase 3: PFS 7.7 vs. 3.0 mo with chemotherapy. ORR 65% vs. 20% with chemotherapy (10)

(continued)

Genetic Abnormality	Prevalence	Clinical Experience with Targeted Agent
		Ensartinib (ALK inhibitor): • Phase 1/2: PFS 25.8 vs. 12.7 mo with crizotinib. ORR 75% vs. 67% with crizotinib. 24 mo OS 78% in both ensartinib and crizotinib (11)
BRAF		**Dabrafenib ± Trametinib** (BRAF V600E) (BRAF and MEK inhibitors): • Cohort Trial: pts w/ previously treated BRAF V600E-mutant ORR 63%, CR 2, PR 36; pts w/ previously untreated BRAF V600E-mutant 61%, CR 1, PR 21 (12)
EGFR	12%–15% (mutation in exon 19 or 21)	**Osimertinib** (EGFR inhibitor): • Phase 3 (in pts with exon 19 or L858R allele mutations): OS 38.6 vs. 31.8 mo in pts treated with either gefitinib or erlotinib; PFS 18.9 vs. 10.2 mo in pts treated with either gefitinib or erlotinib (13) **Erlotinib** (EGFR inhibitor): • Phase 3 (in pts with exon 19 or 21 deletions or exon 21 mutations): RR 60%–70% vs. 15%–20% with standard chemotherapy. PFS 9.7 vs. 5.2 mo (14) • Phase 3 (in pts with exon 19 or exon 21 L858R mutations): PFS 13.1 vs. 4.6 mo with chemotherapy. ORR 83% vs. 36% with chemotherapy (15) • Phase 3: PFS 11.0 vs. 5.5 mo with chemotherapy. OS 26.3 vs. 25.5 with chemotherapy. ORR 62.7% vs. 33.6% with chemotherapy (16)

Genetic Abnormality	Prevalence	Clinical Experience with Targeted Agent
		Gefitinib (EGFR inhibitor): • Phase 3 (IMPRESS): RR 70%, PFS 10.8 vs. 5.4 mo with chemotherapy, OS 31 vs. 24 mo (17) **Cetuximab** (EGFR inhibitor): • Phase 2 (with cisplatin/vinorelbine): RR 35% vs. 28% with cisplatin/vinorelbine alone, PFS 5.0 vs. 4.5 mo, OS 8.3 vs. 7.3 mo (18) **Afatinib** (EGFR inhibitor): • Phase 3 (LUX-Lung 3) (with pemetrexed): PFS 11.1 vs. 6.9 mo with cisplatin/pemetrexed; PFS 13.6 vs. 6.9 mo in exon 19 del and L858R (19) **Dacomitinib** (EGFR inhibitor): • Phase 3 (exon 19 deletion or exon 21 L858R): OS 34.1 vs. 26.8 mo with gefitinib (20)
EGFR	Untreated EGFR-mutated tumors: <5% (21) Erlotinib/gefitinib-resistant EGFR-mutated tumors: 50% (22,23)	**Osimertinib** (EGFR inhibitor): • Phase 3: 61% RR in T790M; PFS 18.9 vs. 10.2 mo for standard of care (SOC) in exon 19/L858R (24)

(continued)

Genetic Abnormality	Prevalence	Clinical Experience with Targeted Agent
EGFR	Exon 20 insertion mutations: 4%–9.2% (25,26)	**Mobocertinib** (EGFR inhibitor) (FDA approved 2021): • Phase 1/2: ORR 28%, DOR 17.5 mo, OS 24.0 mo (27) **Poziotinib** (EGFR inhibitor): • Phase 2: RR 73%; inhibits exon 20 insertions over T790M due to compound size and flexibility (28)
EGFR		**Necitumumab** (EGFR inhibitor) (FDA approved in combination with gemcitabine and cisplatin in metastatic squamous NSCLC): • Phase 3 (SQUIRE): OS 11.5 vs. 9.9 mo with gemcitabine/cisplatin alone, PFS 5.7 vs. 5.5 mo with gemcitabine/cisplatin alone, ORR 31% vs. 29% with gemcitabine/cisplatin alone (29)
EGFR	EGFR S768I, L861Q, and G719X mutations	**Afatinib**—pooled post hoc analysis of three trials in which afatinib was compared with platinum-based chemotherapy as initial treatment for those with *EGFR* mutations; clinical benefit was lower in patients with de novo Thr790Met and exon 20 insertion mutations compared with those with *EGFR* S768I, L861Q, or G719X mutations. • Phase 3 (Grp 1: pt mutations/duplications in exons 18–21; Grp 2: Thr790 met mutation in exon 20; Grp 3: exon 20 insertions): PFS 10.7 mo, 1.2–8.3 mo, 2.7 mo respectively. OS 19.4, 14.9, 9.2 mo. ORR 71.1%, 14.3%, 8.7%, respectively (30)

Genetic Abnormality	Prevalence	Clinical Experience with Targeted Agent
EGFR	Exon 20 insertion	**Amivantamab-vmjw** (FDA approved 2021) (EGFR-MET bispecific antibody): • Phase 2: PFS 8.3 mo. OS 22.8 mo, ORR 40% with CR 3 pts, 29 pts PR, SD 39 pts (31)
HER 2 mutation	Approximately 1%–3% of NSCLC tumors	**Ado-Trastuzumab Emtansine:** • Phase 2 (18 pts with *HER2*-mutant advanced lung cancer with a median of two prior lines of systemic therapy): ORR 57%, PFS 5.0 mo, DOR 4.0 mo (32) **Trastuzumab Deruxtecan**· • Phase 1: administered to 42 patients with HER2-positive NSCLC, RR 62% (33)
KRAS	24% (mutation)	**Sotorasib** (FDA approved 2021) (KRAS-G12C inhibitor): • Phase 1 NSCLC (59 pts): PR 19 pts, 33 pts SD. PFS 6.3 mo (34) • Phase 2: ORR 37.1%; CR 4 pts, PR 42 pts, SD 54 pts (35) **Selumetinib** (MEK inhibitor): • Phase 3: PFS 3.9 mo in patients treated with Selumetinib + docetaxel vs. 2.8 mo with placebo + docetaxel; OS 8.7 vs. 7.9 mo, respectively; ORR 20.1% vs. 13.7%, respectively (36)

(continued)

Genetic Abnormality	Prevalence	Clinical Experience with Targeted Agent
MET exon 14	Occurs in 3% of lung adenocarcinomas and up to 20% of the relatively rare sarcomatoid-histology NSCLC	Capmatinib (FDA approved 2020) (MET inhibitor): • Phase 2 (GEOMETRY): ORR 32% with 1 or 2 lines previous Tx, 68% with no previous Tx (37) Tepotinib (FDA approved 2021) (MET inhibitor): • Phase 2 (VISION): ORR 46%, DOR 11.1 mo (38) Crizotinib (multikinase inhibitor): • Phase 1/2 (PROFILE): ORR 46%, CR 3 pts, PR 18 pts, SD 29 pts (39)
MET amplification	2%–4% of treatment-naïve NSCLC, and 5%–20% of *EGFR*-mutated tumors that have acquired resistance to EGFR inhibitors	**No current FDA approval for targeted therapy and the ideal methodology for determining level of amplification and appropriate cutoffs for treatment is still an active area of research.** Tepotinib (MET inhibitor): • Phase 2 (PROFILE): ORR 42%, PFS 4.2 mo, PR 10 pts, SD 1 pt (40) Capmatinib (MET inhibitor): • Phase 2: ORR 20%: ORR 47%; in pts with MET Gene Copy Number (GCN) ≥6; PFS in pts with MET GCN ≥6, 9.3 mo (41) Crizotinib (multikinase inhibitor): • Phase 2: ORR 28.9%. CR 2 pts, PR 9 pts, SD 11 pts. PFS 5.1 mo (42)

Genetic Abnormality	Prevalence	Clinical Experience with Targeted Agent
NTRK	<1%	**Larotrectinib** (FDA approved 2018) (TRK inhibitor): • Phase 1/2: ORR 79%, CR 24 pts, PR 97 pts, SD 19 pts (43) **Entrectinib** (FDA approved 2019) (TRK inhibitor): • Phase 1/2 (STARTRK-2, STARTRK-1. ALKA-372-001): ORR 57% across all tumor types (95% CI 43–71), including a 7% complete response rate (44)
PD-1/PD-L1	N/A	**Nivolumab** (anti-PD-1 antibody) (FDA approved): • Phase 2: ORR 14.5%, PFS 1.9 mo (45) • Phase 3: OS 9.2 vs. 6.0 mo with docetaxel, RR 20% vs. 9% with docetaxel, PFS 3.5 vs. 2.8 mo with docetaxel (46) • Phase 1/2, with **ipilimumab** (anti-CTLA-4): ORR 25% vs. 11% Nivo alone, OS 7.9 vs. 4.1 mo Nivo alone (47) **Pembrolizumab** (anti-PD-1 antibody) (FDA approved): • Phase 1: ORR 19.4%, PFS 3.7 mo; in pts with PD-L1-expressing tumors: RR 45.2%, PFS 6.3 mo (48) • Phase 2/3: PFS 3.9 mo (2 mg/kg), 4 mo (10 mg/kg), 4 mo with docetaxel; OS 10.4 mo (2 mg/kg), 12.7 mo (10 mg/kg) vs. 8.5 mo with docetaxel. In pts with PD-L1-expressing tumors: OS 14.9 mo (2 mg/kg), 17.3 mo (10 mg/kg) vs. 8.2 mo with docetaxel; PFS 5.0 mo (2 mg/kg), 5.2 mo (10 mg/kg) 4.1 mo with docetaxel (49) • Phase 2, with **carboplatin** and **pemetrexed**: ORR 55% vs. 29% chemo alone, PFS 13 vs. 8.9 mo chemo alone (50) *(continued)*

Genetic Abnormality	Prevalence	Clinical Experience with Targeted Agent
PD-1/PD-L1	N/A	**Atezolizumab** (anti-PD-L1 antibody) (FDA approved): • Phase 2: OS 12.6 vs. 9.7 mo with docetaxel; increased PFS and ORR observed with increasing PD-L1 expression: PFS 7.8 vs. 3.9 mo with docetaxel, ORR 38% vs. 13% with docetaxel (51) • Phase 3 (OAK): OS 13.8 vs. 9.6 mo with docetaxel; increased OS and ORR observed with increasing PD-L1 expression: OS 15.7 vs. 10.3 mo with docetaxel, ORR 31% vs. 11% with docetaxel (52) • Phase 3, with bevacizumab (anti-VEGF-A) + **carboplatin** + **paclitaxel**: PFS 8.3 vs. 6.8 mo, ORR 64% vs. 48% in atezo + Bev + carboplatin + paclitaxel vs. Bev + carboplatin + paclitaxel, respectively (53) **Consolidation therapy** **Durvalumab** (FDA approved 2020) (anti-PD-L1) after chemoradiotherapy: • Phase 3 (PACIFIC): PFS 16.8 vs. 5.6 mo with placebo, RR 28.4% vs. 16% with placebo (54)

Genetic Abnormality	Prevalence	Clinical Experience with Targeted Agent
RET	1%–2% of adenocarcinomas, and occur more frequently in younger patients and in never-smokers	**Selpercatinib** (FDA approved 2020): • Phase 1/2 (LIBRETTO): ORR 64% in previously treated with platinum chemotherapy, ORR 85% in previously untreated, PFS 16 mo in previously treated group, NE in untreated group (55) **Pralsetinib** (FDA approved 2020): • Phase 1/2 (ARROW): ORR 61% in previously treated with platinum chemotherapy, ORR 70% in previously untreated; CR 5 pts, PR 48 pts and SD 26 pts in previously treated with platinum chemotherapy; CR 3 pts, PR 16 pts, SD 4 pts in previously untreated (56)

(continued)

Genetic Abnormality	Prevalence	Clinical Experience with Targeted Agent
ROS1	1%–2% of NSCLCs via a genetic translocation between *ROS1* and other genes, the most common of which is *CD74*	*ROS1* tyrosine kinase is highly sensitive to the ROS1/MET inhibitor *crizotinib* as well as the ROS1/tropomyosin receptor kinase (TRK) inhibitor *entrectinib*. Crizotinib (ROS1 inhibitor): • Phase 1: ORR 72%, PFS 19.2 mo, CR 3 pts, PR 33 pts (57,58) **Entrectinib (ROS1 inhibitor):** • Phase 1/2: ORR 67.1%, PFS (12 mo), OS (12 mo) 81% (59) Favor entrectinib for patients with central nervous system (CNS) involvement, due to better intracranial penetration Lorlatinib (ROS1 inhibitor) in treatment post-**Crizotinib:** • Phase 1/2: CR 2 pts, PR 12 pts, SD 16 pts. 14 pts with confirmed objective response. DOR 13.8 mo (60) **Repotrectinib (ROS1 inhibitor):** • Phase 1 (TRIDENT-1): ORR 91% in TKI-naïve pts (61) **Taletrectinib (ROS1 inhibitor):** • Phase 1: ORR 33.3% 6 pts (62) • Phase 1: PR 2 pts, SD 2 pts (63) • Phase 1: ORR 66.7% in TKI-naïve pts and 33.3% in crizotinib-pretreated pts; PFS 29.1 and 14.2 mo, respectively (64)

Lung Cancer (SCLC)

Genetic Abnormality	Prevalence	Clinical Experience with Targeted Agent
DLL3		**Rovalpituzumab Tesirine** (anti-DLL3 ADC): • Phase 1: RR 18% of all pts, RR 38% in DLL3+ pts; PFS 2.8 mo for all pts, PFS 4.3 mo for DLL3+ pts vs. 2.2 mo for DLL3– pts (65)
PARP	N/A	**Veliparib** (PARP inhibitor): • Phase 2, with **temozolomide**: ORR 39% veliparib + TMZ vs. 14% placebo + TMZ; OS 8.2 mo veliparib + TMZ vs. 7 mo placebo + TMZ (66) • Phase 2, with **cisplatin** + **etoposide**: PFS 6.1 mo for CE + V vs. 5.5 mo for CE + placebo; OS 10.3 for CE + V vs. 8.9 mo for CE + P (67) **Talazoparib** (PARP inhibitor): • Phase 1: 2/23 pts with confirmed PRs • ECIST confirmed partial responses and 3/23 with SD lasting more than 24 wk (clinical benefit rate of 25%) (68)
PD-1/PD-L1	N/A	**Nivolumab** (anti-PD-1 antibody): • Phase 1/2: ORR 10%; PFS 1.4 mo (69) • Phase 1/2 with **ipilimumab** (anti-CTLA-4): 1 mg/kg Nivo + 3 mg/kg Ipi: ORR 23%, PFS 2.6 mo; 3 mg/kg Nivo + 1 mg/kg Ipi: ORR 19%, PFS 1.4 mo (70) **Pembrolizumab** (anti-PD-1 antibody): • Phase 1b: ORR of 33% in PD-L1-expressing SCLC (71)

Lymphoma

Actionable Target	Abnormality	Clinical Experience with Targeted Agent
AKT	Key signaling pathway	**Perifosine** (AKT inhibitor): HL: • Phase 2 perifosine with sorafenib: ORR 28% in rr-HL (1) **Afuresertib** (AKT inhibitor): CLL: • Phase 2: afuresertib plus ofatumumab: OR 50% (CR 3.6%), PFS 8.5 mo, OS 34.8 mo (2)
AURKA	Key signaling pathway	**Alisertib** (aurora A kinase inhibitor): TCL: • Phase 3 alisertib vs. investigator's choice: ORR 33% vs. 43%, PFS 3.7 vs. 3.4 mo, OS 9.9 vs. 12.2 mo in rr-PTCL (3)
BCL-2	Translocation/overexpression	**Navitoclax (ABT-263)** (BCL-2 inhibitor): BCL: • Phase 1, with rituximab: ORR 75% in FL, PRR 100% in CLL/SLL in rr-CD20+ lymphoid malignancies (4) **Venetoclax** (BCL-2 inhibitor): CLL: • Phase 2: ibrutinib and venetoclax, at 12 cycles, 88 had complete remission or complete remission with incomplete count recovery, 61% had remission with undetectable minimal residual disease (5)

Actionable Target	Abnormality	Clinical Experience with Targeted Agent
		• Phase 2 (AIM): ibrutinib and venetoclax, CRR 42% at week 16, which was higher than the historical result of 9% at this time point with ibrutinib monotherapy (*p* < 0.001); CR 62% at week 16 and 71% overall (6) CLL: • Phase 2: 65% ORR (7) BCL: • Phase 1: ORR (n = 30) ITT was 97% with 27 (90%) CRs and 2 (7%) PRs; 1 was not evaluable; follow-up is ongoing; of 15 DHL, ORR 93% and CRR 80% (8)
BCL-2	Translocation/ overexpression	**Obatoclax (GX15-070)** (BCL-2 inhibitor): MCL: • Phase 1/2 obatoclax and bortezomib: ORR 31% in rr-MCL (9)
BTK	Key signaling pathway	**Ibrutinib** (BTK inhibitor): DLBCL: • Phase 1/2: ORR 37% in relapsed ABC DLBCL, 5% in relapsed GCB DLBCL (10) • Phase 1 ibrutinib with R-CHOP: ORR 100%; CRR 71% in GCB, 100% in non-GCB tn-DLBCL (11) MZL: • Phase 2: ORR 48%, mDOR NR, PFS 14.2 mo in rr-MZL (12) *(continued)*

Actionable Target	Abnormality	Clinical Experience with Targeted Agent
BTK	Key signaling pathway	BCL: • Phase 1/2a ibrutinib with nivolumab: in rr-BCL, ORR 83.3% for rr-CLL, 66.7% for rr-SLL, 30% for rr-FL, 35.6% for rr-DLBCL, and 60% for RT; PFS 5.5 mo for rr-FL, 3.2 mo for rr-DLBCL, and 3.6 mo for RT (13) HL: • Phase 2 brentuximab vedotin + ibrutinib: ORR 69%, CRR 46% in rr-cHL (14) Nongerminal center B-cell DLBCL: • Phase 3: ibrutinib plus R-CHOP vs. placebo plus R-CHOP, in ITT population, addition of ibrutinib did not increase PFS, OS, ORR (89.3% vs. 93.1%), CRR (67.3% vs. 68.0%); age <60 yr, ibrutinib plus R-CHOP improved EFS, PFS, OS, ORR was 93.6% vs. 94.6%, CRR was 71.2% vs. 69.9%; age ≥60 yr, ibrutinib plus R-CHOP worsened EFS, PFS, and OS (15) CLL: • Phase 2: ibrutinib with venetoclax, at 12 cycles 88% had complete remission or complete remission with incomplete count recovery, and 61% had remission (5) CLL/SLL: • Phase 3: ibrutinib vs. ofatumumab, PFS 44.1 vs. 8.1 mo, ORR with ibrutinib 91%, OS was better with ibrutinib (16) FL and MZL: • Phase 2: estimated 2-yr PFS rate 76%; FL: ORR according to Lugano criteria 97%, CR 78%; MZL: ORR 80%, CR 60% (17)

Actionable Target	Abnormality	Clinical Experience with Targeted Agent
		MCL and CLL: • Phase 1b/2: cirmtuzumab plus ibrutinib, MCL 83% ORR, 33% CR, 50% PR, 17% SD; CLL 88% ORR (92% tn, 86% rr), 3% CR, 85% PR/PR-L, 12% SD (18) R/R DLBCL: • Phase 2: ORR 53.2% and CR 35.9% after 4th cycle; at the end of induction, ORR 35.9% and CR 29.7% (19) R/R DLBCL: • Phase 1b: in response-evaluable patients, ORR 44% (CR 28%); among them, ORR 65% (CR 41%) in non-GCB and 69% in relapsed (n = 16) and 56% in secondary refractory (n = 27) disease (20) **Acalabrutinib (BTK inhibitor):** MCL: • Phase 2: ORR 81%, CRR 40%, mTTR 1.9 mo, mDOR NR, 12-mo PFS 67%, 12-mo OS 87% in rr-MCL (21) R/R MCL: • Phase 2 (ACE-LY-004): at 15.2 mo, OR 81%, CR 40%; at 12 mo, PFS 67%, OS 87% (22) R/R CLL: • Phase 3: acalabrutinib vs. investigator's choice, PFS significantly longer (PFS not reached) vs. 16.5 mo, 12-mo PFS 88% vs. 68% (23) R/R CLL: • Phase 2: ORR 94%, mDOR and PFS not reached; estimated 45-mo PFS rate 62% (24)

(*continued*)

Actionable Target	Abnormality	Clinical Experience with Targeted Agent
BTK	Key signaling pathway	**ONO/GS-4059** (BTK inhibitor): BCL: • Phase 1: ORR 92% in rr-MCL, 35% in rr-non-GCB DLBCL, 96% in rr-CLL (25) **BGB-3111** Zanubrutinib (BTK inhibitor): BCL: • Phase 1b: ORR 58.1% (60.9% in aggressive NHL and 50.0% in iNHL) in rr-BCL (26) MZL: • Phase 2: ORR 56%, CR 20% (27) • Phase 2: CT-based ORR 80%, CR 20% (28) WM: • Phase 3 (ASPEN): vs. ibrutinib: VGPR 28% vs. 19%, MRRs 77% vs. 78%, 18 mo. PFS 85% vs. 84% (29)
CAR-T	Immune surveillance	**CD30 CAR-Ts:** • Phase 1: ORR and CRR 14% (1/7 patients) in rr-HL, ORR and CRR 50% in rr-ALCL (but only 2 patients) (30) R/R HL: • Phase 1/2: ORR in the 32 patients with active disease who received fludarabine-based lymphodepletion was 72%, 59% had CR; 1-yr PFS was 36%, OS was 94% (31).

Actionable Target	Abnormality	Clinical Experience with Targeted Agent
CAR-T	Immune surveillance	**CD19 CAR-T:** • Phase 2 CTL019 (tisagenlecleucel) JULIET: 6-mo ORR 37%, 6-mo CRR 30%, 6-mo OS 64.5% in rr-DLBCL (32) • Phase 1/2 axicabtagene ciloleucel (KTE-C19, ZUMA-1): ORR 82%, CRR 54% after single infusion of axi-cel in rr-BCL (DLBCL, tFL, PMLBCL), best ORR 52%, CR 40%, PR 12% (33) **rr-MCL:** • Phase 2: 93% had objective response; 67% had CR; ITT analysis, 85% had an objective response, 59% had a CR; 12-mo estimated PFS 61%, OS 83% (34) **rr-DLBCL:** • Phase 2: best ORR 52%; 40% had CR, 12% had PR; at 12-mo rate of relapse-free survival was 65% (79% among patients with a CR) (35) **Refractory LBCL:** • Phase 2 (axi-cel): objective response rate 82%, CRR 54%, median follow-up 15.4 mo, CR 40%, 18-mo OS rate 52% (36) **Refractory LBCL:** • Phase 1/2 (axi-cel plus lenzilumab, ZUMA-1): objective response 83%, CR 58%, mDOR 11.1 mo, OS not reached, PFS 5.9 mo (37) **rr-LBCL:** • Phase 1 (lisocabtagene maraleucel, TRANSCEND NHL 001): objective response 73%, CR 53% (38) *(continued)*

Actionable Target	Abnormality	Clinical Experience with Targeted Agent
		rr-LBCL: • Phase 1/2 (axi-cel plus lenzilumab, ZUMA-19): (only abstract) (39) Refractory LBCL: • Phase 2 (axi-cel plus rituximab or lenalidomide, ZUMA-14): (only abstract) (40) LBCL: • Phase 2 (axi-cel, ZUMA-12): centrally confirmed LBCL, ORR 92%, CR 75%; safety analysis set, ORR 93%, CR 80% (41) rr-DLBCL: • Phase 1 (axi-cel, ZUMA-6): ORR 90%, CR 60%, PR 30%; 33% converted to CR at month 6 and month 9 after PR (42)
CAR-T	Immune surveillance	**RNA CAR-T:** • Phase 1: ORR at day 28 was 50%, 1/5 patients had CR, who progressed at 3 mo, in rr-cHL (43) HL: • Early phase 1: at 1 mo, 1 CR, 1 PR, 1 SD, 1 PD (44) **ACTR:** • Phase 1 ACTR087 + rituximab: ORR 50%, CRR 33% in rr-CD20+ BCL (45) R/R nHL: • Phase 1: CR in 3 of 6 patients (46) • DLBCL, MCL, PBMCL, Gr3b FL, or transformed FL subtype: • Phase 1 (ATTCK-20-2): 2 CR, 1 PR (45)

Lymphoma (*continued*)

Actionable Target	Abnormality	Clinical Experience with Targeted Agent
CCR4	Key signaling pathway	**Mogamulizumab** (anti-CCR4 antibody): TCL: • Phase 3 mogamulizumab vs. vorinostat: ORR 28.0% vs. 4.8%, PFS 7.7 vs. 3.1 mo in relapsed CTCL (47) R/R ATL: • Phase 2 mogamulizumab vs. investigator's choice of chemotherapy: ORR 11% vs. 0%, best response 28% vs. 8% (48)
CD19	B-lymphocyte antigen	**Loncastuximab Tesirine (ADCT-402)** (anti-CD19 antibody): BCL: R/R nHL: • Phase 1: at doses ≥120 µg/kg, ORR 59.4%; 40.6% had CR; 18.8% had PR; PFS 5.5 mo, OS 11.6 mo (49)
CD20	B-lymphocyte antigen	**Ofatumumab** (anti-CD20 antibody): FL: • Phase 2 ofatumumab and CHOP: ORR 90%–100%, CRR 62% in untreated FL (50) iNHL: • Phase 2 bendamustine and ofatumumab: ORR 90% in untreated iNHL (51)

(*continued*)

Actionable Target	Abnormality	Clinical Experience with Targeted Agent
CD20	B-lymphocyte antigen	DLBCL: • Phase 3 in rr-DLBCL: ORR 38%, CRR 15% for O-DHAP; ORR 42%, CRR 22% for R-DHAP; ASCT completed in 33% of the O arm and 37% of the R arm; 2-yr PFS rate 24% vs. 26%, 2-yr OS rate 41% vs. 38% (52) CLL/SLL: • Phase 3: ibrutinib vs. ofatumumab, PFS 44.1 vs. 8.1 mo • Ibrutinib vs. ofatumumab in the genomic high-risk population with del(17p), TP53 mutation, del(11q), and/or unmutated IGHV status; PFS 44.1 vs. 8.0 mo; ORR with ibrutinib was 91% (16) **Obinutuzumab (GA101)** (anti-CD20 antibody): FL: • Phase 3 G vs. R-based induction and maintenance: 3-yr PFS rate G-chemo 80% vs. 73.3% for R-chemotherapy in untreated FL; ORR 88.5% vs. 86.9% (53,54) iNHL: • Phase 3 G with bendamustine and G maintenance vs. bendamustine: PFS 25.3 vs. 14.0 mo, OS NR vs. 53.9 mo in R refractory iNHL (55)

Actionable Target	Abnormality	Clinical Experience with Targeted Agent
CD20	B-lymphocyte antigen	DLBCL: • Phase 3 G vs. R with ACVBP-14 or CHOP-14: 2-yr PFS rate for aa-IPI 2–3 G-CHOP 56.1%, R-CHOP 51.7%, G-ACVBP 61%, R-ACVBP 58.6% for untreated DLBCL age <60 y: (56) • Phase 3 randomized G-CHOP vs. R-CHOP in untreated DLBCL: 3-yr PFS rate 70% vs. 67%, 3-yr OS rate 81.2% vs. 81.4% (57) BCL: • Phase 2: ORR 32% in rr-DLBCL, ORR 27% in rr-MCL (58) R/R DLBCL: • Phase 1b/2: single-arm pola-BG, CRR 29.6%, OS 10.8 mo • Random cohort: pola-BR vs. BR: IRC-assessed CRR 40.0% vs. 17.5%, IRC-assessed PFS 9.5 vs. 3.7 mo, OS 12.4 vs. 4.7 mo (59) Rituximab-refractory indolent nHL: • Phase 3 (GADOLIN): obinutuzumab with bendamustine vs. bendamustine, PFS in ITT patients 25.8 vs. 14.1 mo, OS was also prolonged; PFS and OS benefits were similar in patients with FL (60). FL: • Phase 3 (GALLIUM): after 41.1 mo median follow-up, PFS was superior for G plus chemo ($p = 0.0016$) (61).

(*continued*)

Actionable Target	Abnormality	Clinical Experience with Targeted Agent
		R/R FL: • Phase 2 (GALEN): 79% evaluable patients achieved an OR at induction end; at 2 yr, PFS 65% OS 87%, CR 38% at induction, best OR in 81% of induction and 84% of treatment groups (62) Rituximab-refractory FL: • Phase 3 (GADOLIN): High obinutuzumab exposure was associated with greater efficacy, particularly longer PFS (63). CLL: • Phase 3 (iLLUMINATE): ibrutinib plus obinutuzumab vs. chlorambucil plus obinutuzumab: PFS significantly greater (not reached) vs. 19 mo (<0.0001), estimated 30-mo PFS rate 79% vs. 31% (64) DLBCL: • Phase 2 (GATHER): OR and CR rates, as determined by investigators/independent radiologic facility, were 82.0/75.0% and 55.0/58.0%, respectively (65)
CD30	Cell-surface marker of some lymphoma cells	Brentuximab Vedotin (anti-CD30 antibody): DLBCL: • Phase 2: ORR 44%, CRR 17% in rr-DLBCL with variable CD30 expression (66) HL: • Phase 3 consolidation with brentuximab after ASCT vs. placebo: 3-yr PFS rate 61% vs. 43% in HL patients at high risk of relapse (67)

Actionable Target	Abnormality	Clinical Experience with Targeted Agent
CD30	Cell-surface marker of some lymphoma cells	TCL: • Phase 2: CRR 66%, 5-yr OS rate 60% in rr-ALCL; patients who achieved CR had 5-yr PFS rate of 57% and 6-yr OS rate of 79%, ORR 66% (68) • Phase 2: ORR 100%, CRR 58%, mDOR 20 wks, in refractory lymphomatoid papulosis (69) PTCL: • Phase 3 (ECHELON-2): A+CHP vs. CHOP: PFS 48.2 vs. 20.8 mo (70) HL: • Phase 3: BV vs. placebo, 5-yr PFS rate 59% vs. 41% (71) cHL: • Phase 2: OR and complete remission rates after initial BV lead-in dose were 18 (82%) of 22 and 8 (36%) of 22, respectively, and 40 (95%) of 42 and 34 (90%) of 42, respectively, after six cycles of AVD among 42 response-evaluable patients (72) nHL: • Phase 2: disease control rate 16/33, including 6 CR and 3 PR; PFS 1.9 mo and OS 6.1 mo (73) PTCL: • Phase 2: (only abstract) (74) PTCL: • Phase 1: 5-yr PFS and OS rates 52% and 80%; 50% remained in remission at the end of the study, with PFS ranging from 37.8+ to 66.0+ mo (75)

(continued)

Actionable Target	Abnormality	Clinical Experience with Targeted Agent
		DLBCL: • Phase 2: ORR 97% with 80% PET-negative CR; CD30+ vs. CD30–, CR 92% vs. 69%; CR rates were similar between ABC and GCB subtypes (76).
CD52	Lymphoid cell antigen	**Alemtuzumab** (anti-CD52 antibody): CLL: • Phase 3 alemtuzumab with fludarabine and cyclophosphamide vs. fludarabine and cyclophosphamide: 3-yr PFS rate 53% vs. 37% in untreated CLL with high-risk features, ORR 88% vs. 78%; 3-yr OS rate improved (85% vs. 76%) but only for patients <65 yr (77) • Phase 2 pentostatin, alemtuzumab, and low-dose rituximab: ORR 56%, CRR 28%, PFS 7.2 mo, OS 34.1 mo in rr-CLL or untreated CLL with 17p13 deletion (78) TCL: • Phase 2 CHO(E)P-14 followed by alemtuzumab consolidation: ORR 60.9%, CRR 58.5%, 3-yr OS rate 62.5% in untreated PTCL (79) • Phase 2 alemtuzumab, fludarabine, cyclophosphamide, and doxorubicin: ORR 63%, PFS 11.8 mo, and OS 25.9 mo in ND PTCL, OS 6.1 mo in rr-PTCL (80) PTCL: • Phase 3 (DSHNHL2006-1B/ACT-2): A-CHOP vs. CHOP, CR/CRu rate 60% vs. 43%, 72% vs. 66%, 3-yr EFS rate 27% vs. 24%, PFS rate 28% vs. 29%, OS rate 37% vs. 56% (81) TCL, NK cell lymphoma: • Phase 1/2: ORR 83.3%, OS 20.2 mo, PFS 6.6 mo (82)

Actionable Target	Abnormality	Clinical Experience with Targeted Agent
Checkpoint inhibition	Immune evasion	**Nivolumab** (anti-PD-1 monoclonal antibody): NHL and CLL • Phase 1/2a: ibrutinib and nivolumab: OR in CLL/SLL 61%, FL 33%, DLBCL 36%, Richter's transformation 65% (83) HL: • Phase 2 nivolumab induction followed by nivolumab AVD in ND advanced stage cHL: results pending (84); advanced cHL: objective response rate 84% with 67% CR, 9-mo PFS rate 92% (85) • Phase 2: ORR 81.3%, CRR 44.4%, 6-mo PFS rate 60%, 6-yr OS rate 100%, CR 4 in rr-cHL previously treated with brentuximab vedotin (86) cHL: • Phase 2 (CheckMate 205): objective response rate 84%, with 67% achieving complete remission; with a minimum follow-up of 9.4 mo, 9-mo modified PFS rate 92% (85) R/R PMBCL: • Phase 2 (CheckMate 436): nivolumab plus BV: at a median follow-up of 11.1 mo, ORR 73%, with a 37% complete remission rate per investigator and ORR 70%, with a 43% complete metabolic response rate per independent review (87) R/R cHL: • Phase 2 (CheckMate 205): objective response rate 69% overall and 65% to 73% in each cohort, mDOR 16.6 mo, PFS 14.7 mo (88) (*continued*)

Actionable Target	Abnormality	Clinical Experience with Targeted Agent
		R/R DLBCL: • Phase 2: PFS 1.9 mo and OS 12.2 mo in the auto-HCT-failed cohort and 1.4 mo and 5.8 mo in the auto-HCT-ineligible cohort (89) HL: • Phase 2 (ACCRU): brentuximab vedotin plus nivolumab, 48% of patients achieved a complete metabolic response and 13% achieved a partial metabolic response (ORR 61%) (90) **Pembrolizumab** (anti-PD-1 monoclonal antibody): RR NK/T-cell lymphoma: • Named-patient off-label basis: CR in 5/7 patients, PR in 2/7 (91) R/R cHL: • Phase 3 (KEYNOTE-204): pembrolizumab vs. BV: PFS 13.2 vs. 8.3 mo (92) HL: • Phase 2: ORR 69%, CRR 22.4% in rr-cHL (93)
Checkpoint inhibition	Immune evasion	PMBCL: • Phase 1b: ORR 41%, mDOR NR, OS NR in rr-PMBCL (94) FL: • Phase 2 pembrolizumab + rituximab: ORR 64%, CRR 48% in rr-FL (95)

Actionable Target	Abnormality	Clinical Experience with Targeted Agent
		R/R HL: • Phase 1/2 (KEYNOTE-051): rr-HL, of 15 patients 2 had CR and 7 had PR; thus, 9 patients achieved an objective response; solid tumors and other lymphomas, of 136 patients, 8 had PR, objective response was 5.9% (96) DLBCL: • Phase 2: overall, 59% of patients were alive and progression-free at 18 mo, which did not meet primary endpoint; 18-mo OS 93% (97) **Ipilimumab** (anti-CTLA-4 monoclonal antibody): Lymphoma: • Phase 1 nivolumab and ipilimumab: ORR 74% in rr-HL, 20% in rr-BCL, 9% in rr-TCL (98)
Folate	Key signaling pathway	**Pralatrexate** (antifolate): PTCL: • Phases 1 and 2: ORR 45%, CRR 10%, PFS 5 mo, OS NR in rr-PTCL (99) rr-TCL: • Phase 1: pralatrexate plus romidepsin, ORR 57% across all patients and 71% in PTCL (100) rr-cutaneous TCL: • Phase 1/2: response rate 60%; CR 4, PR 14 PFS 12.8 mo (101) *(continued)*

Actionable Target	Abnormality	Clinical Experience with Targeted Agent
HAT (EP200, CREBBP)	Mutation	**Vorinostat** (HDAC inhibitor): FL: • Phase 2: ORR 49%, PFS 20 mo in rr-FL (102) BCL: • Phase 2: ORR 47% in rr-FL, 22% in rr-MZL, 0% in rr-MCL (103) iNHL: • Phase 2 vorinostat and rituximab: ORR 46%, 67% in tn-iNHL; 41% for rr-iNHL; PFS 29.2 mo in ND and rr-iNHL (104) MCL: • Phase 2 vorinostat with fludarabine, mitoxantrone, and dexamethasone: ORR 77.8%, PFS 9.3 mo in rr-MCL (105) TCL: • Phase 1/2 lenalidomide in combination with vorinostat and dexamethasone: ORR 25%, PFS 2.2 mo, OS 6.7 mo in rr-PTCL (106) • Phase 1 vorinostat-CHOP: CRR 93%, 2-yr PFS rate 79%, 2-yr OS rate 81% in tn-PTCL (107) Cutaneous TCL: • Phase 3 (MAVORIC): Mogamulizumab vs. vorinostat: PFS 7.7 vs. 3.1 mo (108) DLBCL: • Phase 1/2 (SWOG S0806): vorinostat with R-CHOP, 2-yr PFS estimate 73%, OS estimate 86% (109)

Actionable Target	Abnormality	Clinical Experience with Targeted Agent
HAT (EP200, CREBBP)	Mutation	**Panobinostat** (HDAC inhibitor): DLBCL: • Randomized phase 2 panobinostat with or without rituximab: ORR 28%, rituximab did not increase response in relapsed DLBCL (110) HL: • Phase 2: ORR 27%, PFS 6.1 mo, 1-yr OS rate 78% in rr-HL after autologous SCT (111) R/R cHL: • Phase 1/2: for Phase 2, CR 82% for P-ICE and 67% for ICE (112) **Belinostat (PXD101)** (HDAC inhibitor): TCL: • Phase 2: ORR 25.8%, CRR 10.8%, PFS 1.6 mo, OS 7.9 mo in rr-PTCL (113) • Phase 2: ORR 25% in rr-PTCL and ORR 14% in rr-CTCL (114) **Romidepsin** (HDAC inhibitor): TCL: • Phase 2 gemcitabine and romidepsin (GEMRO regimen): ORR 30%, CRR 15%, 2-yr PFS rate 11.2%, 2-yr OS rate 50% in rr-PTCL (115)

(*continued*)

Actionable Target	Abnormality	Clinical Experience with Targeted Agent
HAT (EP200, CREBBP)	Mutation	R/R TCL: • Phase 1: pralatrexate plus romidepsin, ORR 57% across all patients and 71% in PTCL (100) PTCL: • Phase 2: response rates, PFS, and OS were not statistically different for younger vs. older patients (116) **Depsipeptide (Romidepsin) (FK228)** (HDAC inhibitor): TCL: • Phase 2: ORR 30% in rr-Sezary syndrome (117)
HDAC	Key signaling pathway	**Mocetinostat** (HDAC inhibitor): BCL: • Phase 2: ORR 18.9%, PFS 1.8–22.8 mo in responders for rr-DLBCL; ORR 11.5%, PFS 11.8–26.3 mo in responders for rr-FL (118)
Immunomodulation	Microenvironment/ inflammation/ immune surveillance/ angiogenesis	**Lenalidomide** (stimulates T cells, promotes G1 cell cycle arrest and apoptosis, inhibits TNF-α/VEGFbFGF/ angiogenesis): DLBCL: • Phase 3 lenalidomide vs. placebo maintenance in untreated DLBCL 60–80 yr old after 6–8 cycles of R-CHOP: PFS NR vs. 58.9 mo, mOS NR in either group, 2-yr OS rate 87% vs. 89% (119)

Actionable Target	Abnormality	Clinical Experience with Targeted Agent
		• Phase 2 lenalidomide maintenance: 1-yr PFS rate 64% ± 11% for GCB DLBCL and 67% ± 11% for non-GCB DLBCL in untreated DLBCL, tFL, and relapsed DLCBL not eligible for ASCT (120)
		• Phase 2 lenalidomide with R-CHOP: ORR 98%, CRR 80%, 24-mo OS 78% in untreated nongerminal center DLBCL (121)
		• Phase 2 lenalidomide and R-CHOP21: ORR 92%, CRR 86% in untreated DLBCL elderly patients (122)
		• Phase 2 lenalidomide and rituximab: ORR 33%, PFS 3.7 mo, mOS 10.7 mo in rr-DLBCL and tFL (123)
Immunomodulation	Microenvironment/ inflammation/ immune surveillance/ angiogenesis	HL: • Phase 2: ORR 19% in rr-cHL (124) CLL/SLL: • Phase 2 bendamustine and rituximab with lenalidomide maintenance: PFS 18.3 mo in rr-CLL/rr-SLL (125) FL: • Phase 3 lenalidomide + rituximab vs. rituximab: ORR 59% vs. 37%, PFS 9.5 vs 6.7 mo, 1-yr OS rate 83.1% vs. 76.6% in high-risk, relapsed FL (126) • Phase 2 three-arm randomized trial with (a) BR then MR, (b) BVR then MR, (c) MR with lenalidomide: 3-yr PFS rate 76% vs. 81% vs. 74% in untreated high-risk FL, OS 87%, 90%, 84% (127)

(continued)

Actionable Target	Abnormality	Clinical Experience with Targeted Agent
Immunomodulation	Microenvironment/ inflammation/ immune surveillance/ angiogenesis	**iNHL:** • Phase 2 lenalidomide and rituximab: CRR 87% and ORR 98% in untreated FL; CRR 67% and ORR 89% in untreated MZL; CRR 23% and ORR 80% in untreated SLL (128) • Phase 2 lenalidomide and rituximab: ORR 74%, CRR 44%, PFS 12.4 mo in rr-iNHL (129) **MCL:** • Phase 2: ORR 28%, PFS 4.0 mo, mOS 20.9 mo in rr-MCL (130) • Phase 2 lenalidomide and rituximab: ORR 92%, CRR 64%, 2-yr PFS rate 85%, 4-yr PFS rate 69.7%, 2-yr OS rate 97% in untreated MCL (131,132) **TCL:** • Phase 2: ORR 26%, CRR 8%, PFS 4 mo, mOS 12 mo in rr-TCL other than mycosis fungoides and untreated TCL not candidate for combination chemotherapy (133) **R/R indolent lymphoma:** • Phase 3: lenalidomide plus rituximab vs. placebo plus rituximab: PFS 39.4 vs. 14.1 mo ($p < 0.001$) (134) **R/R DLBCL:** • Phase 2: tafasitamab plus lenalidomide, 43% had a CR, 18% had a PR (135) • **CC-122** (cereblon modulating agent) (pleiotropic pathway modifier):

Actionable Target	Abnormality	Clinical Experience with Targeted Agent
		BCL: • Phase 1b CC-122 + obinutuzumab: ORR 66%, CRR 29%, PFS 336 d in rr-BCL (DLBCL, FL, MZL) (136) R/R nHL: • Phase 1: 34% had CR, 34% had PR, 12% had PD, PFS 16.2 mo (137)
JAK/STAT	Key signaling pathway	**Pacritinib (SB1518)** (Janus kinase inhibitor): Lymphoma: • Phase 1: ORR 14% at the highest dose level in relapsed lymphoma (138) **Ruxolitinib** (JAK1/JAK2 inhibitor): R/R HL: • Phase 2: mDOR 7.7 mo, PFS 3.5 mo, OS 27.1 mo (139)
mTOR	Key signaling pathway	**Temsirolimus** (mTOR inhibitor): DLBCL: • Phase 2 temsirolimus with R-DHAP: ORR 82%, CRR 25.6% in rr-DLBCL (140) BCL: • Phase 2 temsirolimus with bortezomib: ORR 16.7% in rr-DLBCL, 57% in rr-MCL, 56% in rr-FL (141)

(continued)

Actionable Target	Abnormality	Clinical Experience with Targeted Agent
mTOR	Key signaling pathway	MCL: • Phase 4 temsirolimus 175/75 vs. 75 mg: ORR 27.7% vs. 20.9%, PFS 4.3 vs. 4.5 mo in rr-MCL (142) • Phase 3 ibrutinib vs. temsirolimus: ORR 72% vs. 40%, PFS 14.6 vs. 6.2 mo in rr-MCL (143) • Phase 3 temsirolimus vs. investigator's choice: ORR 22% vs. 2%, OS 12.8 vs. 9.7 mo in rr-MCL (144) MCL: • Phase 3: ibrutinib vs. temsirolimus: PFS 15.6 vs. 6.2 mo; ORR 77% vs. 47%; CR 23% vs. 3%; OS 30.3 vs. 23.5 mo (145) **Everolimus** (mTOR inhibitor): HL: • Phase 2: ORR 47%, mTTP 7.2 mo in relapsed HL (146) BCL: • Phase 2: ORR 20%, PFS 5.5 mo in rr-MCL (147) • Phase 2: ORR 25%, PFS 14 mo in rr-MZL (148) • Phase 2: everolimus plus rituximab, ORR 38%, 1-yr OS rate 37% in relapsed DLBCL (149) TCL: • Phase 2 everolimus with CHOP: ORR 90%; PFS 11 mo; 2-yr OS rate 70% in tn-PTCL; CRR 100% in tn-AITL, 63% in tn-PTCL-NOS, 29% in ALK-negative tn-ALCL (150) • Phase 2: ORR 44%, PFS 4.1 mo in relapsed TCL; OS 10.2 mo (151)

Actionable Target	Abnormality	Clinical Experience with Targeted Agent
		iNHL: • Phase 2: ORR 35%, CRR 4%, mTTR 2.3 mo, mDOR 11.5 mo, PFS 7.2 mo in rr-iNHL (152)
mTOR	Key signaling pathway	HL: • Phase 1 everolimus with panobinostat: CRR 15% in rr-HL, ORR 43% (153) R/R lymphoma: • Phase 1/2 trial: everolimus with lenalidomide, ORR 27% (154)
NF-κB	Key signaling pathway	Bortezomib (proteasome/NF-κB inhibitor): DLBCL: • Phase 2 VR-CAP vs. R-CHOP, ORR 93.4% vs. 98.6% ($p = 0.11$), no difference in PFS or OS in tn-non-GCB DLBCL (155) FL: • Phase 3 bortezomib + rituximab vs. rituximab alone: PFS 12.8 vs. 11.0 mo in relapsed FL (156) iNHL: • Phase 2 bortezomib-R-CHOP: ORR 100%, 4-yr PFS rate 83%, 4-yr OS rate 93% in tn-FL, MZL, SLL (157) MCL: • Phase 3 R-CHOP vs. VR-CAP: CRR 42% vs. 53%, PFS 14.4 vs. 24.7 mo, 4-yr OS rate 54% vs. 64% in tn-MCL not eligible for SCT (158) *(continued)*

Actionable Target	Abnormality	Clinical Experience with Targeted Agent
NF-κB	Key signaling pathway	• Phase 2 of R-CHOP with bortezomib induction followed by bortezomib maintenance: ORR 83% following maintenance therapy, 5-yr PFS rate 28%, 5-yr OS rate 66% in tn-MCL (159) • Phase 2 CHOP vs. CHOP-bortezomib: ORR 47.8% vs. 82.6%, OS 11.8 vs. 35.6 mo, difference of PFS nonsignificant in relapsed MCL (160) • Phase 2 VcR-CVAD with maintenance rituximab: ORR 95%, 3-yr PFS rate 72%, 3-yr OS rate 88%, no substantial difference in PFS or OS between patients treated with maintenance rituximab vs. ASCT in tn-MCL (161) • Phase 2 VcR-CVAD induction chemotherapy followed by maintenance rituximab: CRR 77%, 3-yr PFS rate 63%, 3-yr OS rate 86% in untreated MCL (162) TCL: • Phase 2 bortezomib with CHOP: CRR 65%; ORR 76%, 87% for PTCL-NOS/AITL/ALCL; 3-yr PFS rate 35%; 3-yr OS rate 47% in untreated PTCL (163) MCL: • Phase 3: VR-CAP vs. R-CHOP: at a median follow-up of 82.0 mo, OS 90.7 vs. 55.7 mo ($p = 0.001$) (164) MCL: • Phase 2 (CALGB/Alliance 50403): PFS >4 yr ($p < 0.001$); 8-yr PFS estimates in the BC arm 54.1% and 64.4% in the BM arm (165)

Actionable Target	Abnormality	Clinical Experience with Targeted Agent
		MCL: • Phase 2: 24-mo PFS rate 70%, 4-yr OS rate of patients who did not have or had detectable molecular residual disease in the blood at completion of treatment 86.6% and 28.6%, respectively ($p < 0.0001$) (166)
PI3K	Key signaling pathway	Idelalisib (p110δ PI3K inhibitor): iNHL: • Phase 2: ORR 54% in FL, SLL 61%, MZL 47%; PFS 11.0 mo; OS 20.4 mo in refractory iNHL (167) MCL: • Phase 1: ORR 40%, PFS 3.7 mo in rr-MCL (168) rr-CLL: • Phase 3 (ASCEND), acalabrutinib vs. investigator's choice, PFS (16.5 mo) 14.0 vs. 17.1 mo, 12-mo PFS rate 88% vs. 68% (23) Relapsed CLL: • Phase 3: idelalisib plus rituximab vs. placebo plus rituximab, OS 40.6 vs. 34.6 mo; IDELA/R-to-IDELA, PFS 20.3 mo, ORR 85.5% (169) Duvelisib (IPI-145; p110δ and p110γ PI3K inhibitor): TCL: • Phase 1 duvelisib + romidepsin (a) or duvelisib + bortezomib (b): (a) ORR 50%, mTTR 51 d; (b) ORR 53%, CRR 20%, mTTR 52 d in rr-TCL (170) *(continued)*

Actionable Target	Abnormality	Clinical Experience with Targeted Agent
PI3K	Key signaling pathway	NHL: • Phase 1 DR, DBR, DB: ORR 64% in relapsed NHL, 92% in relapsed CLL; PFS 13.7 mo in relapsed NHL; NHL and CLL, ORR 71.8%, PFS 13.7 mo (171) rr-CLL/SLL: • Phase 3: duvelisib vs. ofatumumab: PFS 13.3 vs. 9.9 mo, ORR 74% vs. 45% (172) iNHL: • Phase 2: ORR 47.3%, PFS 9.5 mo (173) iNHL: • Phase 1: PFS 14.7 mo, 24-mo OS rate 71.7% (174) **Voxtalisib** (pan-class I PI3K inhibitor and mTORC1 inhibitor): Lymphoma: • Phase 1: ORR 18.8% in rr-lymphoma, 41.3% in FL, 11.9% in MCL, 4.9% in DLBCL, 11.4% in CLL/SLL (175) Copanlisib (pan-class I PI3K inhibitor): iNHL: • Phase 2: ORR 59%, CRR 12%, mTTR 53 d, mDOR 22.6 mo, PFS 11.2 mo, OS NR in refractory iNHL (176) **INCB050465** (PI3K-δ inhibitor): R/R BCL: • Phase 1/2: objective response rates were 71% in FL, 78% in MZL, 67% in MCL, and 30% in DLBCL (177).

Actionable Target	Abnormality	Clinical Experience with Targeted Agent
Syk	Key signaling pathway	**Fostamatinib** (Syk inhibitor): BCL: • Phase 1/2: ORR 22% in rr-DLBCL, 10% in rr-FL, 11% in rr-MCL; PFS 4.2 mo (178) **Entospletinib** (Syk inhibitor): Indolent nHL and MCL: • Phase 2: PFS at 16 wks in the MCL cohort 63.9%, PFS at 24 wks in FL 51.5%, LPL/WM 69.8%, MCL 56.6%, and MZL 46.2% (179) R/R CLL: • Phase 2: 16/49 achieved PR and 21/49 had SD; ORR 32.7%, PFS 5.6 mo; 48.8% of patients experienced nodal response (180).
Syk	Key signaling pathway	**Dasatinib** (SRC inhibitor): CLL: • Phase 2: ORR 20%, OS 27 mo in rr-CLL (181) R/R nHL: • Phase 1/2: objective response rate 29%, PFS 3 mo, OS 22.4 mo (182)

(*continued*)

Actionable Target	Abnormality	Clinical Experience with Targeted Agent
XPO1	Key signaling pathway	**Selinexor (CRM1 inhibitor):** R/R DLBCL: • Phase 2 (SADAL): ORR 28%, 12% CR, 17% PR (183)

ABC, activated B-cell like; A-CHOP, alemtuzumab, cyclophosphamide, doxorubicin, vincristine, prednisone; A+CHP, brentuximab vedotin, cyclophosphamide, doxorubicin, prednisone; ACTR, autologous T lymphocytes expressing antibody-coupled T-cell receptors; ACVBP, doxorubicin, cyclophosphamide, vindesine, bleomycin, prednisone; AITL, angioimmunoblastic T-cell lymphoma; AKT, serine threonine protein kinase; ALCL, anaplastic large-cell lymphoma; ASCT, autologous stem cell transplantation; ATL, adult T-cell leukemia/lymphoma; AURKA, aurora kinase A; auto-HCT, autologous hematopoietic cell transplantation; AVD, doxorubicin, vinblastine, dacarbazine; BC, bortezomib consolidation; BCL, B-cell lymphoma; BCL-2, B-cell lymphoma 2; BM, bortezomib maintenance; BR, bendamustine rituximab; BTK, Bruton tyrosine kinase; BV, brentuximab vedotin; BVR, bendamustine, bortezomib, rituximab; CAR, chimeric antigen receptor; cHL, classic Hodgkin lymphoma; CHOP, cyclophosphamide, doxorubicin, vincristine, and prednisone; CLL, chronic lymphocytic leukemia; CR, complete response; CREBBP, CREB binding protein; CRR, complete response rate; CRu, complete response unclassified; CTCL, cutaneous T-cell lymphoma; DB, duvelisib bendamustine; DBR, duvelisib bendamustine rituximab; Del, deletion; DHAP, dexamethasone, high-dose cytarabine, cisplatin; DHL, double-hit lymphoma; DLBCL, diffuse large B-cell lymphoma; DOR, duration of response; DR, duvelisib rituximab; EFS, event-free survival; FL, follicular lymphoma; G-, obinutuzumab; GCB, germinal center B cell; HAT, histone acetyltransferases; HL, Hodgkin lymphoma; IBR, ibrutinib, bendamustine, rituximab; ICE, Ifosfamide, carboplatin, and etoposide; IDELA, idelalisib; IGHV, immunoglobulin heavy chain variable region; iNHL, indolent non-Hodgkin lymphoma; IPI, international prognostic index; IRC, independent review committee; ITT, intent-to-treat; JAK, Janus kinase; LBCL, large B-cell lymphoma; LPL, lymphoplasmacytoid lymphoma; MCL, mantle cell lymphoma; mDOR, median duration of response; mo, month(s); mOS, median overall survival; MR, maintenance rituximab; MRR, major response rate; mTORC1, mTOR complex 1; mTTP, median time to progression; mTTR, median time to response; MZL, marginal zone lymphoma; NF-κB, nuclear factor kappa-light-chain-enhancer of activated B cells; NHL, non-Hodgkin lymphoma; NOS, not otherwise specified; NR, not reached; OR, overall response; ORR, overall response rate; OS, overall survival; PD, progressive disease; PET, positron emission tomography; PFS, progression-free survival; P-ICE, panobinostat, ifosfamide, carboplatin, etoposide; PI3K, phosphoinositide 3-kinase; PMECL, primary mediastinal large B-cell lymphoma; pola-BR, polatuzumab vedotin, bendamustine, rituximab; PR, partial response; PRR, partial response rate; PTCL, peripheral T-cell lymphoma; R, rituximab; R-CHOP, rituximab, cyclophosphamide, doxorubicin, vincristine, and prednisone; R-DHAP, rituximab dexamethasone, cytarabine, cisplatin; rr-, relapsed and/or refractory; RT, Richter transformation; SCT, stem cell transplantation; SD, stable disease; SLL, small lymphocytic lymphoma; STAT, signal transducer and activator of transcription; Syk, spleen tyrosine kinase; TCL, T-cell lymphoma; tFL, transformed follicular lymphoma; tn, treatment naïve; VcR-CVAD, rituximab, bortezomib, modified hyper-cyclophosphamide, doxorubicin, vincristine, dexamethasone; VGPR, very good partial response; VR-CAP, bortezomib, rituximab, prednisone, cyclophosphamide, doxorubicin; WM, Waldenström macroglobulinemia; XPO1, nuclear export protein.

Actionable Target	Abnormality	Clinical Experience with Targeted Agent
BCMA	Overexpression	**Ide-cel (bb2121)** (BCMA chimeric antigen receptor [CAR] T cell): • Phase 1 trial ide-cel ORR 85% in all pts, PFS 11.8 mo (1) **Cilta-cel (LCAR-B38M)** (BCMA chimeric antigen receptor [CAR] T cell): • Phase 1 trial cilta-cel ORR 94.8%, 6 mo PFS 87.4% (2) **Belantamab mafodotin** (BCMA antibody–drug conjugate): • Phase 2 trial belantamab mafodotin: ORR 31% (3) • Phase 1 trial belantamab mafodotin, pomalidomide, dexamethasone: ORR 86.2% (4) **Teclistamab** (BCMA × CD3 Bispecific Antibody): • Phase 1 trial teclistamab: ORR 63.8% (5)
CD38	Overexpression	**Daratumumab** (anti-CD38 monoclonal antibody): • Phase 2 trial daratumumab monotherapy: ORR 29%, PFS 3.7 mo (6) • Phase 3 trial daratumumab, lenalidomide, dexamethasone (PFS, not reached) vs. lenalidomide, dexamethasone (PFS 18.4 mo) (7) • Phase 3 trial daratumumab, bortezomib, dexamethasone (12-mo PFS 77.5%) vs. bortezomib, dexamethasone (12-mo PFS 29.4%) (8) • Phase 2 trial daratumumab, pomalidomide, and dexamethasone: ORR 60%, PFS 8.8 mo, OS 17.5 mo (9) • Phase 3 trial daratumumab, carfilzomib, and dexamethasone (PFS, not reached) vs. carfilzomib, dexamethasone (PFS 15.8 mo) (10) • Phase 2 trial (newly diagnosed myeloma) of daratumumab, bortezomib, lenalidomide, dexamethasone (sCR 62.6%, 24-mo PFS 95.8%) vs. bortezomib, lenalidomide, dexamethasone (sCR 45.4, 24-mo PFS 89.8%) (11)

Actionable Target	Abnormality	Clinical Experience with Targeted Agent
		Isatuximab (anti-CD38 monoclonal antibody): • Phase 2 trial isatuximab monotherapy: ORR 24% (12) • Phase 3 trial isatuximab, pomalidomide, dexamethasone (PFS 11.5 mo) vs. pomalidomide, dexamethasone (PFS 6.5 mo) (13) • Phase 3 trial isatuximab, carfilzomib, dexamethasone (PFS not reached) vs. carfilzomib, dexamethasone (PFS 19.5 mo) (14)
Fc receptor-homolog 5 (FcRH5)	Overexpression	**BFCR4350A, FcRH5/CD3 T-Cell-Engaging Bispecific Antibody:** • Phase 1 trial BFCR4350A monotherapy: ORR (51.7%) (15)
GPRC5D	Overexpression	**Talquetamab, G-Protein-Coupled Receptor Family C Group 5 Member D (GPRC5D) × CD3 Bispecific Antibody:** • Phase 1 trial talquetamab monotherapy: ORR 78% (16)
SLAMF7 (CS1)	Overexpression	Elotuzumab (anti-SLAMF7 monoclonal antibody): • Phase 1 trial elotuzumab monotherapy, ORR 0%, SD 27% (17) • Phase 3 trial elotuzumab, lenalidomide, dexamethasone (PFS 19.4 mo, ORR 79%) vs. lenalidomide, dexamethasone (PFS 14.9 mo, ORR 66%) (18) • Phase 2 trial elotuzumab, pomalidomide, dexamethasone (PFS 10.3 mo) vs. pomalidomide, dexamethasone (PFS 4.7 mo) (19)

(*continued*)

Actionable Target	Abnormality	Clinical Experience with Targeted Agent
t(11;14)	Translocation defining sensitivity to BCL-2 targeted therapies	**Venetoclax** (BCL-2 inhibitor): • Phase 1 trial venetoclax monotherapy: ORR in t(11;14) 40%, ORR in non-t(11;14) 6% (20) • Phase 3 trial venetoclax, bortezomib, dexamethasone (PFS 22.4 mo, NR in t(11;14) subgroup) vs. bortezomib and dexamethasone (PFS 11.5 mo, 9.9 mo in t(11;14) subgroup) (21)
XPO1	Key signaling pathway	**Selinexor** (selective inhibitor of nuclear export): • Phase 2 trial selinexor, dexamethasone: ORR 26%, PFS 3.7 mo (22) • Phase 3 trial selinexor, bortezomib, dexamethasone (PFS 13.9 mo) vs. bortezomib, dexamethasone (PFS 9.4 mo) (23)

Actionable Target	Abnormality	Prevalence (%) (1,2)	Clinical Experience with Targeted Agent
BRAF	Mutation	2 (low-grade serous) (1) 4 (endometrioid) 1 (clear cell) 10 (mucinous)	**Selumetinib** (MEK inhibitor): • Phase 2: CR 2%, PR 13%, SD 65% low grade only (2) **Binimetinib** (MEK inhibitor): • Phase 3 (vs. physician's choice chemotherapy in low-grade serous): Terminated early due to futility (3) • Phase 1b (with weekly paclitaxel): RR 17% (4) **Trametinib** (MEK inhibitor): • Phase 3: RR 26%, PFS improved vs. standard of care (median 13.0 vs. 7.2 mo; HR 0.48; 95% CI, 0.36–0.64; $p <$ 0.0001), low grade only (5)
KRAS	Mutation	0–12 (high-grade serous) 19–35 (low-grade serous) (1) 4–10 (endometrioid) 5–16 (clear cell) 40–60 (mucinous)	
BRCA1/2	Mutation	10–20 (high-grade serous)	**Olaparib** (PARP inhibitor): • Phase 2: RR 41% in BRCA+, 24% in BRCA– (6) • Phase 2 (with cediranib vs. olaparib alone, platinum sensitive): PFS 17.7 vs. 9 mo with olaparib alone (7) • Phase 2 (BRCA+): RR 34% (8)

(continued)

Actionable Target	Abnormality	Prevalence (%) (1,2)	Clinical Experience with Targeted Agent
			Phase 2 (with carboplatin/paclitaxel vs. carboplatin/paclitaxel alone, platinum sensitive): PFS 12.2 vs. 9.6 mo with chemo alone, $p = 0.0012$ (9)
			• Phase 1 (with vistusertib): RR 20% (10)
			• Phase 3 (vs. placebo, maintenance for platinum-sensitive recurrence): PFS 19.1 vs. 5.5 mo (for placebo) (11)
			• Phase 1b (with alpelisib): PR 36%, SD 50% (12)
			• Phase 3 (vs. placebo, upfront maintenance in BRCA+): PFS NE vs. 13.8 mo (placebo) (13)
			• Phase 3 (with bevacizumab vs. placebo and bevacizumab, upfront maintenance): 22.1 vs. 16.6 mo (placebo) (14)
			Iniparib (PARP inhibitor):
			• Phase 2 (with carboplatin/gemcitabine): RR 71% in platinum-sensitive pts, 32% in platinum-resistant pts (15,16)
			• Phase 2 (BRCA+): RR 0%, SD 8.3% (17)
			Veliparib (PARP inhibitor):
			• Phase 2 (BRCA+): RR 26% (18)
			• Phase 2 (with cyclophosphamide vs. cyclophosphamide alone, BRCA+): RR 10.8% vs. 18.4% in cyclophosphamide alone (19)

Actionable Target	Abnormality	Prevalence (%) (1,2)	Clinical Experience with Targeted Agent
			• Phase 1/2 (BRCA+): RR 65.7% (20) • Phase 3 (with chemo and continued as maintenance vs. placebo w/ chemo and placebo maintenance): PFS 23.5 vs. 17.3 mo (placebo) (21) **Rucaparib** (PARP inhibitor): • Phase 2 (BRCA+): RR 65% (22) **Niraparib** (PARP inhibitor): • Phase 2 (vs. with bevacizumab): PFS 11.9 vs. 5.5 mo (for niraparib alone) (23) • Phase 2: ORR 28% (24) • Phase 3 (vs. placebo, upfront maintenance): PFS 13.8 vs. 8.2 mo (placebo) (25)
Cell Cycle Checkpoint Kinases/p53 mutation			**Adavosertib** (Wee1 inhibitor): • Phase 2 (with carboplatin, platinum resistant): RR 27%, SD 41% (26) • Phase 2 (with gemcitabine vs. gemcitabine alone in platinum resistant): PFS 4.6 vs. 3 mo (chemo alone) (27) **Berzosertib** (ATR inhibitor): • Phase 2 (with gemcitabine vs. gemcitabine alone in platinum resistant): PFS 22.9 vs. 14.7 wks (chemo alone) (28) **Prexasertib** (CHK1/2 inhibitor): • Phase 2: PR 29% (29)

(*continued*)

Actionable Target	Abnormality	Prevalence (%) (1,2)	Clinical Experience with Targeted Agent
EGFR	Amplification	17–73 (low-grade serous) (1) 10 (endometrioid) 50 (clear cell) 9 (mucinous) 74 (sex cord stromal)	**Gefitinib** (EGFR inhibitor): • Phase 2: RR 4%, SD 15% (30) • Phase 1/2 (with oxaliplatin/vinorelbine): RR 24% in platinum-resistant pts, 90% in platinum-sensitive pts, high grade only (31) • Phase 2 (with carboplatin/paclitaxel): RR 19% in platinum-resistant pts, 62% for platinum-sensitive pts, high grade only (32)
	Mutation	15 (endometrioid) 50 (clear cell) 9 (mucinous)	**Erlotinib** (EGFR inhibitor): • Phase 2: PR 6%, SD 44% high grade only (33) • Phase 1b (with carboplatin/docetaxel): CR 22%, PR 30% high grade only (34) • Phase 3 (front-line maintenance vs. observation): No improvement in PFS or OS (35) **Cetuximab** (EGFR inhibitor): • Phase 2: RR 4%, SD 36% (36) • Phase 2 (with carboplatin): CR 11%, PR 21%, SD 29% high grade only (37)
ER	Expression	58 (low-grade serous) (40)	**Anastrozole** (hormone receptor inhibitor): • Phase 1 (with everolimus): RR 22% (38) • Various hormonal therapies: RR 9% low grade only (39)
PR	Expression	43 (low-grade serous) (40)	

Actionable Target	Abnormality	Prevalence (%) (1,2)	Clinical Experience with Targeted Agent
Folate receptor alpha (FRα)	Upregulation	90 (41)	**Farletuzumab** (FRα inhibitor): • Phase 1: SD 36% (42) • Phase 2 (with carboplatin/taxane): RR 70% (43) • Phase 1b (with carboplatin/pegylated liposomal doxorubicin, platinum sensitive): RR 73.3%, SD 26.7% (44) **Mirvetuximab** (FRα inhibitor): • Phase 1 (platinum resistant): RR 40% (45)
HER2	Amplification	11 (low grade) (1) 41 (clear cell) 45 (mucinous)	**Trastuzumab** (HER2 inhibitor): • Phase 2: CR 2%, PR 5%, SD 39% (46) **Pertuzumab** (HER2 inhibitor): • Phase 2: PR 4%, SD 7% high grade only (47)
	Mutation	6 (low grade) (1)	• Phase 2 (with carboplatin/paclitaxel or gemcitabine): RR 74% high grade only (48) • Phase 3 (with physician choice chemo vs. chemo alone, platinum resistant): PFS 4.3 vs. 2.6 mo in chemo-alone arm, p = NS (49) **Lapatinib** (HER2 inhibitor): • Phase 1 (with carboplatin): PR 27%, SD 27% high grade only (50) • Phase 2 (with topotecan): PR 14%, SD 48% high grade only (51) • Phase 2: RR 0% (52) (*continued*)

Actionable Target	Abnormality	Prevalence (%) (1,2)	Clinical Experience with Targeted Agent
MAPK			**Ralimetinib** (MAPK inhibitor): • Phase 1b/2 (with gemcitabine/carboplatin vs. chemo alone): PFS 10.3 vs. 7.9 mo (chemo alone), OS 29.2 vs. 25.1 mo (chemo alone) (53)
Notch Pathway			**Demcizumab** (DLL4 inhibitor): • Phase 1b (with paclitaxel): ORR 21%, CBR 42% (54)
PD-1/PD-L1	Expression	74.2 PD-1 (carcinosarcoma) 31.4 PD-L1 (carcinosarcoma) 68.6 PD-1 (serous) 12.9 PD-L1 (serous) 68.2 PD-1 (endometrioid) 9.1 PD-L1 (endometrioid)	**Pembrolizumab** (PD-1 inhibitor): • Phase 1b: ORR 11.5%, SD 23% (55) • Phase 2 (with PLD): CBR 52.2%, ORR 26.1% (56) • Phase 2: PFS 2.1 mo, ORR 10% for CPS ≥ 1 (57) • Phase 2 (with bevacizumab and cyclophosphamide): ORR 47.5%, CBR 95% (58) **Avelumab** (PD-L1 inhibitor): • Phase 1b: ORR 10.7%, PR 9.7% (59)

Actionable Target	Abnormality	Prevalence (%) (1,2)	Clinical Experience with Targeted Agent
PD-1/PD-L1	Expression	46 PD-1 (clear cell) 7 PD-L1 (clear cell) 30 PD-1 (mucinous) 9 PD-L1 (mucinous) 33 PD-1 (granulosa cell) 77.8 PD-L1 (granulosa cell)	**Nivolumab** (PD-1 inhibitor): • Phase 2: PR 14.8%, SD 40.7% (60) • Phase 2 (with bevacizumab): ORR 28.9%, PFS 8 1 mo (61) **Durvalumab** (PD-1 antibody): • Phase 1/2 (with olaparib): RR 17% (62) • Phase 1/2 (with cediranib): RR 50% (62) • Phase 2 (with folate receptor alpha vaccine TPIV200): PR 3.7%, SD 33.3% (63)
	Microsatellite instability	13	
PIK3CA	Amplification	68 (high-grade serous) 20 (low-grade serous) 20 (endometrioid) 20 (clear cell)	**MKC-1** (AKT/tubulin inhibitor): • Phase 2: SD 37% (64) **Perifosine** (AKT/PI3K inhibitor): • Phase 1 (with docetaxel): RR 5%, SD 14% high-grade serous only (65) **Alpelisib** (PI3K inhibitor): • Phase 1b (with olaparib): PR 36%, SD 50% (12)

(*continued*)

Actionable Target	Abnormality	Prevalence (%) (1,2)	Clinical Experience with Targeted Agent
	Mutation	2 (low-grade serous) 20 (endometrioid) 20–34 (clear cell)	**Temsirolimus** (mTOR inhibitor): • Phase 2: RR 9%, SD 24% (66) • Phase 2: Trial terminated due to lack of efficacy (67) • Phase 2 (frontline with carboplatin and paclitaxel in clear cell): RR 54% in the USA/Korea and 73% in Japan (68) • Phase 2 (with trabectedin in clear cell): RR 15%, SD 29% (69) **Everolimus** (mTOR inhibitor): • Phase 2 (with bevacizumab): 6-mo PFS 28%, RR and SD not reported (70) **Vistusertib** (mTORC1/2 inhibitor): • Phase 1 (with olaparib): RR 20% (10) **Afuresertib** (AKT inhibitor): • Phase 1/2 (with carboplatin/paclitaxel): RR 32.1% (71)
PTEN	Protein loss	45 (high grade) 24 (endometrioid)	
	Mutation	33 (endometrioid) 3 (clear cell)	
SRC			**Dasatinib** (SRC inhibitor): • Phase 2: RR 0% high grade only (72) • Phase 2 (with carboplatin/paclitaxel): RR 40%, CR 15%, PR 25%, SD 50% high grade only (73)

Actionable Target	Abnormality	Prevalence (%) (1,2)	Clinical Experience with Targeted Agent
			Saracatinib (SRC inhibitor): • Phase 2 (with carboplatin/paclitaxel): RR 53% (74) • Phase 2 (with weekly paclitaxel vs. weekly paclitaxel alone in platinum resistant): RR 29% in saracatinib arm vs. 43% in taxane-only arm, p = NS (75)
WNT Pathway			**Ipafricept** (WNT inhibitor). • Phase 1b: ORR 75.7%, PFS 10.3 mo, OS 33 mo (76)
VEGFR	Expression		**Bevacizumab** (VEGF inhibitor): • Phase 2: CR 4%, PR 16%–18%, SD 28%–40% all grades (77) • Phase 2: PR 17%, SD 78% (78) • Phase 2 (with metronomic cyclophospha-mide): PR 24% (79) • Phase 2 (with carboplatin/liposomal doxoru-bicin): CR 15%, PR 57%, SD 20% (80) • Phase 3 (with carboplatin/paclitaxel): PFS 11.2 vs. 10.3 mo with chemo alone (81) • Phase 3 (with carboplatin/paclitaxel): PFS 24.1 vs. 22.4 mo with chemo alone (82) *(continued)*

Actionable Target	Abnormality	Prevalence (%) (1,2)	Clinical Experience with Targeted Agent
			• Phase 3 (with carboplatin/gemcitabine): PFS 12.4 vs. 8.4 mo with chemo alone (83) • Phase 2 (with everolimus): 6-mo PFS 28%, RR and SD not reported (84)
VEGFR	Expression		Phase 2 (with carboplatin/paclitaxel vs. carboplatin/paclitaxel alone, front-line neo-adjuvant): Rate of optimal surgery 77.7% vs. 86.4% favoring the bevacizumab arm (85) **Aflibercept** (VEGF inhibitor): • Phase 2: PR 5%, SD 18% (47) • Phase 1/2 (with docetaxel): CR 24%, PR 34%, SD 24% (86) • Phase 2 (2 vs. 4 mg/kg, platinum resistant): CBR 12.3% at 2 mg/kg and 11% at 4 mg/kg (87) **Cediranib** (VEGFR inhibitor): • Phase 2: PR 17%, SD 13% • Phase 3 (with carboplatin/paclitaxel): PFS 12.6 vs. 9.4 mo with chemo alone, OS 20.3 vs. 17.6 mo (88) • Phase 2: RR 26%, SD 51% for platinum sensitive; RR 0%, SD 66% for platinum resistant (89)

Actionable Target	Abnormality	Prevalence (%) (1,2)	Clinical Experience with Targeted Agent
			• Phase 2 (with olaparib vs. olaparib alone, platinum sensitive): PFS 17.7 vs. 9 mo with olaparib alone (7) **Ramucirumab** (VEGF inhibitor): • Phase 2: RR 5%, SD 56.7% (90)
VEGFR	Expression		**Sorafenib** (VEGFR/RAF inhibitor): • Phase 2: PR 3%, SD 34% (91) • Phase 1/2 (with topotecan): PR 17%, SD 47% high grade only (92) • Phase 2 (with gemcitabine): PR 5%, SD 23% high grade only (93) • Phase 2 (with carboplatin/paclitaxel vs. carboplatin/paclitaxel alone): RR 69% vs. 74% for chemo-only arm, p = NS (94) • Phase 2 (alone vs. with carboplatin/paclitaxel): RR 15% vs. 61% for the chemo arm, p = 0.014 (95) • Phase 2 (with topotecan vs. topotecan alone): PFS 6.7 vs. 4.4 mo in topotecan alone, OS 17.1 vs. 10.1 mo in topotecan alone (96)

(*continued*)

Actionable Target	Abnormality	Prevalence (%) (1,2)	Clinical Experience with Targeted Agent
			Sunitinib (VEGFR/PDGFR/RET/KIT/FLT3 inhibitor): • Phase 2: PR 3%, SD 53% (97) • Phase 2: RR 8.3% (98) **Pazopanib** (VEGFR/PDGFR/KIT inhibitor): • Phase 2: PR 18%, SD 56% (99) • Phase 2 (with weekly paclitaxel vs. pazopanib alone, platinum resistant): PFS 6.35 vs. 3.49 mo in chemo alone, $p = 0.0002$ (100) • Phase 2 (with weekly gemcitabine vs. gemcitabine alone): PFS 5.3 vs. 2.9 mo (chemo alone) (101) **Apatinib** (VEGFR-2 inhibitor) • Phase 2: ORR 41.4%, PFS 5.1 mo, OS 14.5 mo (102) • Phase 2 (with etoposide): ORR 54% (103)
VEGFR	Expression		**Vanucizumab** (VEGF-A/Ang-2 inhibitor): • Phase 1: RR 29%, SD 54% (104)

Actionable Target	Abnormality	Prevalence (%)	Clinical Experience with Targeted Agent
ATM, PALB2	Loss (ATM), Mutation (ATM, PALB2)	14%–16% have alterations in DDR genes (including ATM and PALB2) (1)	**Olaparib** (PARP inhibitor): • Phase 2: PFS 5.7 mo; OS 13.6 mo in patients with advanced, previously treated PDAC with DDR genetic alterations (2)
BRCA2	Mutation	10 (3)	**Olaparib** (PARP inhibitor): • Phase 2: ORR 22%, SD for ≥8 wk 35% (4) • Phase 3 vs. placebo: PFS 7.4 vs. 3.8 mo in patients with either BRCA1 or BRCA2 genetic alteration or both (5)
KRAS	G12C mutation	1% (6)	**Sotorasib (AMG510)** (KRASG12C inhibitor): • Phase 1: 1 patient with PR for 4.4 mo (7)
MSI-H, dMMR	Mutation/ expression		**Dostarlimab-gxly** (PD-1 inhibitor) (FDA approved 2021): • Phase 1: ORR 41.6%, CR 9.17%, 32.5% PR, DOR 34.7 mo (95.4% with duration ≥ 6 mo) (8) **Pembrolizumab** (PD-1 inhibitor) (FDA approved 2018): • Phase 2 (KEYNOTE-158): ORR 34.3% pts, DOR ≥ 24 mo 77.6%, PFS 4.1 mo, OS 23.5 mo (9)

(continued)

Actionable Target	Abnormality	Prevalence (%)	Clinical Experience with Targeted Agent
NTRK	Fusion	0.67 (10)	Entrectinib (FDA approved 2019) (TRK inhibitor): • Phase 1/2 (STARTRK-2, STARTRK-1, ALKA-372-001): ORR 57% across all tumor types (95% CI 43–71), including a 7% complete response rate, RR 67% in pancreatic cancer pts (11) Larotrectinib (FDA approved 2018) (TRK inhibitor): • Phase 1/2: ORR 75% for multiple tumor types, including pancreatic cancer (12) • Phase 1/2: ORR 79% across all tumor types, CR 24 pts, PR 97 pts, SD 19 pts, RR 50% in pancreatic cancer pts (13)
RET	Fusion		**Pralsetinib (BLU 667)** (RET inhibitor): • Phase 1/2: ORR 50% and responses were observed in all 3 patients with pancreatic cancer (14).

Genetic Abnormality	Prevalence (%)	Clinical Experience with Targeted Agent
Androgen receptor	50 (mutation) (1) 25–30 (amplification) (2)	**All therapies are approved in conjunction with continued androgen deprivation therapy (ADT)** **Castrate-Sensitive Setting (M1):** Abiraterone (17 alpha-hydroxylase/C17,20-lyase inhibitor): • Phase 3 data showing median OS were not estimable and 34.7 mo in the abiraterone acetate and placebo arms, respectively (HR 0.621; 95% CI: 0.509, 0.756; $p < 0.0001$) (3) Apalutamide (androgen receptor antagonist): • Phase 3 data showing 2-yr OS were greater with apalutamide than with placebo (82.4% in the apalutamide group vs. 73.5% in the placebo group; hazard ratio for death, 0.67; 95% CI, 0.51–0.89; $p = 0.005$) (4). Enzalutamide (androgen receptor antagonist): • Phase 3 data showing overall survival at 3 yr were 80% (based on 94 events) in the enzalutamide group and 72% (based on 130 events) in the standard-care group, hazard ratio, 0.67; 95% confidence interval (CI), 0.52–0.86; $p = 0.002$ (5) **Castrate-Resistant Setting:** Apalutamide: • Phase 3 data showing improved OS for apalutamide compared with placebo (HR 0.75; 95% CI 0.59–0.96; $p = 0.0197$) *(continued)*

Genetic Abnormality	Prevalence (%)	Clinical Experience with Targeted Agent
		Darolutamide (androgen receptor antagonist): • Phase 3 data showing OS at 3 yr were 83% (95% confidence interval [CI] = 80%–86%) in the darolutamide group and 77% (95% CI = 72%–81%) in the placebo group (hazard ratio [HR] = 0.69, 95% CI = 0.53–0.88; $p = 0.003$) (6) **Enzalutamide**: • Phase 3 data for M0 castrate-resistant disease showing significantly improved OS over placebo: Median OS was 67.0 mo (95% confidence interval [CI], 64.0 to not reached) in the enzalutamide group and 56.3 mo (95% CI, 54.4–63.0) in the placebo group (hazard ratio for death, 0.73; 95% CI, 0.61–0.89; $p = 0.001$) (7) • Phase 3 data for M1 castrate-resistant disease as well show significantly improved OS over placebo regardless of prior chemotherapy status (8) **Abiraterone**: • Phase 3: OS 14.8 vs. 10.9 mo with placebo, PSA RR 29% vs. 6%, ORR 14% vs. 3% (9)
Immunotherapy	N/A	**Sipuleucel-T** (cellular immunotherapy consisting of autologous PBMCs cultured with recombinant human protein PAP-GM-CSF) (FDA approved for asymptomatic or minimally symptomatic metastatic CRPC): • Phase 3: OS 25.8 vs. 21.7 mo ($p = 0.032$); no difference in TTP (10) • Phase 3: OS 25.9 vs. 21.4 mo ($p = 0.01$); no difference in TTP (11)

Genetic Abnormality	Prevalence (%)	Clinical Experience with Targeted Agent
MSI-H, dMMR	Mutation/ expression	**Dostarlimab-gxly** (PD-1 inhibitor) (FDA approved 2021): • Phase 1: ORR 41.6%, CR 9.17%, 32.5% PR, DOR 34.7 mo (95.4% with duration ≥6 mo) (12) **Pembrolizumab** (PD-1 inhibitor) (FDA approved 2018): • Phase 2 (KEYNOTE-158): ORR 34.3% pts, DOR ≥ 24 mo 77.6%, PFS 4.1 mo, OS 23.5 mo (13)
Mutations in DNA Damage Response (DDR) genes (e.g., *BRCA1/2, ATM, PALB2*)	Germline and/ or somatic mutations occur in up to 25% of pts with metastatic disease (14,15)	PARP inhibition, **olaparib** for any DDR gene, **rucaparib** for *BRCA1/2* defects only in castrate-resistant setting. Responses to PARPi almost exclusively driven by *BRCA2* defects and *BRCA*-adjacent genes (16). Moreover, defects in DDR genes may also predict response to immune checkpoint blockade (17). All therapies are in conjunction with continued ADT.
RB1, TP53, PTEN (Presence of at least two of these defects molecularly defines aggressive variant prostate cancer [AVPC])	Ongoing studies to determine prevalence in castrate-resistant prostate cancer	**Carboplatin/cabazitaxel:** • Combination improved the median PFS over cabazitaxel alone from 4.5 mo (95% CI 3.5–5.7) to 7.3 mo (95% CI 5.5–8.2; hazard ratio 0.69, 95% CI 0.50–0.95, $p = 0.018$), with greatest benefit in men with AVPC signature (18). **AKT Blockade plus AR signaling blockade for PTEN loss**: Abiraterone acetate/prednisone plus **ipatasertib** vs. placebo showed PFS was 18.5 mo with the experimental combination vs. 16.5 mo with placebo in the PTEN-loss subgroup of patients with metastatic castration-resistant prostate cancer ($p = 0.0335$) (12,19).

Actionable Targets	Abnormality	Prevalence (%)	Clinical Experience with Targeted Agent
BRAF	Mutation	4	**Dabrafenib** (BRAF inhibitor): • Case report: SD for 8+ mo (first report of BRAF+ GIST) (1)
ETV6-NTRK3	Fusion	1.7	Larotrectinib (NTRK inhibitor): • Case report: PR for 4+ mo in WT GIST (2)
KIT	Mutation	85 (3)	Imatinib (KIT/BCL/ABL/PDGFR inhibitor): • Phase 2: PR 83% for KIT exon 11 mutations vs. 47.8% for KIT exon 9 mutations, no KIT or PDGFR mutations (3) Sunitinib (KIT/PDGFR/VEGFR/RET/FLT3 inhibitor): • Phase 1/2: PR 37% for KIT exon 9 mutations vs. 5% for KIT exon 11 mutations; CB 25% for PDGFRA mutations, 56% for WT KIT and PDGFRA (4) • Phase 3: PFS 27.3 vs. 6.4 wk with placebo, PR 6.8% vs. 0%, ≥22-wk SD 17.4% vs. 1.9% (4) Dasatinib (KIT/PDGFR/ABL/SRC inhibitor): • Phase 2: PR 32%, >6-mo PFS 21% (5) Sorafenib (KIT/VEGFR/PDGFR/BRAF inhibitor): • Phase 2: PR 13%, SD 55% (6)

Actionable Targets	Abnormality	Prevalence	Clinical Experience with Targeted Agent
			Regorafenib: • Phase 2: RR 12%, SD 65% (7) • Phase 3: PFS 4.8 vs. 0.9 mo for placebo, RR 4.5% vs. 1.5%, SD 71.4% vs. 33.3% (8) **Ripretinib:** • Phase 3: PFS 6.3 mo (95% CI 4.6–6.9) vs. 1.0 mo for placebo (9) **Avapritinib** (KIT/PDGFRA inhibitor): • Phase 1: PDGFRA D842V-mutant population, 88% OR; 95% CI 76–95 with 9% CR, 79% PR, 13% SD (10) **Pazopanib** (KIT/VEGFR/PDGFR inhibitor): • Phase 2: PFS 1.91 mo (95% CI 1.61–5.19). OS 10.7 mo (95% CI 3.9–NR) (11)
NTRK	Fusion		**Entrectinib** (TRK inhibitor): • Phase 1/2 (STARTRK-2, STARTRK-1, ALKA-372-001): ORR 57% across all tumor types (95% CI 43–71), including a 7% complete response rate (12) **Larotrectinib** (TRK inhibitor): • Phase 1/2: ORR 79% across all tumor types, CR 24 pts, PR 97 pts, SD 19 pts. RR 100% in GIST pts (13)

Location of KIT and PDGFR mutations in GIST (prevalence %): KIT exon 9 (18.1%), KIT exon 11 (66.9%), KIT exon 13 (1.6%), KIT exon 17 (1.6%), PDGFR exon 12 (0.8%), PDGFRA exon 18 (3.9%), no mutations in KIT or PDGFR (7.1%). KIT and PDGFRA mutations are mutually exclusive (1,4).

Actionable Targets	Tumor	Prevalence (%)	Clinical Experience with Targeted Agent
ASP-SCR1-TFE3 (ASPL-TFE3)	Alveolar soft tissue sarcoma (ASPS)		**Sunitinib** (KIT/PDGFR/VEGFR/RET/FLT3 inhibitor): • Case series: PR in 5/9 pts and SD in 3/9 pts with PFS of 17 mo (14) • Case series: PR in 6/15 pts and SD in 8/15 pts with PFS of 19 mo (15) **Cediranib** (VEGFR/KIT inhibitor): • Phase 2: RR 35%, SD 60% at 24 wk (16) • Randomized phase 2: RR 21%, SD 68%, PFS was 10.8 mo (17)
CDK amplification	Liposarcoma (well-differentiated and dedifferentiated only)	90	**Palbociclib** (CDK4/CDK6 inhibitor): • Phase 2: PFS 57.2% at 12 wk, PFS 17.9 wk, CR in 1 pt lasting >2 yr (18)
COL1A1–PDGFB gene fusion	Dermatofibrosarcoma protuberans (DFSP) Fibrosarcomatous (FS)-DFSP	96	**Imatinib** (KIT/BCL/ABL/PDGFR inhibitor): • Case studies: Transient response in 1 pt before rapid progression, PR in 1 pt for 6+ mo (19) • Exploration study: CR 50%, of 2 pts with metastatic disease, PR in pt with gene fusion and no response in pt without gene fusion (20)

Actionable Targets	Tumor	Prevalence (%)	Clinical Experience with Targeted Agent
			• Pooled analysis of 2 phase 2 trials; PR 45.9%, SD 25%, median TTP 1.7 yr, 1-yr OS rate 87.5% (21) • Case series: 10 pts with FS-DFSP; 8 PR, 1 SD, 1 PD; median PFS 11 mo (22)
COL6A3–CSF1 gene fusion	Tenosynovial giant cell tumor/pigmented villonodular synovitis	30–60	**Pexidartinib** (CSF1R, KIT, and FLT3-internal tandem duplication inhibitor): • Phase 3: Pexidartinib had ORR 39% at week 25, 15.1% with improvement of range of motion from baseline (23) • Pooled analysis of 3 pexidartinib-treated cohorts: of 130 pts, RECIST ORR 60%, 6-mo RECIST ORR 62%, 18-mo RECIST ORR 92% (24) **Imatinib** (KIT/BCL/ABL/PDGFR inhibitor): • Case study: CR for 7 mo, progression after treatment interruption, CR after reintroduction for 14+ mo (25) • Retrospective study: RR 19% (5/27 pts), SD 74% (26)

(*continued*)

Actionable Targets	Tumor	Prevalence (%)	Clinical Experience with Targeted Agent
EML4-ALK DCTN1-ALK RANBP2-ALK	Inflammatory myofibroblastic tumor	50	**Crizotinib** (ALK/ROS1 inhibitor): • Case report: PR in 1 pt for 6+ mo (27) COG Phase 1: 3 of 7 pts (all 3 received >11 cycles on study) (28) **Crizotinib** (ALK inhibitor): • Case report, with **pazopanib (VEGFR inhibitor)**: PR in 1 pt for 6+ mo (29) **Ceritinib** (ALK inhibitor): • Phase 1: 1 pt with PR (30) **Alectinib** (ALK inhibitor): • Case report: PR in 1 pt for 4+ mo (31)
EWS–FLI1 gene fusion EWS–ERG gene fusion	Ewing	85	**Ganitumab** (AMG 479, IGF-1R inhibitor): • Phase 2: PR 5%, SD 37%, clinical benefit (PR + SD ≥ 24 wk) in 11% (32) **R1507** (IGF-1R inhibitor): • Phase 2: RR 10% with median duration of response of 29 wk and median survival of 7.6 mo (33) **Cixutumumab** (IGF-1R inhibitor): • Phase 2, with **temsirolimus** (mTOR inhibitor): PR 15%, PFS 6 wk, OS 16.2 mo (34)

Actionable Targets	Tumor	Prevalence (%)	Clinical Experience with Targeted Agent
IGF-1R dysregulation	Solitary fibrous tumor (SFT)	100	**Figitumumab** (IGF-1R inhibitor): • Phase 1, with everolimus (mTOR inhibitor): PR in 1/4 pt with SFT for 12+ mo, SD 2/4 pts (35)
INI1/ SMARCB1	Epithelioid sarcoma		**Tazemetostat** (EZH2 inhibitor): • Phase 2: ORR 15% (95% CI 7–26), PFS 5.5 mo (IQR 1.9–7.4), OS 19.0 mo (95% CI 11.0–NR) (36) • Phase 2: ORR 15%, PFS 5.5 mo, 26% SD, OS 19.0 mo, DOR not reached (37)
KDR/VEGF aberrations	Angiosarcoma	90	**Bevacizumab** (VEGF inhibitor): • Phase 2: RR 17%, SD 50%, med TTP 26 wk (38) • Case report: Pt with KDR and FLT4 amplifications showed SD 6 mo and clear improvement of nonmeasurable disease site (skin) (39)
KIAA1549– BRAF gene fusion	Spindle cell sarcoma	Unknown	**Sorafenib** (BRAF/VEGFR/PDGFR/RET inhibitor): • Phase 1, with temsirolimus (mTOR inhibitor) + bevacizumab (VEGF inhibitor): PR 1/1 pt (40)

(*continued*)

Actionable Targets	Tumor	Prevalence (%)	Clinical Experience with Targeted Agent
MDM2 Amplification	Well-differentiated (WD) liposarcoma, dedifferentiated (DD) liposarcoma	>90% of WD/DD liposarcoma	**MK-8242** (MDM2 inhibitor): • Phase 1: 41 pts with WD/DD liposarcoma pts with MDM2 amplification and wild-type TP53 had 3 PR, 31 SD, and 27 pts had median PFS of 237 d (41) **Milademetan** (DS-3032b): • Phase 1: 53 pts with WD/DD liposarcoma with MDM2 amplification and wild-type TP53 had 2 PR, 34 SD, median PFS 7.4 mo (42)
MET	ASPS, clear cell sarcoma	73% expression of ASPS (37)	**Crizotinib** (ALK/ROS1 inhibitor): • Phase 2: ASPS pts with MET+ disease had prolonged 1-yr OS (97.4%) (43) • Phase 2: CCS pts with MET+ disease with RR 3.8%, PFS 131 d, OS 277, and CCS pts with MET disease had no responders (44)

Actionable Targets	Tumor	Prevalence (%)	Clinical Experience with Targeted Agent
NTRK	Fusion		**Larotrectinib** (TRK inhibitor), **Entrectinib** (TRK/ALK/ROS1 inhibitor): • Pooled data: ORR 87% (95% CI 77–94) with larotrectinib vs. 46% (95% CI 19–75) with entrectinib, PFS 28.3 (95% CI 16.8–NE) with larotrectinib vs. 11.0 (95% CI 6.5–15.7) with entrectinib, OS 44.4 mo (95% CI 44.4–NE) with larotrectinib vs. 16.8 mo (95% CI 10.6–20.9) with entrectinib (45) • Phase 1/2 (STARTRK-2, STARTRK-1, ALKA-372-001): ORR 57% across all tumor types (95% CI 43–71), including a 7% complete response rate (12) • Phase 1/2: ORR 79% across all tumor types, CR 24 pts, PR 97 pts, SD 19 pts (13)
PD-1, PD-L1	Soft tissue sarcomas, bone sarcomas	Variable (depends on histology)	**Nivolumab** (anti-PD-1) ± **Pazopanib** (VEGFR inhibitor): • Retrospective series: 3/28 pts with PR (dedifferentiated chondrosarcoma, epithelioid sarcoma, and maxillary osteosarcoma) (46) **Pembrolizumab** (anti-PD-1): • Phase 2: RR 18%. STS PFS at 12 wk was 55% (47)

(continued)

Actionable Targets	Tumor	Prevalence (%)	Clinical Experience with Targeted Agent
			Nivolumab (anti-PD-1) ± **Ipilimumab** (anti-CTLA-4): • Phase 2 (noncomparative, randomized): Nivolumab had ORR 5%, median PFS 1.7 mo. Nivolumab + ipilimumab had ORR 16%, median PFS 4.1 mo (48)
RANKL	Giant cell tumor of bone	N/A	**Denosumab** (RANKL inhibitor): • Phase 2: RR 86% (elimination of 90% of giant cells or no radiologic progression of target lesion up to week 25) (49) • Pooled data: 43/97 pts had advanced/metastatic disease. All had radiographic benefit with median duration of 54 mo; 40% pts discontinuing therapy had progression after median of 8 mo (50).
TSC1/2 (mTOR pathway)	PEComa, pseudomyogenic-hemangioendo-thelioma (PMH)	100% for PEComa/unknown for PMH	**Fyarro (Nab-Sirolimus)** (mTOR inhibitor): • Phase 2: ORR 39%, SD 52%; median PFS 6 mo 71%; pts with TSC2 loss-of-function mutations had ORR 89% (51) **Sirolimus** (mTOR inhibitor): • Case studies: RR 3/3 pts with PEComas exhibiting loss of TSC2 protein expression and mTORC1 activation, 1 pt also had loss of TSC1 (52)

Actionable Targets	Tumor	Prevalence (%)	Clinical Experience with Targeted Agent
			Everolimus/Sirolimus (mTOR inhibitors): • Case studies: CR 3/5 pts, PR 1/5 pts, TSC aberrations in 4/5 pts (53) **Everolimus** (mTOR inhibitor): • Case report: Response in pt with PMH with TSC1 mutation (54)
TSC2 mutation (mTOR pathway)	Lymphangioleiomyomatosis		**Sirolimus** (mTOR inhibitor): • Phase 1/2: Improvement of FEV1 compared with placebo in pts with primary pulmonary disease (55)
VEGFR (angiogenesis)	All soft tissue sarcomas	N/A	**Pazopanib** (VEGFR/PDGFR/KIT inhibitor): • Phase 3: PFS 4.6 vs. 1.6 mo with placebo, OS 12.5 vs. 10.7 mo, PR 6% vs. 0%, SD 67% vs. 38% (56) • 12 patients treated with Pazopanib previously treated with Crenigacestat (NOTCH inhibitor): PFS 6.0 mo (95% CI 2.2–12.0) (57)

COSMIC database: Other ALK fusions have been identified for inflammatory myofibroblastic tumor including ATICALK, CARS-ALK, CLTC-ALK, PPF1BP1-ALK, SEC31A-ALK, TPM3-ALK, and TPM4-ALK.

Actionable Target	Abnormality	Prevalence (%)	Clinical Experience with Targeted Agent
BRAF	Mutation	44–48 (1,2)	**Vemurafenib** (BRAF V600E) (BRAF inhibitor): • Phase 3: RR 48% vs. 5% dacarbazine; OS 13.6 vs. 10.3 mo with dacarbazine (3,4) **Dabrafenib** (BRAF V600E) (BRAF inhibitor): • Phase 3: RR 50%, PFS 5.1 vs. 2.7 mo with dacarbazine (5) **Dabrafenib ± Trametinib** (BRAF V600E, BRAF V600K) (BRAF and MEK inhibitors): • Phase 3: RR 67%, PFS 9.3 vs. 8.8 mo with dabrafenib (6) • Phase 3: RR 64%, PFS 11.4 vs. 7.3 mo with vemurafenib (7) **Vemurafenib ± Cobimetinib** (BRAF V600) (BRAF and MEK inhibitors): • Phase 3: RR 68%, PFS 9.9 vs. 6.2 mo with vemurafenib (8) **Encorafenib ± Binimetinib** (BRAF V600E, BRAF V600K) (BRAF and MEK inhibitors): • Phase 3: RR 63% vs. 40%, PFS 14.9 vs. 7.3 mo, OS 33.6 vs. 16.9 mo with vemurafenib (9) **Dabrafenib ± Trametinib** (BRAF V600E, BRAF V600K) (adjuvant): • Phase 3: 5-yr RFS 52% vs. 36% with placebo, 5-yr distant RFS 65% vs. 54% with placebo (10)

Actionable Target	Abnormality	Prevalence (%)	Clinical Experience with Targeted Agent
			Dabrafenib ± Trametinib (neoadjuvant III–IV, if oligomet): • Phase 2: EFS 19.7 mo with neoadj/adj D/T vs. 2.9 mo with upfront surg and adj therapy (11)
CTLA-4	Immune checkpoint	N/A	**Ipilimumab** (metastatic): • Phase 3: RR 11% vs. 1.5% with gp100, OS 10.0 vs. 6.4 mo with gp100 (12) **Ipilimumab** (adjuvant): • Phase 3: 5-yr OS 65.4% vs. 54.4% with placebo (13)
KIT (exons 9, 11, 13, 17, 18)	Mutation	17%–21% in mucosal, 11%–23% in acral, and 2% in cutaneous (14–16)	**Imatinib** (BCR-ABL kinase, PDGFR and KIT inhibitor): • Phase 2: RR 4.8% (17) • Phase 2: RR 16% (18) • Phase 2: PFS 3.5 mo, RR 23.3% (19) • Phase 2: RR 29% (20) **Dasatinib** (BCR-ABL kinase, PDGFR, and KIT inhibitor): • Phase 2: RR 5.9% (21) **Nilotinib** (BCR-ABL kinase, PDGFR, and KIT inhibitor): • Phase 2: RR 26.2% (22) (*continued*)

Actionable Target	Abnormality	Prevalence (%)	Clinical Experience with Targeted Agent
NRAS	Mutation	23 (11)	**Binimetinib** (MEK 1/2 inhibitor): • Phase 3: RR 15%, PFS 2.8 vs. 1.5 mo with dacarbazine (23) **Binimetinib** ± **LEE011** (ribociclib-CDK4/6 inhibitor): • Phase 1: RR 43% (24) **Binimetinib** ± **Ribociclib** (CDK4/6 inhibitor): • Phase 1: RR 25% (25)
NTRK	Fusion		**Entrectinib** (FDA approved 2019) (TRK inhibitor): • Phase 1/2 (STARTRK-2, STARTRK-1, ALKA-372-001): ORR 57% across all tumor types (95% CI 43–71), including a 7% complete response rate (26) **Larotrectinib** (FDA approved 2018) (TRK inhibitor): • Phase 1/2: ORR 79% across all tumor types, CR 24 pts, PR 97 pts, SD 19 pts. RR 43% in melanoma pts (27)

Actionable Target	Abnormality	Prevalence (%)	Clinical Experience with Targeted Agent
PD-1	Immune checkpoint	N/A	**Nivolumab (metastatic):** • Phase 3 (treatment-naïve, BRAF WT): 1-yr OS 72.9% vs. 42.1% with dacarbazine, PFS 5.1 vs. 2.2 mo with dacarbazine (28) **Ipilimumab ± Nivolumab:** • Phase 3: 3-yr OS 58% vs. 52% with nivolumab and 34% with ipilimumab (29) **Nivolumab (adjuvant):** • Phase 3: RFS at 12 mo 70.5% with nivo and 60.8% with ipi (30). 4 yr RFS 51.7% with nivo and 41.2% with ipi, 4-yr OS 77.9% with nivo and 76.6% with ipi (31)
PD-1	Immune checkpoint	N/A	**Ipilimumab ± Nivolumab (neoadjuvant):** • Phase 1b: 2 doses neoadj + 2 adj with RR 80% (32) • Phase 2: 2 doses neoadj Ipi/Nivo × 3 doses pre-op vs. Nivo × 4 doses pre-op followed by adj Nivo × 6-mo RR 73% in combination arm and RR 25% with Nivo (33) **Pembrolizumab (anti-PD-1):** • Phase 3: RR 32.9% vs. 11.9% with ipilimumab. Estimated 6-mo PFS 46.4% vs. 26.5% for ipilimumab (34) • Phase 2 (progression on Ipi ± BRAF/MEK inhibition): 6-mo PFS 34% vs. 16% with chemo (35)

Actionable Target	Abnormality	Prevalence (%)	Clinical Experience with Targeted Agent
PD-1/PD-L1	N/A	N/A	**Cemiplimab** (PD-1 inhibitor): • Phase 2: 29% RR for locally advanced/metastatic (1) **Nivolumab** (PD-1 inhibitor): • Case report: Ongoing near CR at 4+ mo; high mutational burden (>50 mut/MB); 19 functional alterations in tissue NGS, as well as *PDL1/PDL2/JAK2* amplification (2)
PTCH1	Mutation	39	**Vismodegib** (Hedgehog inhibitor): • Phase 2: RR for metastatic 30%, RR for locally advanced 43%, including CR in 21% (3) **Sonidegib** (Hedgehog inhibitor): • Phase 2: RR for metastatic 15%, RR for locally advanced 43% (2 pts) (4)
SMO	Mutation	12	

Actionable Target	Abnormality	Prevalence	Clinical Experience with Targeted Agent
PD-1/PD-L1	N/A	N/A	**Cemiplimab** (PD-1 inhibitor): • Case report: Durable CR ongoing 16+ mo (5) • ORR (PR + CR, including unconfirmed) 52% (12/23; 4 uPR, 5 PR, 2 CR, 1 uCR); disease control rate (ORR + SD) 70% (16/23, including 4 SD); 3 pts not yet evaluable. PFS and OS not yet reached; only 1 pt experienced PD during REGN2810 treatment after initial response (6). **Nivolumab** (PD-1 inhibitor): • Phase 2: Unresectable/metastatic ORR 54.5%, DCR 77% (7) **Pembrolizumab** (PD-1 inhibitor): • Phase 2: Unresectable/metastatic disease ORR 34%, DCR 52.4%, median PFS 6.9 mo. Median DOR and OS not reached (8)

Actionable Target	Abnormality	Prevalence	Clinical Experience with Targeted Agent
PD-L1	Expression	N/A	**Avelumab** (PD-L1 inhibitor): • Phase 2: RR 32% (CR 9%, PR 23%), responses ongoing in 23/28 pts at time of analysis (9) Pembrolizumab (PD-1 inhibitor): • Phase 2: RR 56% (CR 16%, PR 40%) (10)

Actionable Target	Abnormality	Prevalence (%)	Clinical Experience with Targeted Agent
MSI-H, dMMR	Mutation/ expression		**Dostarlimab-gxly** (PD-1 inhibitor) (FDA approved 2021): • Phase 1: ORR 41.6%, CR 9.17%, 32.5% PR, DOR 34 7 mo (95.4% with duration ≥ 6 mo) (1) **Pembrolizumab** (PD-1 inhibitor) (FDA approved 2018): • Phase 2 (KEYNOTE-158): ORR 34.3% pts, DOR ≥ 24 mo 77.6%, PFS 4.1 mo, OS 23.5 mo (2)

Actionable Target	Abnormality	Prevalence	Clinical Experience with Targeted Agent
KIT	Mutation	10%	**Imatinib** (KIT/PDGFR/BCR-ABL inhibitor): • Phase 2: 5/6 pts with KIT+ per IHC had PD; 1 pt had SD with a >50% decline in serum AFP for 3 mo before developing PD (1)
PD-1/PD-L1	N/A	N/A	**Nivolumab** (PD-1 inhibitor): • Case report: Response observed in pt with embryonal carcinoma (2) **Pembrolizumab** (PD-1 inhibitor): • Phase 2: 3 pts had SD 10.9/5.5/4.5 mo, PFS 5.6 mo (95% CI 1.5–4.5), OS 10.6 mo (3)

Actionable Target	Abnormality	Prevalence (%)	Clinical Experience with Targeted Agent
Angiogenesis	Overexpression	N/A	**Sorafenib** (KIT/RAF/VEGFR/PDGFR inhibitor): • Case reports: PR (>15 mo) (1), PR (>9 mo) (2) in thymic carcinoma **Sunitinib** (VEGFR/PDGFR/RET/KIT/FLT3 inhibitor): • Pilot study: PR in 3 of 4 pts with thymic carcinoma (2, 18, and 22 mo) (3) • Phase 2: Thymic carcinoma: PR 26%, SD 65%. Thymoma: PR 6%, SD 75% (4)
EGFR	Overexpression	69 (5)	**Gefitinib** (EGFR inhibitor): • Phase 2: RR 4%, SD ≥ 4 mo 23% (6) **Erlotinib** (EGFR inhibitor): • Phase 2: RR 0%, SD 60% in combination with **bevacizumab** (VEGF inhibitor) (7) **Cetuximab** (EGFR inhibitor): • Case report: PR in 2 thymoma pts (after 3 mo of therapy [8]), PR (>12 mo) in 1 thymoma pt (9)
IGFR-1	Expression	100	**Cixutumumab** (IGF-1R inhibitor): • Phase 2: RR 14% (thymoma), 0% (thymic) (10)

(*continued*)

Actionable Target	Abnormality	Prevalence (%)	Clinical Experience with Targeted Agent
KIT	Mutation	7	**Imatinib** (KIT inhibitor): • Phase 2: SD 29% thymoma pts (>38 mo in 1 pt) (11) • Case report: PR (6 mo) in 1 thymoma pt (12)
PD-1/PD-L1	N/A	N/A	**Nivolumab** (PD-1 inhibitor): • Phase 2: Thymic carcinoma: SD 73%, SD ≥ 24 wks 33%. PFS 3.8 mo, OS 14.1 mo (13) • Case report: Thymic carcinoma: DOR 9 mo in 1 pt. Thymoma: DOR 14 mo 1 pt (14) **Pembrolizumab** (PD-1 inhibitor): • Phase 2: CR 3%, PR 20%, SD 53% (15) • Phase 2: Thymic carcinoma: ORR 19%, PFS 6.1 mo, PR 19%, SD 54%. Thymoma: ORR 29%, PFS 6.1 mo, PR 29%, SD 71% (16)

Actionable Target	Abnormality	Prevalence	Clinical Experience with Targeted Agent
MSI-H, dMMR	Mutation/ expression		**Dostarlimab-gxly** (PD-1 inhibitor) (FDA approved 2021): • Phase 1: ORR 41.6%, CR 9.17%, 32.5% PR, DOR 34.7 mo (95.4% with duration ≥ 6 mo) (1) **Pembrolizumab** (PD-1 inhibitor) (FDA approved 2018): • Phase 2 (KEYNOTE-158): ORR 34.3% pts, DOR ≥ 24 mo 77.6%, PFS 4.1 mo, OS 23.5 mo (2)
VEGFR2	N/A	N/A	**Lenvatinib*** (VEGFR2 inhibitor) (FDA approved for differentiated thyroid cancer): • Phase 3: CR 1.5%, PR 63.2%, SD 23%, PD 6.9%, PFS 18.3 mo (3) **Sorafenib*** (RAF/VEGFR inhibitor): • Phase 3: PR 13%, SD 67%, PFS 10.8 mo (4)*

*FDA approved for differentiated thyroid cancer; Phase 3 trial in TKI naïve.

Thyroid Cancer (Papillary, Follicular, and Hurthle Cell Carcinoma)

Actionable Target	Abnormality	Prevalence (%)	Clinical Experience with Targeted Agent
BRAF (papillary)	Mutation	52	**Vemurafenib** (BRAF inhibitor): • Phase 2: VEGFR naïve, PR 38.5%, SD 57.7%, PD 3.8%, PFS 18.2 mo; previous VEGFR treated, PR 27.3%, SD 63.6%, PD 4.5%, PFS 8.9 mo (5) **Dabrafenib** (BRAF inhibitor): • Phase 1: RR 33% (6) **Dabrafenib ± Trametinib** (BRAF V600E) (MEK inhibitor): • Phase 2: single-agent dabrafenib: PR 45%; 40% SD, PFS 11.4 mo; dual treatment: PR 38%, 41% PR, PFS 15.1 mo Difference in PFS was not statistically different (7).
MSI-H, dMMR	Mutation/ expression		**Dostarlimab-gxly** (PD-1 inhibitor) (FDA approved 2021): • Phase 1: ORR 41.6%, CR 9.17%, 32.5% PR, DOR 34.7 mo (95.4% with duration ≥6 mo) (1) **Pembrolizumab** (PD-1 inhibitor) (FDA approved 2018): • Phase 2 (KEYNOTE-158): ORR 34.3% pts, DOR ≥24 mo 77.6%, PFS 4.1 mo, OS 23.5 mo (2)

Actionable Target	Abnormality	Prevalence (%)	Clinical Experience with Targeted Agent
NTRK1/3	Fusion	2	**Larotrectinib** (FDA approved 2018) (TRK inhibitor): • Phase 1/2 subanalysis: CR 10%, PR 81%, SD 10% (8) • Phase 1/2: ORR 79%, CR 24 pts, PR 97 pts, SD 19 pts for all tumor types, RR 79% for thyroid cancer pts (9) **Entrectinib** (FDA approved 2018) (TRK inhibitor): 1 of 5 thyroid cancer patients achieved a response (10)
PIK3CA (follicular)	Mutation	7	**Everolimus** (mTOR inhibitor)*: • Phase 2: PR 5%, SD 76% (11)
PTEN (follicular)	Loss	8	
RET	Fusion	11	Selective RET inhibitors: **Selpercatinib**: • Phase 2: RET fusion thyroid cancer (including 2 ATC patients) 79% ORR (12) **Pralsetinib**: • Phase 2: RET fusion thyroid cancer 91%. No ATC patients included (13).

*Included follicular, papillary, anaplastic, and medullary thyroid cancer.

Actionable Target	Abnormality	Prevalence (%)	Clinical Experience with Targeted Agent
MSI-H, dMMR	Mutation/ expression		**Dostarlimab-gxly** (PD-1 inhibitor) (FDA approved 2021): • Phase 1: ORR 41.6%, CR 9.17%, 32.5% PR, DOR 34.7 mo (95.4% with duration ≥ 6 mo) (1) **Pembrolizumab** (PD-1 inhibitor) (FDA approved 2018): • Phase 2 (KEYNOTE-158): ORR 34.3% pts, DOR ≥ 24 mo 77.6%, PFS 4.1 mo, OS 23.5 mo (2)
RAS	Mutation	10 HRAS, 3 KRAS	**Cabozantinib** (RET inhibitor): • Phase 3: PFS 47 wk in treatment arm vs. 8 wk in placebo in RAS mutated pts (14)*

Actionable Target	Abnormality	Prevalence (%)	Clinical Experience with Targeted Agent
RET	Mutation	43% in sporadic disease Nearly 100% in hereditary disease	**Vandetanib*** (RET inhibitor): • Phase 3: PR 46%; PFS 31 mo (estimated), OS > 27 mo (median) (15) **Cabozantinib*** (RET inhibitor): • Phase 3: PR 28%; PFS 11 mo, OS 21 mo (14) **Lenvatinib (E7080)** (VEGFR inhibitor): • Phase 2: PR 49%, SD > 6 mo 27% (3) Selective RET inhibitors: **Selpercatinib*:** • Phase 2: treatment-naïve cohort: ORR 73%; CR 11%, PR 61%, SD 23%, PD 2% (12) • Previously treated cohort: ORR 69%; CR 9%, PR 60%, SD 25%, PD 2% (12) **Pralsetinib*:** • Phase 2: treatment-naïve cohort: ORR 74%; CR 5%, PR 68%, SD 26%, PD 0% (16) • Previously treated cohort: ORR 60%; CR 2%, PR 58%, SD 36%, PD 4% (16)

*FDA approved for medullary thyroid cancer.

Actionable Target	Abnormality	Prevalence (%)	Clinical Experience with Targeted Agent
BRAF	Mutation	40	**Vemurafenib** (BRAF inhibitor): • CR 1/7, PR 1/7, PD 4/7, NE 1/7 (7) **Dabrafenib*** (BRAF inhibitor) + **trametinib** (MEK inhibitor): • FDA approved based on phase 2: ORR 69%; CR 6%, PR 63%, SD 19%; OS of 86 wks (17)
MSI-H, dMMR	Mutation/ expression		**Dostarlimab-gxly** (PD-1 inhibitor) (FDA approved 2021): • Phase 1: ORR 41.6%, CR 9.17%, 32.5% PR, DOR 34.7 mo (95.4% with duration ≥ 6 mo) (1) **Pembrolizumab** (PD-1 inhibitor) (FDA approved 2018): • Phase 2 (KEYNOTE-158): ORR 34.3% pts, DOR ≥ 24 mo 77.6%, PFS 4.1 mo, OS 23.5 mo (2)
NTRK1/3	Fusion	Very rare	**Larotrectinib***: • Phase 1/2 subanalysis (n = 7): PR 29%, SD 14%, PD 43% (9)
PIK3CA	Mutation	12	**Everolimus** (mTOR inhibitor): • SD with regression of tumor in 1/6 pts (11)
PTEN	Protein loss	11	
RET	Fusion	Very rare	Selective RET inhibitors: **Selpercatinib***: • Phase 2: only 2 ATC patients, one with PR (12)

*FDA approved for anaplastic thyroid cancer or for fusion-specific solid tumors.

Actionable Target	Abnormality	Prevalence (%) (1)	Clinical Experience with Targeted Agent
AKT	Mutation	2–3 (endometrioid)	**MKC-1** (AKT/tubulin inhibitor): • Phase 2: RR 0%, SD 44% (2) **MK-2206** (AKT inhibitor): • Phase 2: PR 6%, PFS 2 mo, OS 8.4 mo (3) **Capivasertib** (AKT inhibitor): • Phase 1 (with olaparib): PR 50% (4) **GSK2141795** (AKT inhibitor): • Phase 1 (with trametinib): PR 4% (5) **Temsirolimus** (mTOR inhibitor): • Phase 2: RR 4%–14%, SD 28%–69% (6) • Phase 2 (with megace/tamoxifen vs. temsirolimus alone): RR 22% vs. 14% in the combination arm (7) • Phase 2 (with chemo vs. chemo + bevacizumab): RR 55% (8) **Everolimus** (mTOR inhibitor): • Phase 2: SD 43% (9) • Phase 2, with letrozole: RR 21%, SD 21% (10) • Phase 2 (with letrozole and metformin): RR 29%, SD 38% (11)
PTEN	Mutation	43 (endometrioid) 0–11 (non-endometrioid)	
	Protein loss	80 (endometrioid) 5 (non-endometrioid)	
PIK3R1	Mutation	43 (endometrioid) 12 (non-endometrioid)	
PIK3CA	Mutation	30–40 (endometrioid) 20 (non-endometrioid)	
	Amplification	2–4 (endometrioid) 46 (non-endometrioid)	

(continued)

Actionable Target	Abnormality	Prevalence (%) (1)	Clinical Experience with Targeted Agent
			Ridaforolimus (mTOR inhibitor): • Phase 2: RR 11%, SD 18% (12) • Phase 2: RR 8%, SD 58% (13) • Phase 2 (vs. physician choice chemo): RR 0% vs. 4% with chemo, p = NS; SD 35% vs. 17% with chemo, p = 0.021 (14) **Vistusertib** (mTORC1/2 inhibitor): • Phase 1 (with olaparib): RR 27% (15) **Sapanisertib** (mTORC1/2 inhibitor): • Phase 2 (with chemo vs. chemo alone): ORR 24% vs. 18% for chemo alone, CBR 80% vs. 58% for chemo alone (16) **LY023414** (mTOR/PI3K inhibitor): • Phase 2 (in pts with PI3K pathway mutations): PR 14.3%, SD 35.7% (17) **Pilaralisib** (PI3K inhibitor): • Phase 2: RR 6% (18)
BRCA1/2	Mutation	13 (endometrioid)	**Iniparib** (PARP inhibitor): • Phase 2 (with paclitaxel/carboplatin): RR 23.5%, SD 35% in carcinosarcoma only (20) **Olaparib** (PARP inhibitor): • Phase 1 (with vistusertib): RR 27% (15) • Phase 1 (with capivasertib): PR 50% (21)
PARP	Overexpression	50 (endometrioid) 85.7 (carcinosarcoma) (19)	

Actionable Target	Abnormality	Prevalence (%) (1)	Clinical Experience with Targeted Agent
EGFR	Overexpression	46 (endometrioid) 34 (non-endometrioid)	**Erlotinib** (EGFR inhibitor): Phase 2: RR 12.5%, SD 47% (22) **Gefitinib** (EGFR inhibitor): • Phase 2: RR 3%, SD 15% (23) **Cetuximab** (EGFR inhibitor): • Phase 2: RR 5%, SD 10% (9)
HER2	Overexpression	3–10 (endometrioid) 32 (non-endometrioid)	**Trastuzumab** (HER2 inhibitor): • Phase 2: RR 0%, SD 40% (24) • Phase 2 (with chemo vs. chemo alone): PFS 8 mo (chemo alone) vs. 12.6 mo (25) **Lapatinib** (HER2 inhibitor): • Phase 2: RR 3%, SD 23% (26)
KRAS	Mutation	10–30 (endometrioid) 0–10 (non-endometrioid)	**Selumetinib** (MEK inhibitor): • Phase 2: RR 6%, SD 26% (22) **Trametinib** (MEK inhibitor): • Phase 1 (with GSK2141795): PR 4% (5)

(*continued*)

Actionable Target	Abnormality	Prevalence (%) (1)	Clinical Experience with Targeted Agent
Microsatellite instability		15–30 (endometrioid) (27) 0–5 (non-endometrioid) (28)	**Pembrolizumab** (PD-1 inhibitor): • Phase 2: RR 56% (n = 5), CBR 89% (1)
PD-1/PD-L1	Expression	80 PD-1 (carcinosarcoma) 22 PD-L1 (carcinosarcoma) 68 PD-1 (serous) 10 PD-L1 (serous) 78 PD-1 (endometrioid) (32) 40 PD-L1 (endometrioid) (32)	• Phase 2: RR 13%, PR 12.5% (29) • Phase 2 (with lenvatinib): ORR 35.5% in MSS tumors (30) **Nivolumab** (PD-1 inhibitor): • Phase 2 (vs. with cabozantinib): ORR 25% for combo vs. 16.7%, SD 44.5% for combo vs. 11.1% (31)
P53	Mutation	>90 (serous)	**Adavosertib** (Wee1 inhibitor): • Phase 2: RR 29.4%, 6-mo PFS 58.7% (33)
VEGFR	Overexpression Increased expression associated with poor prognosis (34)		**Bevacizumab** (VEGF inhibitor): • Phase 2: RR 13.5%, SD 40% (35) • Phase 2 (with carboplatin/ paclitaxel): RR 73% (34) **Aflibercept** (VEGF inhibitor): • Phase 2: RR 7%, SD 32% (36)

Actionable Target	Abnormality	Prevalence (%) (1)	Clinical Experience with Targeted Agent
			Sunitinib (VEGFR/PDGFR/RET/KIT/FLT3 inhibitor): • Phase 2: RR 15%, SD 25% (19) • Phase 2: RR 18.1%, SD 18.1% (32) **Cediranib** (VEGFR inhibitor): • Phase 2: RR 12.5% (27) **Nintedanib** (PDGFR/FGFR/VEGFR inhibitor): • Phase 2: RR 9.4% (28) **Cabozantinib** (MET/VEGFR/TIE2/RET/AXL/KIT inhibitor): • Phase 2: RR 11.1% (37) • Phase 2 (with nivolumab vs. nivolumab alone): ORR 25% vs. 16.7% for nivolumab alone, SD 44.5% vs. 11.1% for nivolumab alone (31) **Brivanib** (VEGF/FGFR inhibitor): • Phase 2: RR 18.6% (38) **Lenvatinib** (pan-RTK inhibitor) • Phase 2: ORR 21%, PFS 5.6 mo, OS 10.6 mo (39) • Phase 2 (with pembrolizumab): ORR 35.5% in MSS tumors (40)

Carcinogenesis from the Perspective of Targeted Therapy and Immunotherapy

In this section, we will discuss elements of cellular biology and immunology that have given insight into personalized genomically based treatment and fuel the latest revolution in the systemic treatment of cancer. Early developments included alkylating agents derived from mustard gas chemical weapons from World Wars I and II, antimetabolites that caused disruption of cellular metabolism, naturally occurring *Streptomyces* fungus antibiotics such as adriamycin and rapamycin, the serendipitous discovery of platinum anticancer properties, computer-designed targeted agents, and Dr. Jim Allison's elucidation of the T-cell receptor (TCR) that unlocked the secret of immune checkpoint inhibition. Finally, the remarkable capability of molecular engineering has produced amazing new tools such as antibodies with double or even triple specificity, antibody drug conjugates (ADCs—"smart-bombs" that can deliver toxic agents to specific antigens on cancer cells), as well as strategic combinations of immune stimulators capable of producing durable benefits in settings such as melanoma, thyroid cancer, and mesothelioma that were once considered untreatable.

Despite the above progress, cancer remains a formidable enemy with marked heterogeneity—especially the gastrointestinal cancers such as advanced colorectal and pancreatic carcinoma. Cancers are actually perverse "pseudo-organs" that continue to evolve genomically (just like adding new "apps" to a smartphone). A wide variety of elements—blood vessels, connective tissue, inflammatory cells, together with tumor stem cells—make up the tumor environment. We need to consider cancer as the process of carcinogenesis rather than a static collection of nodules or tumors.

In order to help navigate the new world of precision oncology, we have created a "word cloud" to serve as a primer for the vocabulary needed for a modern precision oncology tumor board discussion (Figure 2.1).

Tumor biology is a fundamental aspect of the discussion regarding an advanced cancer treatment patient. **Germline cells** pass on their genetic material to their offspring and account for some of the most challenging family cancer syndromes such as Li–Fraumeni and BRCA 1 and 2. It is widely recognized that there are marked genetic and molecular differences present in a single tumor. This heterogeneity may well account for mixed responses in the same patient. **Subclones** move DNA segments from a parent vector to a destination vector. A key element in genomic testing requires determining whether a genetic difference is a normal variant or a pathologic oncogene

Figure 2.1

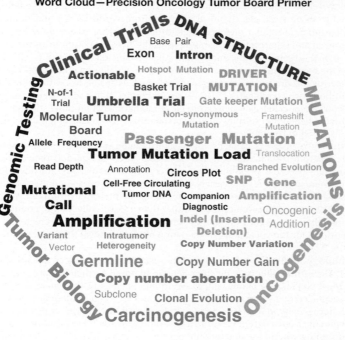

Word Cloud—Precision Oncology Tumor Board Primer

that provides a target for new drugs. **Vectors** such as **plasmids, cosmids,** and **phage** are the new cellular vehicles used to deliver DNA fragments for molecular engineering.

Clonal evolution is the process by which a tumor gives rise to a population of cells with different mutations or molecular characteristics compared to the parent stem cell. Tumors may have aberrations in the number of genes as well as variations in the number of copies of the particular gene among different individuals.

Clinical trials have evolved in a number of important ways. An **actionable gene** is a tumor alteration expected or predicted to affect the response to treatment. **Basket trials** test new drugs in different cancers with the same mutation or biomarker. This is the concept of **genomically informed** treatment. **Molecular tumor boards** provide a team environment to formulate personalized treatment for individual patients. An **"N of 1"** trial tests a particular treatment in a single patient. **Umbrella trials** are designed so that patients with cancer from the same site (e.g., breast, lung, colon, etc.) may receive different drugs based on the specific tumor genomic alterations or "fingerprints" of their cancer.

The structure of DNA was first elucidated in 1952 following the now-famous Photo #51, an X-ray diffraction image taken by Raymond Gosling, a graduate student working under Rosalind Franklin at King's College London. This primitive image allowed Watson and Crick to brilliantly deduce the helical structure of DNA. **Exons** are any part of the gene encoding mature RNA and ultimately proteins. **Introns** are DNA or RNA "inert" segments that act as "spacers," which do not code for proteins and are discarded during RNA production.

The ability to carry out genomic analysis on preserved biopsy material has been an absolute game-changing development. Numerous laboratories are able to carry out detailed "fingerprinting" to interrogate the makeup of the cancer genetic drivers and provide targets for computer-designed drugs. Genes can be amplified with numerous copies in a single cell. **Annotation** is the process of investigating the various elements present in the genome including gene location and function. Some genetic lesions do not occur in active sites and therefore are judged nonactionable. **Cell-free circulating tumor** DNA provides the source of genetic analysis referred to as **liquid biopsies**. **Liquid biopsies** promise to revolutionize sequential evaluation of patient status. A **circos plot** is an informative method of displaying relationships between genes in a colorful circular format. **Companion diagnostics** are tests used to match the patient to a specific drug treatment such as the HercepTest for HER2 amplified breast cancer. The **read depth** is the number of times a particular base is detected during sequencing. Tumor **mutation load** is the number of acquired mutations per million bases (Mb) in a single tumor where ≥10 m/Mb is considered important.

A variety of mutations are recognized. **Driver mutations** give a cancer cell a fundamental growth advantage and may serve as a target for drug treatment. **Frameshift** mutations result from insertion or deletion of a nucleotide resulting in an aberrant sequence. **Gatekeeper mutations** are harmful alterations in genes that normally prevent growth of cancerous cells, such as adenomatous polyposis coli (APC). **Hotspot mutations** are clustered at a specific "business" site in the gene presumed to drive carcinogenesis. **Nonsynonymous mutations** alter the amino acid sequence of a protein. **Passenger mutations** do not initiate cancer but may impact mitochondrial DNA, immunogenicity, chemotherapy response, or even which genes are turned on (**epigenetics**).

Finally, **branched evolution** is the process by which tumors evolve genomically and can acquire resistance in a nonlinear (tree-like) pattern. When segments are inserted or deleted from a gene these are referred to as **indels**. **Oncogene addiction** is the process by which a tumor becomes dependent on a single molecule or pathway (KIT mutation in gastrointestinal stromal tumors [GIST]). **Single nucleotide polymorphisms ("SNiPs")** are substitutions of a single nucleotide at a specific position in the genome present in 1% or more of the population. **Translocations** are mutations in which chromosomal segments break and reattach to a different site.

Starting with the groundbreaking work of Garth Nicholson on the model of cell membranes—called the fluid mosaic model—researchers have recognized a relation between the extent of chromosomal mutation, variation, or instability in repetitive short DNA sequences (microsatellites, aka MSI, or short tandem repeats) and genetic and immunologic heterogeneity. Examples of MSI are TATATATATATA (dinucleotide) or GTC GTC GTC GTC GTC GTC (trinucleotide). These motifs act as "fillers" and do not have coding function, but they are important in terms of genetic "fingerprinting," forensic medicine, and paternity testing. Microsatellites are involved in the risk of developing cancer; and are thought to affect the likelihood of response to immunotherapy and checkpoint inhibitors (Krontiris et al., 1993; Singer and Nicolson, 1972).

Clonogenic elements, together with the inflammatory and stromal mesenchymal elements, "hijack" many of the normal processes of inflammation and tissue repair, produce an entire tumor microenvironment, parasitize the host, and then create life-threatening complications. Malignant functions are acquired in many ways and at various points in the cell cycle (Figure 2.2).

The seminal article "Hallmarks of Cancer: The Next Generation" (Hanahan and Weinberg, 2011) provides a continuing evolution in our understanding. It is useful to consider five common themes in the initiation and development of carcinogenesis. These are also shown in Figure 2.3.

1. **Individual Genetic Risk.** Genetic predisposition is either due to sporadic or familial germline traits or due to decreased or defective DNA damage repair with loss of tumor suppressor function. These include BRCA-1 and -2-related breast and ovarian cancers, familial colon cancers or melanomas, and other cancer families (see familialcancerdatabase.nl). Over the years, we have encountered a number of families where cancers are common and are still awaiting a genetic explanation.

2. **Carcinogens.** Carcinogens are ubiquitous in the environment and lead to mutations, chromosomal translocations, deletions, or fusion products that produce uncontrolled growth unless the cellular surveillance and repair systems remove or fix them. An underappreciated aspect includes continued promotion by prolonged exposure. For example, among patients with tobacco-associated lung cancer, small cell cancer is usually seen in very heavy long-term smokers. This forms another rationale for a benefit to smoking cessation even in patients with metastatic cancer (Davis et al., 2009).

3. **Chronic Inflammation.** Inflammation and the presence of lymphocytes, granulocytes, macrophages, mast cells, and their cytokines provide growth factors that appear to intensify cancer development. This helps provide the rationale for decreased death from colon cancer in individuals taking aspirin and other anti-inflammatory agents.

4. **Proliferative Advantage.** Cellular metabolism becomes reprogrammed (The Warburg Hypothesis) to support the energy needs for immortalized cell growth and give cancer cells a deadly proliferative advantage.

5. **Evasion of Immune Surveillance.** Malignant cells employ a variety of camouflage tactics and inhibitors of T-cell function to evade the immune surveillance system and allow cancers to grow and spread. **James Allison was awarded the 2018 Nobel Prize for discovering how to**

Figure 2.2

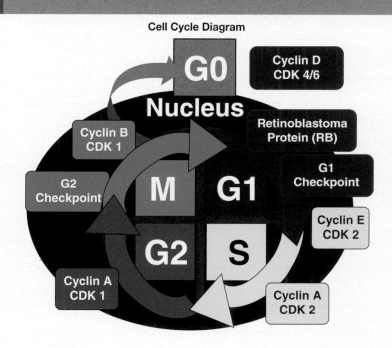

Cell Cycle Diagram

Figure 2.3

167

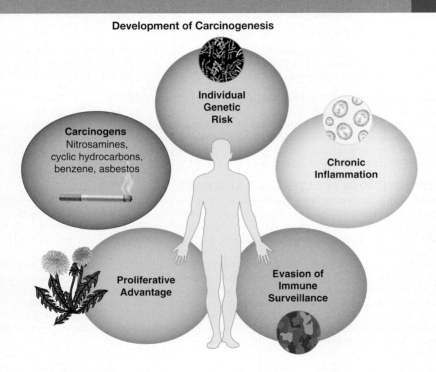

Development of Carcinogenesis

remove these "brakes" and inhibit negative immune regulation: https://www
.nobelprize.org/prizes/medicine/2018/allison/facts/

Processes Cancers Use to Grow

Unfortunately, cancers are very nimble, have the ability to change their behavior, contain many redundant pathways, and often develop resistance to even the most elegant gene-based therapy.

Fourteen important processes that contribute to the growth of cancers are shown in Figure 2.4.

CELL SIGNALING AND THE DEFECTS CONTRIBUTING TO CARCINOGENESIS

It is humbling, indeed, to realize that even a simplified diagram of the "Signal Transduction Roadmap" of cell signaling consists of numerous types of membrane receptors, cytoplasmic systems, and nuclear factors (see Section 3—Signal Transduction Roadmap on p. 231). These systems and the cell cycle regulators are discussed in Section 3.

METABOLISM, GLYCOLYSIS, AND THE WARBURG HYPOTHESIS

Normal energy production favors glucose in the cytoplasm and pyruvic acid in the mitochondria. Under anaerobic conditions, glycolysis predominates. Otto Warburg (1930, 1956a, 1956b) first observed that cancer cells can carry out "aerobic glycolysis" to get more glucose into the cell and compensate for the much lower efficiency of ATP production than that by mitochondrial oxidative phosphorylation.

The basis of the positron emission tomography (PET) scan is that cancer cells can sequester fluorodeoxyglucose and "light up" the cancer. This is accomplished at least in part by upregulating glucose transporters such as GLUT1 (Jones and Thompson, 2009). Glycolysis is also upregulated by rat sarcoma virus (RAS) oncoprotein signaling and hypoxia, which drive up levels of HIF1α and HIF2α transcription factors (Semenza, 2010a, 2010b). Shown in Figure 2.5 is a sequence of PET scans exhibiting dramatic improvement in a large liver metastasis with a hypermetabolic rim that became "cold" in December 2017.

Figure 2.4

169

The Microenvironment and Therapeutic Targeting

1. Cell Signaling	5. Inflammatory Cytokines	9. Genetic Instability
2. Aerobic Glycolysis	6. Ignoring Stop Signals	10. Autophagy and Necrosis
3. Lost Contact Inhibition	7. Cell Cycle Control	11. Immune Monitoring
4. Proliferative Advantage	8. Loss of Senescence	12. Resistance Mutations

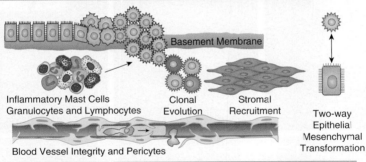

Basement Membrane

Inflammatory Mast Cells
Granulocytes and Lymphocytes

Clonal
Evolution

Stromal
Recruitment

Two-way
Epithelial
Mesenchymal
Transformation

Blood Vessel Integrity and Pericytes

13. Angiogenesis	14. Metastasis—Vascularization, Capillary Invasion, Hematogenous Spread, Embolization, Organ Arrest, Endothelial Adherence, Parenchymal Extravasation, Microenvironment Development, Proliferation, Clinically Evident Metastases

Figure 2.5

Positron Emission Tomography Scan Before and After

GastroIntestinal Stromal Tumor (GIST)

20 Feb 2018

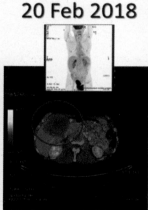

06 Sep 2017   28 Dec 2017   19 Feb 2018

Excess glycolysis also allows glycolytic intermediates to incorporate nucleosides and amino acids that are needed for the growth of new cells. Some cancers actually have a hybrid complementary energy system:

1. Glucose-dependent ("Warburg effect") cells that secrete lactate and
2. Other cells that use the lactate and the citric acid cycle (Kennedy and Dewhirst, 2010).

Because tumors can have fluctuating degrees of hypoxia due to abnormal neovasculature, this provides another way that cancers survive and grow.

Gliomas and other human cancers can develop gain-of-function mutations in the isocitrate dehydrogenase 1/2 (IDH) enzymes, producing elevated oxidation and stability of the HIF1 transcription factors (Reitman and Yan, 2010; Yen et al., 2010). Glutamine (GLU) is a nonessential amino acid that is consumed by proliferating cells far more than other amino acids. Glutaminase removes an amide group that produces glutamic acid, which, in turn, loses its amine group to form α-ketoglutarate.

Ultimately, GLU contributes to the supply of oxaloacetate, citrate, nicotinamide adenine dinucleotide phosphate (NADPH), and carbon molecules—all critical to mitochondrial energy production. GLU is sequestered in the cell by solute carrier (SLC) transporters and serves as a nitrogen donor for nucleotide synthesis mediated by the *c-MYC* oncogene GLU also activates mTORC1, the mammalian target of rapamycin complex 1. Taken together, these observations form a strong argument that cancer cells can be highly GLU dependent ("addicted") and inhibiting GLU-mediated metabolism with glutaminase is an intriguing strategy and therapeutic tactic (Naing et al., 2019; Wise and Thompson, 2010).

LOSS OF CONTACT INHIBITION

Normal tissue growth and repair depends on cells responding to negative growth signals and knowing when to stop when they come into contact with each other. Keloids are macroscopic examples of wounds that "heal too much" when this recognition does not occur. One of the earliest microscopic signs of cell transformation is this "heaping up" of cells (Figure 2.6).

There are several ways in which normal cells respond to negative growth signals. Merlin, STK11, and TGFb are three examples of growth controls that may be mutated in various cancers (Hanahan

Figure 2.6

The Microenvironment and Therapeutic Targeting

Epithelial cells sitting on the basement membrane oriented with a top and bottom in tight formation with cell bridges (adhesion molecules).

2. Glycolysis Conversion

3. Loss of Contact Inhibition

4. Proliferative Advantage

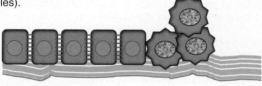

1. Normal Cell Signaling

Transformed cells with nuclear changes, conversion to aerobic glycolysis, and loss of contact inhibition—growing heaped up to begin to form a tumor.

and Weinberg, 2011). Merlin, the neurofibromatosis 2 (*NF2*) gene product, promotes contact inhibition and cell-to-cell bonds (NF2-YAP signaling) by coupling cell surface adhesion molecules (e.g., E-cadherin) to transmembrane receptor tyrosine kinases (RTKs) (e.g., the epidermal growth factor receptor [EGFR]) and blocks mitogenic signals (Wu et al., 2019).

Serine/threonine kinase 11 (STK11), also known as liver kinase B1 (LKB1) or renal carcinoma antigen NY-REN-19, is an epithelial polarity protein that maintains epithelial structural integrity. Germline mutations in this gene have been associated with Peutz–Jeghers syndrome, an autosomal dominant disorder characterized by the growth of polyps in the gastrointestinal tract, pigmented macules on the skin and mouth, and other neoplasms. Somatic mutations of the *LKB1* gene have been found in lung, cervical, breast, intestinal, testicular, pancreatic, and skin cancers. *LKB1* can block *MYC* oncogene function (Partanen et al., 2009).

Transforming growth factor beta (TGF-β) is a multipurpose cytokine activity that exists in three isoforms. It is part of a superfamily that includes inhibins, activin, anti-Müllerian hormone, bone morphogenic protein, decapentaplegic, and Vg-related protein 1. TGF-β is known for its antiproliferative effects (Vander Ark et al., 2018). However, in many late-stage tumors, TGF-β signaling changes from suppression of cell proliferation and instead activates a cellular program, termed the *epithelial-to-mesenchymal transition* (EMT) (see "EMT and Metastasis" section on p. 198), seen in high-grade malignancy.

Cancer as a "Pseudo-organ" with Great Proliferative Advantage

ORCHESTRATING THE DEVELOPMENT OF THE TUMOR MICROENVIRONMENT

Displaying a useful graphic depiction of the highly complex network of microenvironmental signaling interactions remains a great challenge, made even more difficult because of tumor progression and the interplay between neoplastic and supporting stromal cells. This model becomes even more complex as cancers metastasize.

Cancer Stem Cells

Cancer stem cells (CSCs) are the "seeds" that develop when normal tissue stem cells undergo transformation. CSCs are often more resistant to chemotherapy and radiation and may also become dormant only to recur even years after initial treatment. What starts as a "clone then may become genetically and phenotypically heterogeneous with variable degrees of differentiation" (Nguyen et al., 2012).

Genome sequencing has revealed striking intratumoral genetic diversity within adjacent areas in the same tumor deposit (Gerlinger et al., 2012). This plasticity helps explain the frequent mutation to resistance seen following dramatic responses to targeted therapy in EGFR-mutated lung cancer and the need for different strategies for V600E BRAF mutations. BRAF-mutated melanoma can be highly sensitive to a single agent, whereas colon may need a "cocktail" of encorafenib, binimetinib, and cetuximab (Kopetz et al., 2019).

Even in the area of BRAF-mutated metastatic melanoma, one of the great oncology success stories, not all patients have a durable benefit. One variable in the therapeutic equation is NRAS with its complex interplay between mTOR, MAP kinase, and the cell cycle (Moore et al., 2020) (Figure 2.7).

Endothelial Cells

Endothelial cells (ECs) form a thin layer on the interior surface of blood and lymphatic vessels throughout the circulatory system. They play a critical role in vascular biology, controlling leakage of proteins and blood cells, protecting against clots, controlling vasoconstriction and dilatation, and supporting the repair and renewal of damaged vessels (Ruggeri et al., 2018).

ECs contain networks of interconnected signaling pathways involving ligands of signal-transducing receptors such as the following:

1. **Notch**, a ubiquitous signaling system found in most multicellular organisms. Notch controls key branch points in embryogenesis and was first discovered as an indentation in the wings of fruit flies in 1914 by John S. Dexter (Morgan, 1917) and sequenced in the 1980s (Kidd et al., 1986).
2. **Fibroblast growth factor (FGF) signaling**. FGFs, discovered in 1973, are "promiscuous" heparin-binding mitogens with a wide range of functions, including mesoderm induction, angiogenesis, keratinocyte organization, and wound healing.

Figure 2.7

175

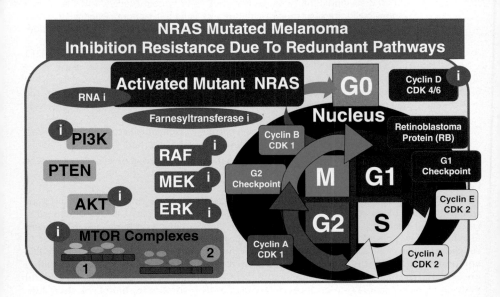

NRAS Mutated Melanoma
Inhibition Resistance Due To Redundant Pathways

3. **Vascular endothelial growth factor (VEGF).** In 1983, Dr. Harold Dvorak and colleagues first showed that tumor cells secreted vascular permeability factor (VPF) and that a blocking antibody to VPF, later named VEGF, could prevent the edema and fluid accumulation that are characteristic of human cancers. VEGF is in part responsible for the abnormal vasculature seen in human tumors (Senger et al., 1983).
4. **Ephrin type A receptor** (encoded by the *EPHA1* gene), a mediator of nervous system development implicated in carcinogenesis
5. **Angiopoietins 1/2**, the ligands for the *t*yrosine kinase *i*mmunoglobulin/*E*GF receptors TIE1 and TIE2. They work intimately with VEGF and are proangiogenic (ANG-1) or cause vessel regression (ANG-2).
6. **Neuropilin** is a membrane-bound co-receptor for VEGF and semaphorins (semaphorins are the 500-amino-acid proteins that bind to plexins and direct axon growth and neurologic development). Neuropilin is encoded by the *NRP-1* gene.
7. **Roundabout homolog 1**, a membrane protein controlling axon guidance and cell adhesions, encoded by *ROBO1*, a member of the immunoglobulin (Ig) gene superfamily

   A number of new experimental agents have been developed to target most of these signals.

Pericytes

Pericytes are specialized, mesenchymal, smooth muscle–like cells with finger-like projections wrapped around blood vessel ECs (see Figure 2.4). Pericytes secrete VEGF as well as antiproliferative ANG-1 ligand for endothelial surface TIE2 receptors. Along with the vascular basement membrane, they prevent hydrostatic pressure–induced leakage and retard cancer cell entry to circulation (Chen et al., 2016). **There are several pathways of communication between the ECs and pericytes. The first is TGF signaling mediated by EC. Angiopoietin and Tie-2 signaling are essential for maturation and stabilization of ECs. Platelet-derived growth factor (PDGF) pathway signaling from ECs recruits pericytes to migrate to developing blood vessels. Sphingosine-1-phosphate (S1P) signaling also aids in pericyte recruitment by communication through G-protein-coupled receptors (GPCRs).**

Communication between ECs and pericytes is vital. Inhibiting the PDGF pathway leads to pericyte deficiency. This causes endothelial hyperplasia, abnormal junctions, and diabetic retinopathy.

A lack of pericytes also causes an upregulation of VEGF, vessel leakage, and bleeding. Angiopoietin 2 can act as an antagonist to Tie-2, destabilizing the ECs, which results in less EC and pericyte interaction. Inhibition of the PDGF pathway by angiopoietin 2 reduces levels of pericytes, leading to diabetic retinopathy.

PDGF inhibition reduces pericyte coverage of tumor vessels and destabilizes vascular integrity and function (Östman, 2017). Stimulating pericyte function, therefore, represents another tactic for metastasis inhibition.

Cancer-Associated Fibroblasts

Fibroblasts often make up a major portion of tumor stroma and seem to function as pawns on the cancer "chessboard." Structural fibroblasts form the supporting structure of normal epithelium. Myofibroblasts express smooth muscle actin (SMA) in wounds and chronic inflammation. Both are seen in very dense fibrous (desmoplastic) cancers (Hanahan and Weinberg, 2011).

Stromal Progenitors

Mesenchymal stem and progenitor cells, labeled and tracked using green fluorescent protein (GFP), have been found to migrate from the marrow into tumors, like new recruits to the battlefield, where they may differentiate and transform further. Tumor-associated stromal cells may then be supplied by local cell growth, conscription of adjacent normal cells, or bone marrow stem cell migration. NCI Protocol NCT00761644, a novel combination of liposomal doxorubicin, bevacizumab, and temsirolimus (scheduled for completion in 2019), tested the strategy of attacking the nucleus (anthracycline), stromal blood vessels (VEGF inhibitor), and cell signaling (mTOR inhibitor) (clinicaltrials .gov) to overcome the large repertoire of tactics cancer cells use to gain a proliferative advantage.

Stem cells can thrive in the absence of growth factors required for normal cells, but if exposed to stimulatory molecules either from themselves (autocrine) or from their neighbors (paracrine), growth accelerates. CSCs can sequester and use glucose far more efficiently and are bolstered by other cellular "recruits" that provide a nurturing protective fibrous infrastructure for cancer colonization. It is this "trifecta" that must be taken into account when devising new targeted therapies for epithelial malignancies because the multiple mutations seen in carcinomas such as non–small cell lung cancers (NSCLCs) with their redundant and nimble cellular systems are not likely to be amenable to long-term control with a single agent. This is in contrast to other diseases such as chronic granulocytic leukemia (CGL) and gastrointestinal stromal tumor (GIST), where imatinib may be effective for many years (Hochhaus et al., 2020).

Almost 11 years of follow-up have shown that the efficacy of imatinib persisted over time and that long-term administration of imatinib was not associated with unacceptable cumulative or late toxic effects (Hochhaus et al., 2017).

INFLAMMATION AND TUMOR PROMOTION

Virtually every tumor deposit contains inflammatory cells ranging from scattered infiltration detectable only with cell type–specific antibodies to dense cellular infiltrates apparent by standard light microscopy (DeNardo et al., 2010). These inflammatory cells supply a whole array of molecules: growth and survival factors, proangiogenic factors, matrix-modifying enzymes that facilitate invasion and metastasis, and inducers of EMT and reactive mutagenic oxygen species (Greten and Grivennikov, 2019). It is quite possible that some of the beneficial effects of chemotherapy actually may be due to decreasing the activity of sensitive, tumor-infiltrating inflammatory cells even when the cancer cells themselves have acquired chemotherapy resistance.

Leukocytes (macrophages, mast cells, neutrophils, and T/B lymphocytes) can be found in most neoplastic lesions and promote tumor progression (i.e., tumors are wounds that never heal) (Dvorak, 1986; Schäfer and Werner, 2008). In the course of normal wound healing and fighting infections, immune inflammatory cells appear transiently and regress in contrast with the chronic inflammation of cancer, which is associated with fibrosis, scarring, aberrant angiogenesis, and neoplasia (Greten and Grivennikov, 2019) (Figure 2.8).

Immune inflammatory cells can release a variety of cytokines that have either tumor-promoting or tumor-killing effects:

1. **Epidermal growth factor (EGF)**
2. **Angiogenic growth factor (VEGF)**
3. **FGF2** (see "FGF" section)
4. **Chemokines**, the 8- to 10-kDa cysteine-containing signaling proteins that induce movement (Greek—*kinos*) or chemotaxis in neighboring responsive cells. Chemokines are classified into

Figure 2.8

The Microenvironment and Therapeutic Targeting

5. Inflammatory Cytokines

 Monocytes

 Neutrophilic Granulocytes

 Eosinophilic Granulocytes

 Mast Cells

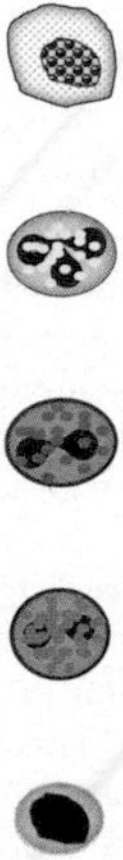

 Lymphocytes

A variety of inflammatory leukocytes are attracted (chemotaxis) and recruited into the stroma of the tumor and recruited by the cancer to produce growth factors/cytokines that stimulate growth. Spindle cells/fibroblasts are also recruited and contribute to the increase in size of the tumor.

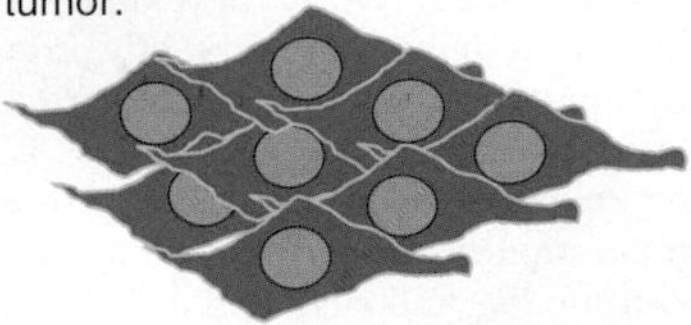

Spindle cells/fibroblasts are also recruited and contribute "scar like," scirrhous (Greek *skirrhos—hard tumor*) quality to the tumor microenvironment and increase the size of the cancer.

subfamilies (CXC, CC, CX3C, and XC). They interact with G-protein-linked trans-membrane receptors.

5. **Cytokines** that amplify the inflammatory state

6. **Metalloproteinases**, zinc-requiring enzymes that degrade extracellular matrix proteins

7. **Cysteine cathepsin** (Greek, *hepsein* "boil," *kata* "down") proteases activated at low pH, usually inside lysosomes (Bergmann and Fruton, 1936)

8. **Heparanase (HPSE)**, which cleaves heparan sulfate heavily glycosylated proteins (proteoglycans, HSPG), has been associated with poor prognosis. Heparan, a close relative of heparin, is made up of sulfated disaccharides and forms the blood vessel interior lining, which must be penetrated for cancer cells to metastasize hematogenously.

All of the above cytokines are potential targets for cancer therapeutic agents. Tumor-infiltrating myeloid cells, expressing macrophage marker CD11b and neutrophil marker Gr1, suppress cytotoxic T-lymphocyte (CTL) and natural killer (NK) cell activity. Recruitment of these myeloid elements may be doubly damaging by directly promoting angiogenesis and tumor progression as well as affording a means to evade immune destruction. Another strategy, therefore, may be to inhibit these promoter cells rather than the CSCs.

Cytokine release syndrome (CRS, also sometimes referred to as cytokine "storm") is a systemic inflammatory response that can be triggered by infections and certain drugs such as monoclonal antibodies and engineered T cells. Cytokine storm implies a rapid dramatic reaction, whereas CRS can occur in a delayed fashion. CRS symptoms include fever, fatigue, loss of appetite, muscle and joint pain, vomiting, diarrhea, rashes, fast breathing, rapid heartbeat, low blood pressure, seizures, headache, confusion, delirium, hallucinations, tremor, and loss of coordination (Figure 2.9).

CRS can also be caused by autologous T cells modified with chimeric antigen receptors (CAR T-cell therapy). CRS is marked by elevated levels of interleukin-6 (IL-6), IL-8 (aka CXCL8), and IL-10 as well as interferon gamma (IFN-γ), colony stimulating factors (CSFs), macrophage inflammatory proteins (MIPs), and others. Important clinical markers of CAR-T induced CRS at 36 hours are fever >38.9°C (102°F) and elevated levels of serum monocyte chemoattractant protein-1 (MCP-1/CCL2).

Figure 2.9

IL-2 Activation Diagram

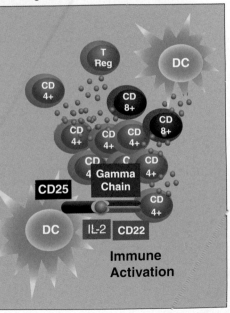

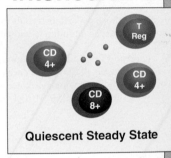

IL-6, MCP-1, and MIP-1 are not produced by CAR T cells, but rather by inflammatory myeloid lineage cells. Some of the life-threatening complications of COVID-19 are attributed to CRS.

Patients with fulminant COVID-19 and acute respiratory distress syndrome (ARDS) have classical serum biomarkers of CRS including elevated C-reactive protein (CRP), LACTIC DEHYDROGENASE (LDH), IL-6, and ferritin.

Treatment for less severe CRS is supportive, addressing the symptoms like fever, muscle pain, or fatigue. Moderate CRS requires oxygen therapy and giving fluids and agents to raise blood pressure. For moderate to severe CRS, the use of immunosuppressive agents like corticosteroids may be necessary, but judgment must be used to avoid negating the effect of drugs intended to activate the immune system.

Tocilizumab, an anti-IL-6 monoclonal antibody, was U.S. Food and Drug Administration (FDA) approved for steroid-refractory CRS and has been used widely in severely ill COVID-19 cases. Lenzilumab, an anti-GM-CSF monoclonal antibody, may also be effective at managing cytokine release by reducing activation of myeloid cells and decreasing the production of IL-1, IL-6, MCP-1, MIP-1, and interferon gamma-induced protein 10 (IP-10).

NECROSIS HAS PROINFLAMMATORY AND TUMOR-PROMOTING POTENTIAL

Many cancers, such as squamous cancer of the lung, demonstrate spontaneous necrosis. During necrosis, in contrast to apoptosis, cells self-destruct and release their contents into the local tissue microenvironment. This results in tumor-promoting inflammation, increased angiogenesis, and proliferation because of cytokines such as IL-1α (Hanahan and Weinberg, 2011).

Cell death by necrosis appears to be under genetic control in some circumstances and, rather than being a random and undirected process, explains why some necrotic cancers can act in a very aggressive fashion and produce a whole array of paraneoplastic complications such as fever, anorexia, and fatigue (Galluzzi and Kroemer, 2008). Tumor lysis syndrome is the most extreme example of the harm that can occur when tumors die too rapidly and liberate toxic, life-threatening organic acids, potassium, and so forth. Finding ways to limit cellular necrosis could be a very effective strategy to limit cancer acceleration.

IGNORING STOP SIGNALS

Many negative feedback loops are in place to limit the growth of normal cells. These include tumor suppressors cyclin-dependent kinase (CDK)-interacting protein and kinase-inhibitory protein (CIP and KIP) and inhibitor of kinase 4/alternative reading frame (INK4a/ARF). The CIP/KIP family includes the genes *p21*, *p27*, and *p57*. They halt cell cycle in G1 phase, by binding to, and inactivating, cyclin–CDK complexes. *p21* is activated by *p53* (which, in turn, is triggered by DNA damage, e.g., because of radiation). *p27* is activated by TGF-β, a growth inhibitor. The INK4a/ARF family includes p16INK4a, which binds to CDK4 and arrests the cell cycle in G1 phase, and p19ARF, which prevents p53 degradation. However, these "stop signals" can be ignored by cancer cells (Figure 2.10), leading to unregulated growth (e.g., RAS mutations with decreased RAS GTPase activity in cellular events that are constantly in the "on" position rather than temporary and short lived) (Schwartz and Shah, 2020).

LOSS OF SENESCENCE AND ACQUISITION OF "IMMORTALITY"

1. From the early days of cell culture research, it was noted that normal cell lines are able to pass through only a limited number of successive cell growth and division cycles. This natural aging—senescence—is associated with distinct processes and entrance into a nonproliferative but viable state. Cytoplasm enlarges, cells lose proliferation markers and accumulate lysosomal β-galactosidase (Collado and Serrano, 2010). Some cancer cells can disable their senescence- or apoptosis-inducing circuitry.

2. **Crisis** is a term for cell death because of genetic damage (*RB1*, *p53*) or nutrient deprivation. Telomeres, composed of multiple tandem hexanucleotide repeats, shorten progressively in cultures of nonimmortalized cells. Eventually, the DNA fuses into nonviable dicentric chromosomes. The lost protective function triggers entrance into crisis.

   Telomerase, the specialized DNA polymerase, which adds repeat segments to the ends of telomeric DNA, is low or absent in normal cells but is expressed at significant levels in human cancer cells.

The Microenvironment and Therapeutic Targeting

Invasive Cancer. The tumor enlarges penetrating the basement membrane. Cancer stem cells (light color) are only a small fraction of the total tumor but represent the key clonal progenitors.

6. Ignoring Stop Signals
7. Loss of Cell Cycle Control
8. Loss of Senescence
9. Genetic Instability and Clonal Evolution

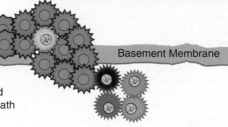

Basement Membrane

Instead of maturing properly and undergoing programmed cell death (apoptosis) the cells become immortalized and continue to accumulate.

Clonal evolution occurs with the stem cells taking on additional genetic changes and more malicious characteristics.

SENESCENCE AS A TARGET FOR CANCER THERAPY

Senescence is one way that cancer cells may "hibernate." Senescence limits tumor progression and could represent a strategy to increase survival using tactics such as TP53 reactivation, inhibition of c-MYC in addicted tumors, or treatment with CDK inhibitors.

INTERPLAY BETWEEN TP53 AND TELOMERASE

The loss of TP53-mediated surveillance of genomic integrity may permit cells to survive chromosomal breakage–fusion–bridge (BFB) cycles, which increase genome mutability. Delayed acquisition of telomerase function first serves to generate tumor-promoting mutations, whereas its later activation stabilizes the mutant genome and then confers "immortality." This is another example of the "bipolar" nature of cellular processes whereby early on a cancer may develop as a result of the absence of a certain function and later the cancer may be promoted by the acquisition of that same function.

ADDITIONAL FUNCTIONS OF TELOMERASE

Telomerase and its catalytic reverse transcriptase (hTERT) are found at multiple sites along chromosomes, not just at the telomeres. This results in other functions: telomerase is a cofactor of the Wnt/β-catenin/lymphocyte enhancer function (LEF) complex (Jung and Park, 2020). (See Chapter 3 Wnt Signaling.) Telomerase can also enhance cell proliferation, RNA polymerase, resistance to apoptosis, and DNA damage repair (Guterres and Villanueva, 2020). This recurring theme of multifunctionality adds complexity to the design of new clinical strategies but could also be exploited to great effect because a telomerase inhibitor could attack cancers in a variety of ways.

GENETIC INSTABILITY

Multistep tumor progression can be portrayed as a sequence of clonal evolution. Given the billions of mitotic events that occur in our body, it is no surprise that additional enabling mutations can occur by chance in an already vulnerable DNA "portfolio." In addition to frank mutation, tumor suppressor genes can be inactivated through "epigenetic" DNA methylation switching and histone modifications (see Figure 2.11) (Panjarian and Issa, 2021). The extraordinary ability of genome maintenance systems to detect and repair defects in the DNA ensures that rates of spontaneous mutation are

Figure 2.11

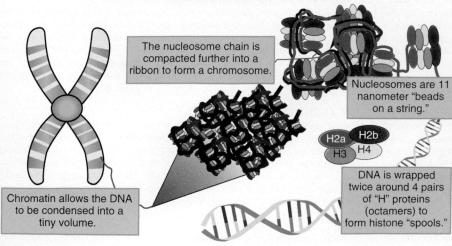

Histone Modification
How DNA Double Helix Turns into Chromosomes

The nucleosome chain is compacted further into a ribbon to form a chromosome.

Nucleosomes are 11 nanometer "beads on a string."

Chromatin allows the DNA to be condensed into a tiny volume.

H2a H2b
H3 H4

DNA is wrapped twice around 4 pairs of "H" proteins (octamers) to form histone "spools."

usually very low during each cell generation (Hanahan and Weinberg, 2011); however, in the course of acquiring the multiple mutant genes needed to orchestrate tumorigenesis, cancer cells often increase the rates of mutation (Negrini et al., 2010; Salk et al., 2016). These genetic changes are brought about through a breakdown in the genomic maintenance machinery.

In addition, the accumulation of mutations can be accelerated by compromising the surveillance systems that normally monitor genomic integrity and force genetically damaged cells into either senescence or apoptosis (Jackson and Bartek, 2009; Merchut-Maya et al., 2019) (Figure 2.10). The role of TP53 is central here, leading to its being called the "guardian of the genome" (Lane, 1992). Tumor suppressors detect and repair damaged DNA. They also inactivate or intercept mutagenic molecules before they have damaged the DNA (Joseph et al., 2020; Negrini et al., 2010).

Telomeres are the caretakers of the chromosomes. Loss of telomeric DNA impairs stability with amplification and deletion of chromosomal segments (Roake and Artandi, 2020). Genome instability is clearly a characteristic that is central in the role of carcinogenesis and the vexing task of dealing with cancers that "change the rules in the middle of the game."

Autophagy and Cell Death
AUTOPHAGY MEDIATES RECYCLING, CELL SURVIVAL, AND DEATH

Cancer cell cytoplasmic vesicles under circumstances of stress or limited nutrients can ingest organelles such as ribosomes and mitochondria, fuse them with lysosomes, and recycle them for energy and growth. Nobel Prize winner Christian de Duve coined this process "autophagy" (see Figure 2.12) (Deter et al., 1967; Klionsky, 2008; Levy et al., 2017).

Beclin-1, a member of the BCL-2 homology domain 3 (BH3), is bound to BCL-2/BCL-xL in an inactive state. When autophagy is triggered, Beclin-1 separates from BCL-2/BCL-xL analogous to the release of BAX and BAK, initiating apoptosis (see Figure 2.13 showing the various Bcl-2 family members).

Other BH3 proteins (e.g., BID, BAD, PUMA) can induce programmed cell death or alternatively induce cell shrinkage, autophagy, and reversible dormancy (Galluzzi et al., 2017). This may explain the persistence and eventual regrowth of some late-recurring tumors, such as melanoma,

Figure 2.12

The Microenvironment and Therapeutic Targeting

10. Autophagy

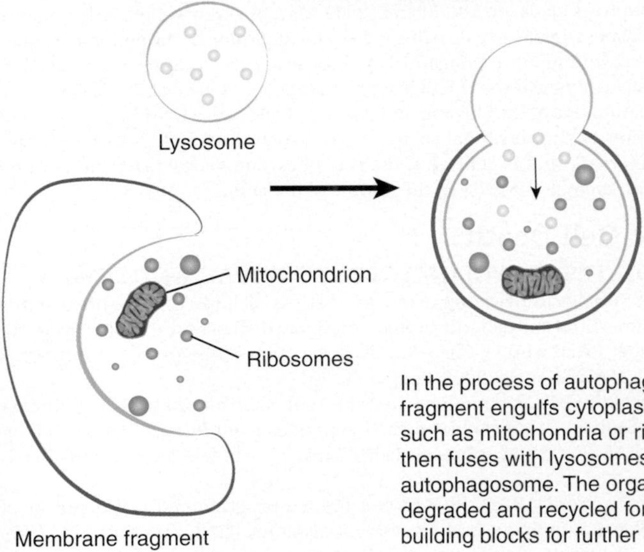

Lysosome

Mitochondrion

Ribosomes

Membrane fragment

In the process of autophagy, a membrane fragment engulfs cytoplasmic organelles such as mitochondria or ribosomes and then fuses with lysosomes to form an autophagosome. The organelles are degraded and recycled for energy and building blocks for further cell growth.

Figure 2.13

189

The Microenvironment and Therapeutic Targeting

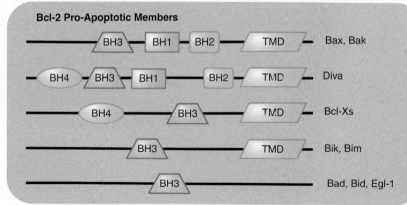

*Modular elements: BH1, BH2, BH3, BH4; Transmembrane Domain (TMD)

following initial therapy. Just as TGF-β signaling can be tumor-suppressing early on and tumor-promoting later, autophagy seems to have variable effects (Apel et al., 2009).

Phosphatidylinositol-3-OH (PI3K), AKT, and mTOR kinases can block both apoptosis and autophagy when survival signals are present and can be downregulated otherwise. It would appear that successful targeting of autophagy will need to take into account the balance between the BH3 regulatory proteins, the BCL-2 family, and the state of activity of PI3K (see Figure 2.13).

IMMUNE MONITORING

Immune surveillance is the process whereby a competent immune system recognizes and eliminates early cancers. This concept is supported by increased cancers such as squamous cancers of the skin and lymphoma in immunosuppressed transplant patients and other individuals with deficient CD8+ CTLs, CD4+ Th1 (T helper) cells, or NK cells (Collins et al., 2019). Figure 2.14 highlights the impediments to immune surveillance. Some immunosuppressed organ transplant recipients have developed donor-derived cancers, suggesting that the transplanted "passenger" cancer cells had been held in check by the donor's immune system (Vidovic and Giacomantonio, 2020).

Colon and ovarian tumors that are heavily infiltrated with CTLs and NK cells have a better prognosis than those that lack such abundant killer lymphocytes (Nelson, 2008; Pagès et al., 2010). In addition, the immunosuppression of HIV can lead to HIV-associated cancers such as non-Hodgkin lymphoma and Kaposi sarcoma (Rabkin et al., 1991). Highly immunogenic cancer cells can be eliminated ("immuno-editing"). In order to be successful, cancer cells must, therefore, limit their immunogenicity. Examples of this "stealth" behavior are to paralyze infiltrating CTLs and NK cells, by secreting TGF-β (Bule et al., 2021; Yang et al., 2010) or recruiting immunosuppressive regulatory T cells (Tregs) and myeloid-derived suppressor cells (MDSCs).

A more detailed discussion of immunotherapy principles is seen later in this section.

RESISTANCE MUTATIONS

Targeted therapies directed against receptor-activated protein kinases have transformed clinical management of many cancers, but keeping a step ahead of inevitable cancer resistance to these drugs is an enormous challenge (see Figure 2.15). Gerard Manning and colleagues reported analysis

Figure 2.14

191

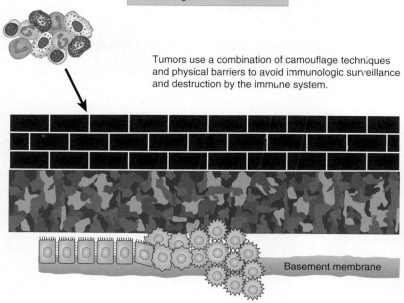

The Microenvironment and Therapeutic Targeting

11. Avoiding Immune Surveillance

Tumors use a combination of camouflage techniques and physical barriers to avoid immunologic surveillance and destruction by the immune system.

Basement membrane

The Microenvironment and Therapeutic Targeting

12. Resistance Mutations

Cancers can be comprised of several different clones, some of which may be sensitive to a given treatment, and some of which may be resistant. There may be initial shrinkage with persistence of the resistant clone. In addition, with time, additional clones can emerge, giving rise to additional resistance to treatment.

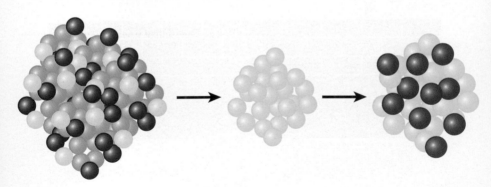

of 518 kinases making up the human "kinome" (Manning et al., 2002), many of which are key targets for interrupting the uncontrolled signaling in cancer cells.

NSCLC harbors activating mutations in a large number of patients in the United States—especially EGFR in nonsmokers (Figure 2.16). The percentages also differ depending on early or later stages of the disease (Skoulidis and Heymach, 2019).

Whereas these mutations in EGFR may confer unique sensitivity to targeted therapy, secondary mutations such as T790M lead to resistance to first-generation EGFR-TKIs after a median of 10 to 14 months, requiring a switch to conventional chemotherapy or, in some cases, newer kinase inhibitors that target other kinases.

The remarkable ability of cancers to devise "workarounds" remains a huge challenge. Cancer cell resistance strategies range from serial mutations in drug-targeted receptors, such as EGFR, to production of proteins from noncancer cells in their surrounding tissues (stroma) that help fuel cancer to grow and metastasize.

Third-generation drugs such as osimertinib (EGF816) are effective in T790M-mutated NSCLC, with an overall response rate of 61% (Janne et al., 2015). Osimertinib was granted breakthrough status in September 2017 on the basis of a large randomized controlled trial compared to gefitinib or erlotinib in first-line EGFR-mutated NSCLC (exon 19 deletion or L858R—The FLAURA Trial).

The NSCLC EGFR story has evolved further with the development of poziotinib for previously refractory exon 20–mutated NSCLC (Kim et al., 2018).

Cancer cells typically express multiple RTKs that mediate signals converging on key downstream cell survival effectors such as PI3K and mitogen-activated protein kinase (MAPK). MAPK cascades, for example, are evolutionarily conserved intracellular signal transduction pathways that respond to various extracellular stimuli and control fundamental cellular processes including growth, proliferation, and differentiation.

The tumor microenvironment can also mediate resistance to cancer therapies by secretion of hepatocyte growth factor (HGF) and MET activation (see MET (also known as HGF receptor) in Section 3), resulting in resistance of BRAF-mutated melanoma. This suggests a role for dual inhibition of RAF and either HGF or MET. Another possibility is to combine different classes of agents such as chemotherapy, vascular inhibitors, and targeted agents such as the liposomal doxorubicin, bevacizumab, and temsirolimus regimen (Wu and Dai, 2017).

Figure 2.16

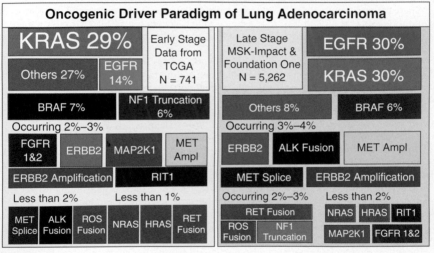

(Adapted from Skoulidis F, Heymach JV. Co-occurring genomic alterations in non-small-cell lung cancer biology and therapy. *Nat Rev Cancer*. 2019;19(9):495–509.)

Angiogenesis is induced surprisingly early during the multistage development of invasive cancers both in animal models and in humans (Figure 2.17). Activation of an "angiogenic switch" helps sustain expanding neoplastic growth (Hanahan and Folkman, 1996).

VEGF-A and members of the FGF family are angiogenesis stimulators, whereas thrombospondin-1 (TSP-1) is an angiogenesis inhibitor. VEGF receptor tyrosine kinases (VEGFR-1,2,3) are regulated by hypoxia and oncogene signaling (Apte et al., 2019). VEGF sequestered in the extracellular matrix can be released and activated by matrix metalloproteinase-9 (MMP-9) (Najafi et al., 2019).

Attempts at producing MMP inhibitors, although conceptually appealing, have had very limited success to date. Tumor blood vessels are tortuous, leaky, and distorted with excessive branching and erratic flow. They also have abnormal EC proliferation and apoptosis (Arneth, 2019). Neovasculature has higher resistance and differing flow characteristics. This begs the question of whether some current treatments have limited success because the drugs are shunted away from the tumor by abnormal vasculature.

GRADATIONS OF THE ANGIOGENIC SWITCH

Tumors exhibit diverse vascular patterns (Hanahan and Weinberg, 2011). They may be highly aggressive tumors with avascular "deserts" (Chapouly et al., 2019) or densely vascularized cancers (e.g., renal). Dominant oncogenes (*RAS* and *MYC*) can upregulate expression of angiogenic factors, whereas TSP-1, fragments of plasmin (angiostatin), and type 18 collagen (endostatin) are angiogenesis inhibitors (Ribatti and Tamma, 2020).

Pericytes (see Figure 2.17) support the neovasculature of most, if not all, tumors (De Palma et al., 2017) and may have a protective role against antitumor drugs. Multiple bone marrow cells (macrophages, neutrophils, mast cells, myeloid progenitors) also play crucial roles in angiogenesis (Nielsen and Schmid, 2017).

Figure 2.17

The Microenvironment and Therapeutic Targeting

Cancers stimulate production of new blood vessels to obtain nutrients. Individual cancer cells can express mesenchymal cell characteristics with loss of head-to-toe orientation, motility into the blood vessels, travel to distant sites, exit from capillaries into a particular organ, and adaptation and colonization of that organ's parenchyma. Finally, the malignant cells can transform back to epithelial characteristics as they form a "mature" metastasis.

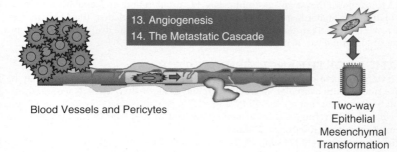

13. Angiogenesis
14. The Metastatic Cascade

Blood Vessels and Pericytes

Two-way
Epithelial
Mesenchymal
Transformation

INVASION AND METASTASIS

The study of invasion and metastasis pioneered by Isaiah "Josh" Fidler (1936–2020) showed that there is a virtual "decathlon" of events required for cancers to spread (Langley and Fidler, 2011):

1. Primary tumor vascularization
2. Local capillary invasion
3. Hematogenous transport
4. Malignant cell embolization
5. Organ arrest
6. Endothelial adherence
7. Extravasation into parenchyma
8. Microenvironment establishment
9. Tumor proliferation
10. Clinically evident metastases

These steps entail local invasion, gaining entry into nearby vessels, mobility through the lymphatic and systemic circulation, escape of cancer cells from vessels into the parenchyma of distant tissues (extravasation), formation of small nodules of cancer cells (micrometastases), and growth of macroscopic tumors in a foreign environment—"colonization" (Figure 2.17).

By the time cancers become evident, there has often been a clinically silent prelude, taking months and even years. This means that preventive interventions are possible, even though transformation has occurred.

Calcium-dependent adherence proteins (cadherins) are transmembrane "Velcro-like" proteins that bind cells tightly together. The various classes of cadherins are designated by a prefix that specifies its affiliated type of tissue. *E-cadherin* forms junctions with adjacent epithelial cells and helps to assemble epithelial cell sheets and maintain the quiescence of the cells within these sheets.

Downregulation or mutational inactivation of E-cadherin promotes metastasis (De Keuckelaere et al., 2018). *N-cadherin* is normally expressed in migrating neurons and mesenchymal cells during organogenesis and is upregulated in many invasive carcinoma cells (Loh et al., 2019).

EMT is a process by which epithelial cells lose their cell polarity and cell–cell adhesion, and gain migratory and invasive properties to become mesenchymal stem cells; these are multipotent stromal cells that can differentiate into a variety of cell types. EMT is essential for numerous developmental processes, including mesoderm formation and neural tube formation (Hanahan and Weinberg, 2011). EMT has also been shown to occur in wound healing, in organ fibrosis, and in the initiation of metastasis for cancer progression (Wei et al., 2020). These transformed epithelial cells can then have the abilities to invade, resist apoptosis, and disseminate (Terry et al., 2017). Snail, slug, twist, and zinc finger E-box-binding homeobox 1/2 (ZEB1/2) are transcription factors that are associated with EMT and the process of cellular migration during embryogenesis and in a number of malignant tumor types. The cells lose their tight junctions and convert from polygonal/epithelial to spindly/fibroblastic shapes. They express matrix-degrading enzymes, increased mobility, and resistance to apoptosis. These are all traits required for invasion and metastasis (Micalizzi et al., 2017).

Cells that undergo EMT give rise to CSCs. Transfection and induction of EMT by activated RAS cause an increase in cancer cells with stem-like properties that are high in CD44 and low in CD24 (Mani et al., 2008). ZEB1 is a protein encoded by the *ZEB1* gene. ZEB1 is capable of conferring stem cell–like properties. These properties conferred by EMT are especially dangerous because they enable the cancer cells to enter the bloodstream and then "set up shop" once they reach their metastatic destination (Mitra et al., 2015).

In one model system, tumor-associated macrophages (TAMs) supply EGF to breast cancer cells, which in turn produce CSFs that reciprocally stimulate the macrophages. This mutual stimulation then promotes dissemination of the cancer (Qian and Pollard, 2010). Because metastasis requires an entire cellular "repertoire," it may be possible to interrupt the metastatic process at a number of steps without actually affecting the primary CSCs themselves.

LOCAL INVASION VERSUS DISTANT METASTASIS

The current model of cancer metastasis also includes signals from the stroma and other cells of the pseudo-organ that induce epithelial cells to become locally invasive. Many squamous cell carcinomas do not appear to have distant metastatic potential but can move through the extracellular matrix, attract inflammatory cells to the area, and "borrow" matrix-degrading enzymes in order to pass through basement membranes and other natural tissue barriers to local spread (Madsen and Bugge, 2015; Qian and Pollard, 2010).

METASTATIC COLONIZATION IS ACTUALLY AN INEFFICIENT PROCESS

Dissemination from a primary tumor to distant organs requires growth in foreign "soil." Thousands of cells can be shed daily from cancers—presumably once they reach a certain size and have a substantial blood supply. Large numbers of circulating cancer cells can be found in many individuals with cancer, yet the number of metastatic sites is usually limited. This leads us to conclude that many micrometastases may never actually become clinically detectable (Talmadge and Fidler, 2010). In fact, it is estimated that tumors can shed millions upon millions of cells per gram of tumor but less than 0.01% manage to extravasate into the tissues. Of those that traverse the capillaries, only a tiny number ever produce clinically meaningful metastatic tumors (Perea Paizal et al., 2021).

WORKING AT A DISTANCE—THE ABSCOPAL EFFECT

One of the most intriguing areas of metastasis biology is the complex interplay between primary tumors and distant metastases—the abscopal effect. For hundreds of years, physicians have noted that removal of a primary tumor can result in changes in the growth rate of distant lesions.

Various case reports have documented postsurgical dormancy or accelerated growth. This strongly implies that primary tumors were producing suppressors or alternatively releasing factors that in some way supported the distant metastases (Demicheli et al., 2019; Folkman, 2002). Radiation of the primary tumor in both human and animal systems has been shown to produce variable distant effects ranging from acceleration to complete tumor regression in a melanoma patient treated with sequential local radiation and ipilimumab immunotherapy (Postow et al., 2012).

Delayed metastases can develop mysteriously years after a primary tumor has been completely resected, especially in cases of breast cancer and melanoma. This may be due to late acquisition of colonization capability (Weidenfeld and Barkan, 2018), failure to activate tumor angiogenesis (Naumov et al., 2008), or immune system suppression (Teng et al., 2008) or may require the time for the chance (stochastic) emergence of numerous requisite colonization programs.

Finally, certain tissue sites may be especially hospitable to circulating cancer cells such as the adrenal gland, a common site for lung cancer spread (Talmadge and Fidler, 2010). The hunt is on to identify the "metastatic signatures" that facilitate the growth and development of macroscopic metastases in specific tissues (Coghlin and Murray, 2010).

IMMUNOGENIC CELL DEATH

When cancer cells are damaged by a number of stressors, including chemotherapeutic drugs, oncolytic viruses, and radiotherapy, a secondary activation of the immune system called immunogenic cell death (ICD) can occur (Figure 2.18).

ICD involves the release of damage-associated molecular patterns (DAMPs) from all parts of the dying tumor cells. This results in tumor-specific immune responses and combined direct cancer cell killing and antitumor immunity. DAMPs include the cell surface exposure of calreticulin (CRT, endoplasmic reticulum) and cytoplasmic heat shock proteins (HSP70 and HSP90 and ATP). High-mobility group box-1 (HMGB1) comes from the nucleus. Dendritic cells engulf and process DAMPS with activation of T4+ and T8+ lymphocytes and eventual immune cell attack. One of the most recent examples of ICD was publication of a promising platinum-containing agent, PT-112, that has shown clinical benefit in lung and prostate cancer. PT-112 induces ICD and also synergizes with immune checkpoint blockers in mouse tumor models (Galluzzi et al., 2020; Yamazaki et al., 2020).

STRATEGIES FOR THE FUTURE AND ORGAN AGNOSTIC THERAPY

Many of the targeted cancer drugs developed to date have been deliberately directed toward specific cellular mutations that are involved in some aspect of the metastatic process. Although dramatic and durable responses can occur in such diseases as chronic myelogenous leukemia and melanoma—and even rare cases of lung cancer—they are frustratingly uncommon. Cancer cells are able to exist and thrive through redundant signaling pathways. As a result, targeted agents inhibiting a single pathway often fail because cancer cells adapt by mutating, activating epigenetic changes, or remodeling their local microenvironment.

Numerous combination regimens have been designed to overcome resistance. One notable example is dabrafenib plus trametinib for BRAF-driven cancer (Hyman et al., 2015; Long et al., 2016).

NTRK FUSION AND GENE-BASED ORGAN AGNOSTIC TREATMENT

Another important development has been the recognition that genomically informed treatment can be organ site "agnostic" in the case of the tropomyosin receptor kinase (NTRK) family, also

Figure 2.18

201

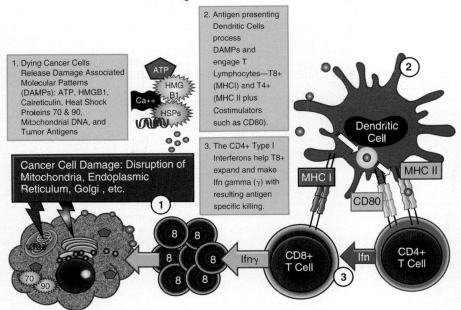

Immunogenic Cell Death

1. Dying Cancer Cells Release Damage Associated Molecular Patterns (DAMPs): ATP, HMGB1, Calreticulin, Heat Shock Proteins 70 & 90, Mitochondrial DNA, and Tumor Antigens

2. Antigen presenting Dendritic Cells process DAMPs and engage T Lymphocytes—T8+ (MHCI) and T4+ (MHC II plus Costimulators such as CD80).

3. The CD4+ Type I Interferons help T8+ expand and make Ifn gamma (γ) with resulting antigen specific killing.

Cancer Cell Damage: Disruption of Mitochondria, Endoplasmic Reticulum, Golgi , etc.

known as neurotrophic tyrosine kinase receptor, encoded by the *NTRK1* gene. These TRK molecules play an essential role in nervous system development. TRK gene fusions define a unique molecular subgroup of cancer patients. Larotrectinib and entrectinib have shown meaningful responses in over 50% of patients with NTRK fusion irrespective of the site of origin (Hong et al., 2020).

In 2017, the FDA approved pembrolizumab for patients with advanced refractory cancer *of any site* on the basis of work that showed a high rate of response in patients with defective DNA repair and increased microsatellite activity (MSI High). This has led the way to an increase in the options for the category of genomically based organ agnostic therapy (Lemery et al., 2017).

THE PARADOX OF ACCELERATED GROWTH RESPONSE TO TARGETED THERAPY

In some settings, targeted agents appear to have paradoxically and tragically induced cancer cells to accelerate growth (Ebos et al., 2009). This hyper-progression has also been observed in rare patients following immune checkpoint inhibitors (Sehgal, 2021).

These cases may also hold important clues to ultimately unraveling the mystery of cancer cell growth and control. Drug development and the design of future treatment protocols will benefit from incorporating the concepts of the multiple biochemical pathways involved in supporting cancer cell growth. These mechanism-guided combinations have already begun to change the cancer treatment landscape with safer, more narrowly acting agents. The role of a glycolysis in malignant growth can be exploited further and resolve the question of how the metabolic machinery can be reprogramming to counteract the cancer-proliferative advantage (Ganapathy-Kanniappan and Geschwind, 2013). Investigational drugs have entered the clinical arena that target many of the molecules and processes listed in this chapter. We are now seeing second- and third-generation agents that will be critical in overcoming acquired cancer cell resistance. Another important area for research is the effect of timing and sequence for combinations of new targeted agents. This will require unprecedented cooperation between pharmaceutical sponsors, regulatory agencies, and clinical investigators.

In November 2017, the FDA approved Foundation Medicine's NGS-based genomic profiling test, FoundationOne CDx (F1CDx). Concurrently, the Centers for Medicare and Medicaid Services (CMS) issued a preliminary national coverage determination for the test and others like it.

The wider availability of genomic testing as *actionable* cancer gene amplification, alterations of function, and novel fusion products will bring new hope to cancer patients and provide avenues of treatment that could only be dreamed of in the past.

The wider availability of genomic testing as *actionable* cancer gene amplification, alterations of function, and novel fusion products will bring new hope to cancer patients and provide avenues of treatment that could only be dreamed of in the past.

The Immune System

TYPES OF IMMUNITY

Immunity can be acquired either actively or passively. Immunity is acquired actively when a person is exposed to foreign substances and the immune system responds. Passive immunity is when antibodies are transferred from one host to another. Both actively acquired and passively acquired immunity can be obtained by natural or artificial means (Frankel et al., 2017; Janeway et al., 2005; Keller and Stiehm, 2000).

Naturally acquired active immunity—when a person is naturally exposed to antigens, becomes ill, and then recovers. Naturally acquired passive immunity—involves a natural transfer of antibodies from a mother to her infant. The antibodies cross the woman's placenta to the fetus. Antibodies can also be transferred through breast milk with the secretions of colostrum.

Artificially acquired active immunity—is done by vaccination (introducing dead or weakened antigen to the host's cell)

Artificially acquired passive immunity—involves the introduction of antibodies rather than antigens to the human body. These antibodies are from an animal or person who is already immune to the disease.

INNATE IMMUNITY

We are all equipped at birth with basic defenses against a number of organisms containing telltale antigens recognizable to our "first responders"—sentinel macrophages and dendritic cells. Toll-like receptors (named in 1996 for the German word for "amazing!"; Satoh and Akira, 2016) are specific for fungi and other microbes. When these pathogen-associated molecular patterns (PAMPs) are encountered, mast cells rapidly release histamine and a variety of leukocytes are attracted by chemokines, including NK cells responding to IFN (Figure 2.19). Vascular ECs swell and "leak" serum and proteins, causing an inflammatory exudate (Figure 2.19) (Uematsu and Akira, 2007).

Innate Immunity

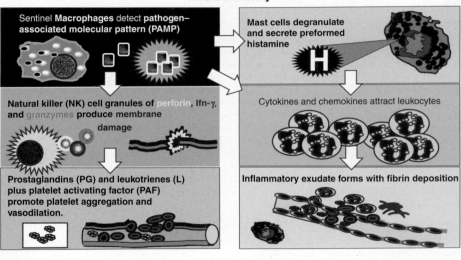

NK cells continue the cascade with release of membrane-damaging perforin granules, IFN-γ, and granzymes, producing further damage. Cellular injury also provokes lipid bilayer inflammatory mediators such as platelet-activating factor (PAF), and arachidonic acids are converted to prostaglandins and leukotriene with more vasodilatation and platelet and fibrinogen activation to form a coagulum designed to control the invader(s). Beutler, Hoffmann, and Steinman won the Nobel Prize in 2011 for the elucidation of innate immunology system. More recently, researchers have also focused on the gut bacterial microenvironment (the "microbiome") as a modulator of the anticancer immune response (Gopalakrishnan et al., 2018).

ADAPTIVE IMMUNITY

If innate immunity is a coarse rapid response team, adaptive immunity (AI) is a more strategic planned response depending on training of the T and B lymphocytes. AI includes highly specialized, systemic cells and processes that eliminate pathogens and produce specific and long-lasting immunologic memory for future exposures to a particular pathogen. AI is the basis of vaccination and is composed of both humoral and cell-mediated components (Janeway et al., 2005; U.S. Department of Health and Human Services, 2007).

The major functions of the adaptive immune system include the following:

1. Recognition of specific "nonself" during antigen presentation
2. Generation of responses tailored to maximally eliminate specific pathogen-infected cells
3. Development of memory B cells and T cells

TOLERANCE AND SURVEILLANCE

The fundamental miracle of the immune system is the ability to distinguish "self" from "nonself." The loss of surveillance, on the one hand, can be highly favorable during pregnancy where specific glycoproteins suppress the uterine immune response and endogenous retroviruses (ERVs) numbering in the dozens (Villarreal, 2001) produce proteins and a placental syncytium that limits exchange of migratory cells from the mother. Cancer cells, on the other hand, also produce a form of tolerance with blockers of programmed cell death (e.g., PD-L1) that helps tumors grow unopposed by what we would hope would be a protective immune system.

LYMPHOCYTES AND RECEPTORS

Early in life, immature cells migrate from the bone marrow to the thymus where they are called thymocytes and ultimately develop into T cells. In humans, approximately 1% to 2% of the lymphocyte pool recirculates each hour to where they encounter specific antigens within the secondary lymphoid tissues. In an adult animal, the peripheral lymphoid organs contain a mixture of B and T cells in at least three stages of differentiation (Wong and Germain, 2018).

Thymus-derived lymphocytes, therefore, are referred to as T cells. There are numerous types of T cells with corresponding subtypes. These include helper CD4+, cytotoxic CD8+, memory T cells, Tregs, innate-like T cells, NK T cells, mucosal-associated invariant T cells, and γδ T cells.

HELPER T-CELL RESPONSES: TH1 AND TH2

Th1 involves production of IFN-γ, which activates the macrophage bactericidal activity and induces B cells to make opsonizing (coating) and complement-fixing antibodies. Th1 responses are focused on intracellular viruses and bacteria (Kitz and Dominguez-Villar, 2017).

The Th2 response includes release of IL-5, which induces eosinophils (Spencer and Weller, 2010) in the clearance of parasites, and IL-4, which facilitates B-cell isotype switching. Th2 is effective against extracellular bacteria, parasites including helminths, and toxins. Most CD4+ helper cells die during the infection process, but a few remain as CD4+ memory cells (Harris and Loke, 2017; Spencer and Weller, 2010).

CTLs induce the death of cells that are infected with viruses (and other pathogens) or are otherwise damaged or dysfunctional.

1. Immature B and T cells from bone marrow or thymus, respectively, have entered the lymphatic system, before any encounter with their particular antigen "partner."
2. Effector cells actively eliminate a pathogen after specific activation.
3. Memory cells persist after an infection and are available for future protection (Flajnik and Kasahara, 2010).

Naive cytotoxic T cells are activated when their TCR strongly interacts with a peptide-bound major histocompatibility complex (MHC) class I molecule. This affinity depends on the type and orientation of the antigen/MHC complex and is what keeps the CTL and infected cell bound together. Once activated, the CTL undergoes a process called clonal selection in which it gains functions and divides rapidly to produce a legion of "armed" effector cells (Alcover et al., 2018).

CTLs are fortunately regulated by "Treg" cells to prevent unwanted autoimmunity, but as they traffic through the body and become activated by a specific strong MHC/antigen signal—often with the help of costimulators and/or CD4+ "helper" T cells, they unleash the cascade of innate immunity events resulting in membrane damage, cell swelling, apoptosis, and destruction (Alcover et al., 2018).

Helper TCRs recognize antigen bound to Class II MHC molecules on antigen-presenting cells. Activated Th1 cells reciprocate with cytokines that affect the antigen presenting cell. Th1 cells do not require as strong a stimulus as cytotoxic T cells, but they provide costimulation that activates killer cells.

Tregs are important suppressors of aberrant immune responses to self-antigens, an important mechanism in controlling the development of autoimmune diseases (Dominguez-Villar and Hafler, 2018).

Follicular helper T cells (Tfh) are uniquely capable of migrating to secondary lymph node follicular B cells and provide positive paracrine signals to generate high-affinity antibodies. Similar to Tregs, Tfh control is necessary for immunologic control because excess Tfh cell numbers can lead to autoantibodies and severe autoimmune disorders (Ma and Phan, 2017).

GAMMA DELTA T CELLS

γδ T cells have features of both innate immunity and AI (Nielsen et al., 2017).

They possess an alternative TCR as opposed to CD4+ and CD8+ γδ T cells and share characteristics of Th1 cells, cytotoxic T cells, and NK cells. They may be considered a component of AI in that they rearrange *TCR* genes via V(D)J recombination and develop "memory." On the other hand, however, the various subsets may also be considered part of the innate immune system. For example, in this setting, large numbers of Vγ9/Vδ2 T cells respond within hours to common microbial molecules and highly restricted intraepithelial Vδ1 T cells respond to damaged or stressed epithelial cells.

B LYMPHOCYTES, IMMUNOGLOBULINS, AND HUMORAL IMMUNITY

B cells are the major cells involved in the creation of antibodies that circulate in blood plasma and lymph (Franchina et al., 2018), known as humoral immunity (*humor* is Latin for "moisture" or "fluid"). Antibodies (also known as immunoglobulins or simply Ig) are large "lobster-like" proteins (two claws, a body, and a tail) used by the immune system to identify and neutralize foreign objects. Mammals have five types of antibodies—IgA, IgD, IgE, IgG, and IgM—designed to handle different kinds of unique antigens and/or specific pathogens (Alberts, 2015).

When antibodies bind to their complementary (cognate) antigen, five different mechanisms occur:

1. Agglutination causes infectious particles to stick together.
2. Complement activation produces inflammation and cell lysis.
3. Antigen coating—opsonization—enhances phagocytosis.
4. Macrophages, eosinophils, and NK cells are recruited to carry out cellular destruction.
5. Bacteria and viruses are blocked from sticking to mucosal membranes.

T cells require an accompanying major histocompatibility molecule (Class I or II) for activation, whereas B cells recognize "naked" antigens (Borghesi and Milcarek, 2006; Horii and Matsushita, 2021).

Once a B cell receives additional signals from a Th2 cell, it further differentiates into a short-lived plasma cell (2–3 days); however, approximately 10% of plasma cells become long-lived antigen-specific memory B cells (Weller and Spencer, 2017).

Throughout life, our memory B and T cells construct a database of immunologic "apps" to protect us in the form of either passive short-term memory or active long-term memory. T cells are useless without antigen presenting cells (e.g., dendritic cells) to activate them, and B cells need help from T cells to function properly (Mami-Chouaib et al., 2018).

CYTOKINES AND SIGNALING

Cytokines (cyto, from Greek *kytos* meaning "cavity," cell + kines, from Greek *kinisi* meaning "movement") are a heterogeneous group of small proteins (~5–20 kDa) that create immune signals within the same cell (autocrine), neighboring cells (paracrine), and/or systemically (endocrine).

Cytokines include the "chemokine families"—IFNS, ILS, lymphokines, and tumor necrosis factors (TNFs). These are generally not hormones or growth factors. Cytokines are produced by macrophages, B lymphocytes, T lymphocytes, and mast cells, as well as ECs, fibroblasts, and various stromal cells. Unlike hormones, cytokines are promiscuous; they may be produced by more than one type of cell or organ site (Nagarsheth et al., 2017).

Cytokines help control the balance between humoral and cell-based immune responses, and they regulate the responsiveness, growth, and development of diverse cell populations. Some cytokines also enhance or inhibit the action of other cytokines (Conlon et al., 2019).

DISCOVERY OF CYTOKINES

IFN-α (type I) was identified in 1957 as a protein that blocked viral replication (U.S. Department of Health and Human Services, 2007). The activity of IFN-γ (type II) was described in 1965. Macrophage migration inhibitory factor (MMIF) was identified simultaneously in 1966 by John David and Barry Bloom.

In 1969, Dudley Dumonde proposed the term *lymphokine* to describe proteins secreted from lymphocytes, and later, proteins derived from macrophages and monocytes in culture were called *monokines*. Ultimately, the term *cytokine* was used to denote this broader class of self-defense proteins. In 1977, Steve Gillis and Kendall Smith reported the discovery of a T-cell growth factor—later named IL-2—that promoted long-term culture of tumor-specific T cells. IL-2 was purified in the late 1970s (Gillis and Smith, 1977; Mier and Gallo, 1980).

Whereas classic hormones circulate in nanomolar (10^{-9} M) concentrations that are relatively constant, cytokines such as IL-6 circulate in picomolar (10^{-12} M) concentrations that can increase up to 1,000-fold during trauma or infection. The widespread source of cytokines—endothelium, epithelium, and macrophages—also differentiates them from a hormone such as insulin that is only produced in the pancreas.

CYTOKINE CLASSIFICATION

Cytokines can be classified on the basis of their function, cell of secretion, or target (Dinarello, 2000):

1. IL is used to denote a protein messenger produced by Th1 cells and targeting leukocytes.
2. Monokines are produced exclusively by monocytes.

3. IFNs "interfere" with protein production and are involved in antiviral responses.
4. CSFS support the growth of cells in semisolid media.
5. Chemokines mediate attraction and movement (chemotaxis) between cells.

Cytokines can be divided structurally into four types (Conlon et al., 2019):

1. The IL-1 family, which primarily includes IL-1 and IL-18
2. The IL-17 family, which promotes proliferation of cytotoxic T cells
3. TGF-β superfamily, including TGF-β types 1, 2, and 3
4. The four-α-helix bundle cytokines, which are divided into three subfamilies (Abel et al., 2018):
   a. The IL-2 subfamily—including erythropoietin (EPO) and thrombopoietin (TPO)
   b. The IFN subfamily
   c. The IL-10 subfamily

FUNCTIONAL CLASSIFICATION

A more useful approach separates cytokines into those that enhance cellular immune responses:
1. Type 1 (TNF, IFN, etc.) (Locksley et al., 2001)
2. Type 2 (TGF, IL-4, IL-10, IL-13, etc.), which favors antibody responses

CYTOKINE RECEPTORS

Cytokine receptors can be classified according to their three-dimensional structure because it relates to their function and drug development (Figure 2.20):

1. Ig superfamily—Ig-like molecules are ubiquitous and include antibodies, adhesion molecules, and some cytokines (IL-1) and certain receptor types.
2. Type 1—The hematopoietic growth factor receptors, whose members have certain conserved motifs in their extracellular amino acid domain. The IL-2 receptor belongs to this group. IL-2Rγ-chain deficiency is directly responsible for the X-linked form of severe combined immunodeficiency (X-SCID) (Aloj et al., 2012).
3. Type 2—The IFN family: receptors for IFN-γ and -δ
4. Type 3—The TNF family, whose members share a cysteine-rich common extracellular binding domain with several other noncytokine ligands like CD40, CD27, and CD30 (Vanamee and Faustman, 2018).

Figure 2.20

211

Cytokine Receptor Superfamilies

Immunoglobulin Superfamily:	Hematopoietic Growth Factors (Type 1):	Interferon (Type 2) Family:
homologous with antibodies and adhesion molecules 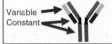 Variable ➡ Constant ➡	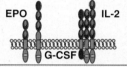 EPO IL-2 G-CSF	Receptors for IFN-β and IFN-γ
Tumor Necrosis Factor Receptor Family (Type 3): 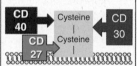	**Seven Transmembrane Helix Family:** Ubiquitous receptors that include the G protein-coupled receptors for hormones and neurotransmitters; also included are CD4 and CCR5, which act as HIV binding proteins	**Interleukin 17 Receptor (IL-17R) Family:** These include an extracellular fibronectin III—like domain and consist of 5 members—A, B, C, D, and E

5. The GPCRs with their seven (hepta—Greek) transmembrane helixes are ubiquitous receptors for hormones and neurotransmitters. This "system" has produced two Nobel Prize winners (Alfred Gilman [1994] and Robert Lefkowitz [2012]). Chemokine receptors, two of which act as binding proteins for HIV (CD4 and CCR5), also belong to this family (https://www.nobelprize.org/prizes/medicine/1994/gilman/biographical/) (https://www.nobelprize.org/prizes/chemistry/2012/lefkowitz/facts/).

6. IL-17R family—This family is distinct from other cytokines. Structural motifs conserved include an extracellular fibronectin III–like domain, a transmembrane domain, and a cytoplasmic domain called "SEFIR" (Zhang et al., 2013). There are five members of this family: IL-17R A–E.

CELLULAR EFFECTS

Each cytokine has a designated cell surface receptor. The effect of a particular cytokine depends on its extracellular titer and the downstream signals activated by receptor binding. Cytokines are characterized by considerable "redundancy" because many cytokines have overlapping or similar function.

Normal tissue integrity is preserved by complex feedback interactions between cytokines and diverse cell types, including adhesion molecules; something can be severely disrupted during carcinogenesis (Dangaj et al., 2013). Oversecretion of cytokines can trigger a dangerous syndrome known as a CRS or cytokine "storm" (Shimabukuro-Vornhagen et al., 2018). This is presumed to have been the cause of severe multisystem organ failure during a British clinical trial of TGN1412, a CD28 agonist antibody, in 2006 (Eastwood et al., 2010) and has also been seen as an uncommon but devastating complication of CAR T-cell therapy as well as COVID-19 (Fajgenbaum and June, 2020) (see Figure 2.9).

ANTIGENS AND ANTIBODIES

Antigens are substances that elicit an adaptive immune response. Pioneering work by Robert S Schwartz (1995) showed that a small number of genes (V(D)J-like "LEGOS") can result in somatic hypermutation to generate a vast number of different antigen receptors that are then uniquely expressed on each individual lymphocyte. Because the gene rearrangement leads to an irreversible change in the DNA of each cell, all progeny of that cell inherit genes that encode the same receptor specificity, including the memory B cells and memory T cells (Parham, 2009).

ANTIGEN PRESENTATION

The adaptive immune response is triggered by recognizing foreign antigen in the cellular context of an activated dendritic cell. Nucleated cells are capable of presenting antigen through the function of MHC molecules. Some cells are specially equipped to present antigen and to prime naive T cells. Dendritic cells, B cells, and macrophages are equipped with special "costimulatory" ligands recognized by costimulatory receptors on T cells and are termed professional antigen presenting cells. Ralph Steinman was notable for being awarded the only posthumous Nobel Prize in 2011 (https://www.nobelprize.org/prizes/medicine/2011/steinman/facts/).

An antibody is made up of two heavy chains and two light chains. The unique variable region allows an antibody to recognize its matching antigen (Alberts et al., 2002). Virtually all proteins and many complex sugars can serve as antigens (Janeway et al., 2005). The parts of an antigen that interact with an antibody molecule or a lymphocyte receptor are called epitopes or antigenic determinants. Most antigens contain a variety of epitopes and can stimulate the production of antibodies, specific T-cell responses, or both. A very small proportion (0.01%) of the total lymphocytes are able to bind to a particular antigen, which suggests that only a few cells respond to each antigen (U.S. Department of Health and Human Services, 2007).

Humans produce more than 1 trillion different antibody molecules to deal with the innumerable pathogens encountered in everyday life, yet the human genome contains fewer than 25,000 genes (Alberts et al., 2002). This extraordinary repertoire is assembled through clonal selection—a vast diversity of unique lymphocytes from information encoded in a small family of genes that undergo V(D)J or combinatorial diversification, in which one gene segment recombines with other gene segments to form a single unique gene. This assembly process generates an almost unlimited diversity of antibodies.

ENDOGENOUS ANTIGENS

Endogenous antigens come from intracellular bacteria and viruses replicating within a host cell. The host cell digests the foreign proteins enzymatically and displays telltale fragments coupled to

MHC. The endogenous antigens are then typically displayed coupled with MHC class I molecules, and this activates CD8+ cytotoxic T cells.

VACCINES

1. Immunization (vaccine) is the deliberate induction of an immune response that represents probably the single most effective public health achievement in modern times. The principle behind immunization is to introduce an antigen, derived from a disease-causing organism, that stimulates the immune system to develop protective immunity against that organism, but that does not itself cause the pathogenic effects of that organism (Baxby, 1999; Pasteur, 1881).

Most viral vaccines are based on live attenuated viruses, whereas many bacterial vaccines are based on acellular components of microorganisms, including harmless toxin components (U.S. Department of Health and Human Services, 2007). Most bacterial vaccines require the addition of adjuvants that activate the antigen presenting cells of the innate immune system to enhance immunogenicity (U.S. Department of Health and Human Services, 2007). Many investigators have tried to develop vaccines against specific cancers. To date, that technology has had only limited success. The COVID-19 pandemic has brought a new vaccine technology using RNA fragments to produce the specific coronavirus protein "spikes" for the immune system to recognize (Miao et al., 2021).

IMMUNE NETWORK THEORY

Immune network theory was developed in 1974 by Niels Jerne and Geoffrey W. Hoffmann and states that the immune system is an interacting network of lymphocytes and molecules that have variable (V) regions. These V regions bind not only to foreign regions but also to other V regions within the system with components connected to each other by V–V interactions. Jerne was awarded the 1984 Nobel Prize for his clonal selection theory, as well as his proposal of the immune network concept (Jerne, 1974).

CHECKPOINT BLOCKADE

Many cancers camouflage themselves from the immune system by producing molecules that inhibit T-cell recognition and activity. Multiple clinically important stimulatory checkpoint molecules are members of the TNF receptor superfamily—CD27, CD40, OX40, GITR, and CD137 (Figure 2.21).

Figure 2.21

215

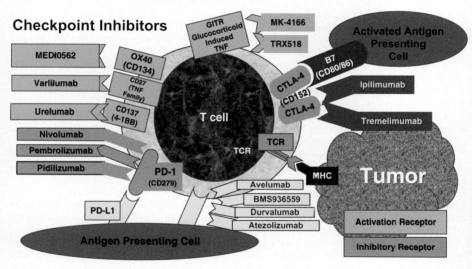

Checkpoint Inhibitors

CD28 and ICOS are two additional stimulatory checkpoint molecules that belong to the B7-CD28 superfamily.

CD27 is vital for T-cell memory and is also a memory marker of B cells (Hendriks et al., 2000). CD27 binds to its ligand, CD70, on lymphocytes and dendritic cells. CDX-1127, an agonistic anti-CD27 monoclonal antibody, has been shown to be effective in the context of TCR stimulation (Lian et al., 2020).

CD28 is constitutively expressed on almost all human CD4+ T cells and on approximately half of all CD8 T cells and promotes T-cell expansion following binding with its two ligands CD80 and CD86 expressed on dendritic cells.

CD40 is found on a variety of immune cells including antigen presenting cells; its ligand is CD154, which triggers T-cell activation and differentiation.

CD122 is the IL-2Rβ subunit and is known to increase proliferation of CD8+ effector T cells (CISION PR Newswire, 2015).

CD137 (aka 4-1BB) is bound by CD137 ligand, resulting in T-cell proliferation. CD137-mediated signaling is also known to protect T cells and, in particular, CD8+ T cells from activation-induced cell death (Mittler et al., 2004).

OX40, also called CD134, has CD252 as its ligand. Like CD27, OX40 promotes the expansion of effector and memory T cells; however, it is also noted for its ability to suppress the differentiation and activity of Tregs and also for its regulation of cytokine production (Croft et al., 2009).

OX40's value as a drug target primarily lies in the fact that it is only upregulated on the most recently antigen-activated T cells within inflammatory lesions. Anti-OX40 monoclonal antibodies have been shown to have clinical utility in advanced cancer. OX40 agonists in development include MEDI0562, MEDI6469, and MEDI6383 (Croft et al., 2009).

GITR, short for glucocorticoid-induced TNFR family–related gene, prompts T-cell expansion, including Treg expansion. The ligand for GITR is mainly expressed on antigen presenting cells. Antibodies to GITR have been shown to promote an antitumor response through loss of Treg lineage stability (Schaer et al., 2013).

ICOS, short for inducible T-cell costimulator, also called CD278, is expressed on activated T cells. Its ligand is ICOSL, expressed mainly on B cells and dendritic cells. The molecule seems to play an important role in T-cell effector function and has spawned a number of new exciting anticancer agents (Wei et al., 2017).

A2AR, short for adenosine A2A receptor, is regarded as an important checkpoint in cancer therapy because adenosine activation of the A2A receptor is a negative immune feedback loop and the tumor microenvironment has relatively high concentrations of adenosine (Leone et al., 2015).

B7-H3, also called CD276, is a coinhibitor, although it was originally understood to be a costimulatory molecule MGA271, and is an Fc-optimized monoclonal antibody that targets B7-H3 (Chapoval et al., 2001).

B7-H4, also called VTCN1, is expressed by tumor cells and TAMs and plays a role in tumor escape (Dangaj et al., 2013).

CTLA-4, short for CTL-associated protein 4 and also called CD152, is the target of ipilimumab (Yervoy), which gained FDA approval in March 2011. Expression of CTLA-4 on Treg cells serves to control T-cell proliferation (Kolar et al., 2009).

IDO, short for indoleamine 2,3-dioxygenase, is a tryptophan catabolic enzyme with immune-inhibitory properties. Another important molecule is TDO, tryptophan 2,3-dioxygenase. IDO is known to suppress T and NK cells, generate and activate Tregs and MDSCs, and promote tumor angiogenesis (Prendergast et al., 2014). IDO inhibitors are under active development.

LAG3, short for lymphocyte activation gene-3, works to suppress an immune response by action to Tregs (Huang et al., 2004) as well as direct effects on CD8+ T cells (Blackburn et al., 2009). BMS-986016 is an anti-LAG3 monoclonal antibody (Grosso et al., 2007).

PD-1, short for programmed death 1 receptor, has two ligands, PD-L1 and PD-L2. This checkpoint is the target of pembrolizumab and nivolumab, among others. These gained FDA approval in September 2014 and has revolutionized the treatment of multiple cancers, including lung, head and neck, and melanoma. An advantage of targeting PD-1 is that it can restore immune function in the tumor microenvironment (Philips and Atkins, 2015).

TIM-3, short for T-cell immunoglobulin domain and mucin domain 3, is expressed on activated human CD4+ T cells and regulates Th1 and Th17 cytokines. TIM-3 acts as a negative regulator of Th1/Tc1 function by triggering cell death on interaction with its ligand, galectin-9 (Das et al., 2017).

VISTA, short for V-domain Ig suppressor of T-cell activation, is primarily expressed on hematopoietic cells so that consistent expression of VISTA on leukocytes within tumors may allow VISTA blockade to be effective across a broad range of solid tumors (Lines et al., 2014).

ENGINEERING T CELLS AND THE IMMUNE SYSTEM

The concept of engineering T cells genetically was developed in the 1980s by Eshhar and colleagues. CAR T cells (Pule et al., 2003) are created by attaching specific variable monoclonal antibody single-chain recognition sites—the "head"—onto effector T cells obtained by apheresis from the patient. Using a retroviral vector by a process called adoptive transfer (Figure 2.22), the "tail" is created. The T cells, which can now recognize specific epitopes on cancer cells, are infused back into the patient (Ecsedi et al., 2021). A remarkable multistep production process is required. See process outline.

1. **The Ectodomain–Receptor Recognition Site**
   a. Almost anything that binds a given target with high affinity can be used as an antigen recognition region.
   b. The most common forms of CARs are fusions of single-chain variable fragments (scFv) fused to intracellular CD3-ζ (zeta—the endodomain attack signal).
   c. The single heavy and light chains are attached by a flexible link.

2. **Retroviral Insertion**
   a. The first destination for this scFv is the endoplasmic reticulum for further processing, and subsequently the construct makes its way to the cell surface.
   b. A signal peptide directs the nascent protein into the endoplasmic reticulum. This is essential if the receptor is to glycosylate and anchor in the cell membrane.

3. **Transmembrane Portion**
   a. Hydrophobic α-helix
   b. The CD3-ζ domain may incorporate the artificial TCR into the native TCR.

4. **Spacer Region**
   a. A spacer region links the antigen-binding domain to the transmembrane domain.
   b. Must be flexible to allow proper orientation for antigen recognition such as the IgG1 hinge region.

5. **Endodomain—The Intracellular Activation Signal**

The intracellular portion starts with the CD3 TCR and has an increasing number of "detonation switches" and costimulators to augment efficacy. There are three immunoreceptor tyrosine-based

Figure 2.22

219

Chimeric Antigen Receptor (CAR) T-Cell Production

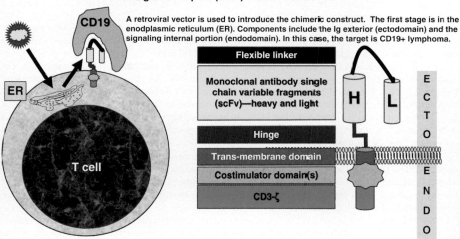

A retroviral vector is used to introduce the chimeric construct. The first stage is in the enodplasmic reticulum (ER). Components include the Ig exterior (ectodomain) and the signaling internal portion (endodomain). In this case, the target is CD19+ lymphoma.

CD19

ER

T cell

Flexible linker

Monoclonal antibody single chain variable fragments (scFv)—heavy and light

Hinge

Trans-membrane domain

Costimulator domain(s)

CD3-ζ

H   L

E C T O

E N D O

activation motifs (ITAMs) commonly used. There are now at least five generations of CAR T cells that even have an "off switch" to deal with immune toxicity caused by the unwanted overstimulation of the immune system. Second-generation CAR T cells: CD28, PX40, 41BB, ICOS (Rudd and Schneider, 2003); third generation: CD3z-CD28-41BB or CD3z-CD28-OX40; fourth generation: nuclear factor of activated T-cell (NFAT) and/or IL-12 mRNA transcripts; and fifth generation: IL2Rβ with JAK-STAT.

Purification and expansion of the CAR T cells can be produced by an eight-residue minimal-peptide sequence (Trp-Ser-His-Pro-Gln-Phe-Glu-Lys) that provides an identification marker for rapid purification and scaling up production as much as 200-fold.

B-cell malignancies that are CD19+ have been a very effective target for this approach. On August 30, 2017, the FDA approved tisagenlecleucel (**Kymriah**™) for childhood acute lymphoblastic leukemia (ALL). **Breyanzi**™ (lisocabtagene maraleucel) and **Yescarta**™ (axicabtagene ciloleucel) were approved for mediastinal and follicular B-cell lymphoma. **Tecartus**™ (brexucabtagene auto-leucel) was approved for relapsed mantle cell lymphoma. **Abecma**™ (idecabtagene vicleucel) is a B-cell maturation antigen (BCMA) directed genetically modified autologous CAR T-cell FDA approved therapy for multiple myeloma.

Small-molecule drug conjugates (SMDCs) have been employed to bind to fluorescein isothiocyanate (FITC) in an effort to create a universal "adaptor molecule" (Liu et al., 2016) to adjust the degree of antitumor activity and provide control of cytokine release and tumor lysis, an "off switch" to stop excess activity, and eventually avoid the need to customize CAR T cells for each unique tumor antigen (Liu et al., 2016).

CAR-modified T cells (CARTs) have shown dramatic activity against leukemia and lymphoma.

CAR T-cell therapy can induce rapid and durable clinical responses but with unique acute toxicities as well, which can be severe or even fatal (Neelapu, 2019).

CRS, the most commonly observed toxicity, has a grading system to allow consistent reporting of the events (Lee et al., 2019):

Grade 1. Fever and constitutional symptoms

Grade 2. Hypotension responding to fluids and/or low-dose vasopressors, moderate organ toxicity

Grade 3. Shock requiring high-dose or multiple vasopressors, hypoxia requiring $\geq 40\%$ FiO_2

Grade 4. Mechanical ventilation or severe organ toxicity

High-dose steroids and tocilizumab, the humanized monoclonal antibody against IL-6R, have made an important difference in the management of CRS as well as growing recognition that severe COVID-19 symptoms can be similar to CRS and might be managed the same way (Fajgenbaum and June, 2020).

NEUROTOXICITY

CAR T-related encephalopathy syndrome (CRES) is the second most common adverse event. Intensive monitoring and prompt management of toxicities are essential. Several institutions have created multidiscipline management teams ("CARTOX") for monitoring, grading, and managing the acute toxicities that can occur in patients treated with CAR T-cell therapy (Neelapu et al., 2017).

When healthy tissues express the same target antigens as the tumor cells, outcomes similar to graft-versus-host disease (GVHD) can occur. One potential solution is to place a "suicide gene" (Casucci et al., 2015) into the modified T cells so that a way exists to trigger apoptosis of the activated CAR T cells. This method has been used safely and effectively in hematopoietic stem cell transplantation (HSCT). Adoption of suicide gene therapy to the clinical application of CART adoptive cell transfer has the potential to alleviate GVHD while improving overall antitumor efficacy (Jin et al., 2016). Rimiducid is a lipid-permeable tacrolimus analogue immune suppressant medication that activates Caspase-9 and has been developed to "kickstart" CAR T-cell suicide to mitigate immune toxicity (Zheng et al., 2021).

ANTIBODY DRUG CONJUGATES AND THE NEW WORLD OF DESIGNER ANTIBODIES

There has been a remarkable acceleration in the appearance of new agents made by deconstructing antibodies and merging them with toxins ("payloads") in an effort to increase immune killing of cancer cells. If an antibody can be visualized as a lobster with two claws, body, and a tail, there are novel drugs entering the clinic that have two different claws (bispecific antibodies such as ZW25 directed against HER2), three claws (trispecific drugs), four claws stuck together without any body or tail to get tumor cells to adhere to lymphocytes (bispecific T-cell engagers—"BITES").

ADCs are now produced by dozens of companies. There are at least 11 approved agents—especially for breast cancer. Trastuzumab emtansine has a HER2 target and a modified maytansine toxin. Sacituzumab govitecan targets the trophoblastic antigen TROP2 and has a topoisomerase inhibitor payload.

We now are benefiting from brilliant efforts to be more strategic and less toxic in the clinic. One such example is IL-15 (Figure 2.23), a more specific "cousin" of IL-2. IL-2 has produced some amazing responses in patients but is also associated with marked toxicity. The hope is that IL-15 can have more specific stimulation of NK and CD8 memory cells and produce benefit with less harm. Figure 2.23 shows a repertoire of IL-15 constructs that have been proposed as possible new weapons.

Figure 2.23

223

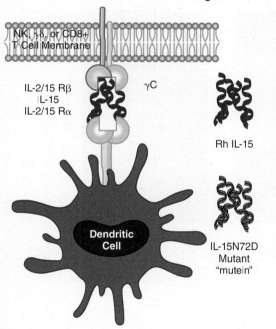

IL-15 Diagram

NK, γδ, or CD8+
T Cell Membrane

IL-2/15 Rβ
IL-15
IL-2/15 Rα

γC

Rh IL-15

**Dendritic
Cell**

IL-15N72D
Mutant
"mutein"

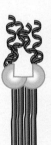

ALT-803
Scaffold
fused to four
single chains
of rituximab

Recombinant
humanized (Rh)IL-15
is produced in
Escherichia coli. IL-
15N72D is a mutant
protein ("mutein")
(asparagine replacing
aspartic residue).
ALT-803 is a fusion of
IL-15N72D plus four
single chains of
rituximab, the
monoclonal
antibody.

Immunology Timeline Legend

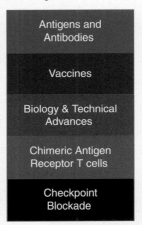

Innate and Adaptive Immunity

Tolerance and Surveillance

FDA Approvals & Milestones

Virology

Lymphocytes & Receptors

Cytokines & Signaling

Antigens and Antibodies

Vaccines

Biology & Technical Advances

Chimeric Antigen Receptor T cells

Checkpoint Blockade

Immunology Timeline I: Before 1980

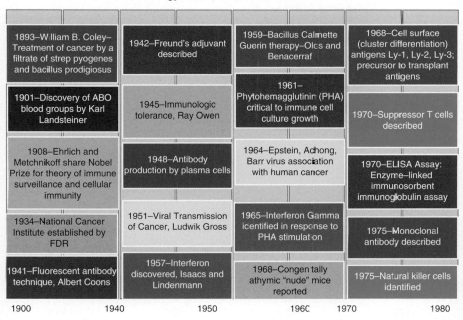

1893–William B. Coley–Treatment of cancer by a filtrate of strep pyogenes and bacillus prodigiosus

1901–Discovery of ABO blood groups by Karl Landsteiner

1908–Ehrlich and Metchnikoff share Nobel Prize for theory of immune surveillance and cellular immunity

1934–National Cancer Institute established by FDR

1941–Fluorescent antibody technique, Albert Coons

1942–Freund's adjuvant described

1945–Immunologic tolerance, Ray Owen

1948–Antibody production by plasma cells

1951–Viral Transmission of Cancer, Ludwik Gross

1957–Interferon discovered, Isaacs and Lindenmann

1959–Bacillus Calmette Guerin therapy–Olcs and Benacerraf

1961–Phytohemagglutinin (PHA) critical to immune cell culture growth

1964–Epstein, Achong, Barr virus association with human cancer

1965–Interferon Gamma identified in response to PHA stimulation

1968–Congenitally athymic "nude" mice reported

1968–Cell surface (cluster differentiation) antigens Ly-1, Ly-2, Ly-3; precursor to transplant antigens

1970–Suppressor T cells described

1970–ELISA Assay: Enzyme–linked immunosorbent immunoglobulin assay

1975–Monoclonal antibody described

1975–Natural killer cells identified

1900   1940   1950   1960   1970   1980

Immunology Timeline II: 1980–2000

1980	1985	1990	1995
1982–Alpha beta T-cell receptor (TCR) described	1987–MHC I HLA-A2 antigen complex presented simultaneously to T cells	1992–ISGF3 proteins define the STAT Family	1996–CTLA-4 antibody melanoma immunity
1983–Simian sarcoma virus sis oncogene encodes PDGF	1989–Hypothesis: Dendritic cells require pathogens for innate immunity	1993–Nuclear factor of activated T cells (NFAT), cyclosporin A and calcineurin, Fos-Jun complex	1996–Toll receptors mediate fungal immunity
1983–Identification of the TCR	1989–Interleukin-12 identified	1995–Natural killer T cells	1997–Tetramer technology monitors vaccine response
1983–Isolation of T-lymphotropic retrovirus (HIV)		1995–CpG oligo nucleotides are TLR9 agonists	1997–Dendritic cells are the link between innate and adaptive immunity
1985–DNA Polymerase Chain Reaction (PCR) developed	1987–Tum antigen, created by a point mutation, results in a protein recognized by CTLs	1995–CD4+CD25+ T regulatory cells IL-2R alpha chains, and autoimmunity	1997–Cancer stem cells
1986–Gamma delta T lymphocytes reported			1997–NY-ESO-1 antigen
	1988–Bcl-2/c-myc and B cell immortality	1996–AID mutator factor role in VJ gene somatic hyper-mutation (SHM)	1997–RANK Ligand a member of the TNF family
1986–Adenovirus E1A binds to RB tumor suppressor protein	1989–CD28 role in T cell co-stimulation	1996–CD4+ T cell tolerance in cancer	1998–Supramolecular activation clusters; the T cell, antigen presenting cell, MHC synapse

Immunology Timeline III: 2000–2015

1995	2000	2005	2015
1998–NF-kappa B/RelFamily	2002–Autologous tumor-derived heat shock protein gp96-peptide complex vaccine	2011–Hallmarks of Cancer add tumor immune evasion and role of inflammation in cancer development	2013–ICOS+ CD4 T cells biomarker for melanoma anti-CTLA-4 therapeutic response.
1998–BCL6 and SHM			
1998–Toll-like receptor (TLR) 4 microbe identification	2003–Indolamine 2,3-dioxygenase (IDO)	2011–CD8+ T cells engineered to recognize NY-ESO-1 antigen induce regressions in synovial sarcoma and melanoma	2013–SIRP alpha CD47 antagonist with tumor specific monoclonal antibodies induces macrophage activation as "one-two punch"
1999–Molecular classification of cancer	2003–E2A-factor binding sequence CAGGTG		
1999–PD-1 knockout autoimmunity	2004–Proteasome peptide splicing	2011–Chimeric anti-human CD30 for HD and anaplastic large cell lymphoma	2013–Incomplete Freund's vaccine adjuvant (Montanide)
	2005–Colon cancer T-cell infiltration		
1999–T-cell receptor (TCR) crystalline structure	2005–TCR signaling microclusters and supramolecular activation clusters	2011–Nobel Prize to Beutler, Hoffmann, and Steinman for innate immunology	2015–Unique tumor-associated macrophages (TAM) suppress infiltrating CTLs; their removal restores reactivity
2001–Crystalline structure of the CTLA-4/B7-1 complex	2004–Proteasome peptide splicing	2012–CD8+ T cells have a tolerance-specific gene profile suggesting epigenetic regulation	2015–Decitabine epigenetic potentiation of NY-ESO-1 ovarian cancer vaccine
2001–Tumor cells expressing NK receptor G2D lignad are destroyed by NK cells in vivo	2004–Proteasome peptide splicing		2015–Bispecific T cell engagers (BiTE) for B cell ALL
2001–Tumor related necrosis factor apoptosis-inducing ligand immune surveillance	2008–Chimeric Antigen Receptor T-cells for B cell lymphomas.	2013–Gut bacteria microenvironment modulation shape the anticancer immune response	2015–Oncolytic melanoma virus therapy approved

Immunology Timeline IV: 2016–2021

2016	2018	2019	2020	2021
2016. Obinutuzumab CD20 Ab for follicular lymphoma	2018. Brentuximab vedotin CD30 antibody-drug conjugate plus chemotherapy for Hodgkin lymphoma (CHL)	Drs. James Allison and Tasuku Honjo–Nobel Prize for Immune Therapy. Dec. 2018	2020. Gardasil 9 vaccine for HPV-related head and neck cancer prevention	2020. Pembrolizumab + chemotherapy triple negative breast cancer (TNBC) expressing PD-L1 (>10%)
2017. Pembrolizumab for solid tumors classified as MSI-hi (high microsatellite instability) or dMMR (deficient DNA mismatch repair)	2018. Blinatumomab bispecific CD19 T cell-engaging Ab for B-cell precursor acute lymphoblastic leukemia (ALL) and minimal residual disease (MRD)	2018. Pembrolizumab for Merkel cell carcinoma (MCC)	2020. Pembrolizumab for adult/pediatric mutational burden-high (TMB-H) solid tumors	2020. Naxitamab-gagk GD-2 antibody plus GM-CSF for neuroblastoma
2017. Tisagenlecleucel for B cell acute lymphoblastic leukemia (B-ALL)	2018. Tisagenlecleucel CD19 CAR T cell therapy for large B cell lymphoma	2019. Pexidartinib CSF-1Ri for tenosynovial giant cell tumor (TGCT)	2020. Pembrolizumab for microsatellite instability-high (MSI-H) or mismatch repair deficient (dMMR) colorectal cancer	2021. Dostarlimab-gxly for uterine cancer or other tumors with dMMR.
2017. Gemtuzumab ozogamicin anti-CD33 antibody-drug conjugate for adult and pediatric CD33-positive acute myeloid leukemia (AML)	2018. "Ipi-Nivo" for CRC with high microsatellite instability (MSI-hi) or deficient DNA mismatch repair (dMMR)	2019. Nivolumab (PD-1) and ipilimumab (CTLA-4i) for hepatocellular carcinoma (HCC)	2020. Brexucabtagene autoleucel CD19 CAR T cells for Mantle cell lymphoma	2021. Cemiplimab(PD-1) hedgehog inhib for basal cell cancer
2017. Axicabtagene ciloleucel CAR-T cell therapy for adult large B cell lymphoma	2018. Nivolumab for metastatic small cell lung cancer (SCLC)	2019. Durvalumab (PD-L1) extensive stage small cell lung cancer with standard chemotherapy	2020. Atezolizumab PD-L1 checkpoint inhibitor + cobimetinib + vemurafenib for BRAF V600 mutated melanoma	2021. Vicleucel anti-BCMA CAR T cell therapy for myeloma
2018. Durvalumab for stable treated unresectable, stage III non-small cell lung cancer (NSCLC)	2018. Cemiplimab (PD-1) for cutaneous squamous cell carcinoma (CSCC),	2019. Atezolizumab and bevacizumab for hepatocellular carcinoma	2020. Nivolumab and ipilimumab PD-1 and CTLA-4 inhibitors for malignant pleural mesothelioma	2021. Amivantamab-specific EGFR/MET antibody exon 20 mutated lung cancer
2016	**2018**	**2019**	**2020**	**2021**

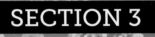

SECTION 3

Molecular Targets and Pathways

An Introduction to the Organization of Cancer Cell Signaling

It is hard to do justice to the exquisite complexity of the cancer cell and to help comprehend the level of intra- and intercell signaling that occurs in the billions of cells in the human body. We have attempted to create an "org chart" to help classify the targets and strategies used to develop precision cancer treatment. There are three broad categories:

A. **Membrane Factors and Receptors (M 1–7)**: Receptor Tyrosine Kinases (RTKs) for Survival Factors, Chemokines and Transmitters, and Growth Factors, the Extracellular Matrix, Fruit Fly Mutations, Death Receptors (DRs), and Cytokine Receptors

B. **Intracellular Systems (1–10)**: Rapamycin, NF-Kappa B, G-Coupled Proteins, Mitogen-Activated Protein (MAP) Kinase (MAPK), SRC, β-Catenin, Caspases, Janus Kinase/Signal Transducer and Transcription (JAK/STAT), and Apoptosis

C. **Nuclear Factors, Cell Cycle Control, and DNA Repair (N)**: MYC, Extracellular Signal–Regulated Kinase (ERK), Cyclins, Retinoblastoma (RB), MDM2, TP53

COLOR KEY

 Agonist

 Antagonist

Signal Transduction Roadmap

M1	Survival Factors/VEGF	C6	β-Catenin/APC
M2	Chemokines/Hormones	C7	Cell Regulators
M3	Growth Factors	C8	Caspases/BCL2
M4	Extracellular Matrix	C9	JAK/STAT
M5	Fruit Fly Receptors	C10	Apoptosis
M6	Death Receptors	N1	Extracell. Reg. Kinases
M7	Cytokines/Interleukins	N2	Cyclins
C1	Rapamycin/mTOR Sys	N3	Retinoblastoma/RB
C2	NF-Kappa B	N4	MYC
C3	G-Proteins/Cyclic AMP	N5	MDM2
C4	RAS→RAF→MAPKinase	N6	TP53/DNA Repair
C5	Sarcoma Gene—SRC	N7	Other Nuclear Factors

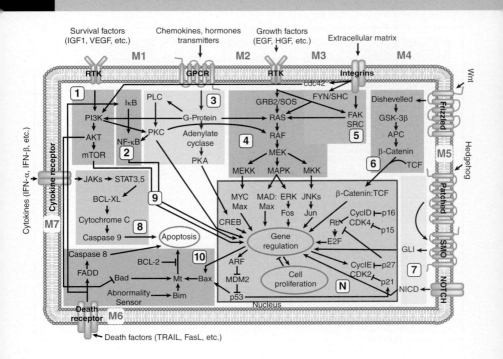

- Vascular endothelial growth factor (VEGF) is one of the most important and prominent proangiogenic factors. VEGF's normal function is to create new blood vessels during embryonic development, new blood vessels after injury, muscle following exercise, and new vessels (collateral circulation) to bypass blocked vessels.
- The VEGF family consists of five members (VEGF-A, -B, -C, -D, and placental growth factor [PlGF]), which transmit signals via three VEGF receptors (VEGFR-1 through VEGFR-3).
- Many human cancers are found to overexpress VEGFs and/or VEGFRs.
  - VEGFR-1 binding by VEGF-B plays a role in the maintenance of newly formed blood vessels.
  - VEGFR-2 activation by VEGF-A binding has been shown to stimulate endothelial cell (EC) mitogenesis and cell migration, leading to cancer progression and metastasis.
  - VEGFR-3 is predominantly expressed in lymphatic vessels. When bound by either VEGF-C or VEGF-D, VEGFR-3 plays a role in lymphangiogenesis and metastatic spread to lymph nodes in a pathologic setting.

Physiology	VEGF-A, -B, -C, -D and PlGF activate VEGFR-1, -2, -3 to promote vascularization
	• during embryogenesis • after injury • after vessel blockage • after exercise
Oncogenic VEGF, VEGFR behaviors	• Overexpressed in many cancers; expression associated with invasiveness, recurrence, prognosis • R2 activation by VEGF-A drives EC division and migration, and thus angiogenesis, cancer progression, metastasis. • R3 activation by VEGF-C, -D promotes metastasis to lymph nodes.

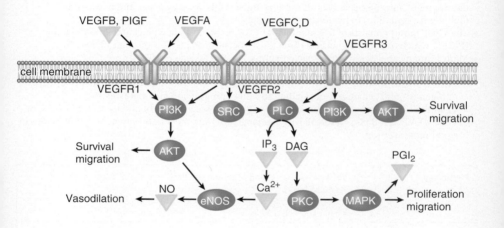

- Fibroblast growth factor receptor (FGFR) family has four highly conserved transmembrane RTKs (FGFR1–4) that differ in their ligand affinities and tissue distribution.
- Fibroblast growth factors (FGFs) include 18 structurally related polypeptides (FGF1–10, FGF16–23) that signal through FGFRs.
- FGFRs can bind canonical FGFs that are in complex with heparan sulfate proteoglycans (HSPGs) in an autocrine and paracrine fashion.
- FGFRs can also bind endocrine FGFs (FGF19, 21, and 23) that are found in circulation, free of HSPGs.
- Once bound to their ligands, FGFRs are induced to dimerize and cross-phosphorylate the tyrosine kinase domain on the cognate receptor.
- Various downstream effector molecules are then recruited, allowing for the activation of signaling events that culminate in regulation of various cellular processes such as cell survival and proliferation, organ development, angiogenesis, and tissue homeostasis, to name a few.
- Each FGFR can be activated by several FGFs; conversely, FGFs can activate more than one receptor.
- Dysregulation of FGFR signaling in cancer may be caused by the following:
  - *FGFR* gene amplifications, activating mutations, translocations, and fusions
  - Amplification of FGF and FGF-related genes
- Dysregulated FGFR signaling may contribute to cancer by the following:
  - Stimulating cancer cell proliferation
  - Driving tumor neovascularization
  - Promoting resistance to anticancer therapies

PHYSIOLOGY

- FGF1–10, FGF16–23 regulate essential cellular processes via FGFR1–4.
- Canonical FGFs elicit paracrine and autocrine effects.
- Others (FGF19, 21, 23) elicit endocrine effects.
- An FGF can trigger multiple FGFRs; an FGFR may engage several FGFs.
- Dysregulated signaling may promote cancer cell proliferation, tumor vascularization, and drug resistance.

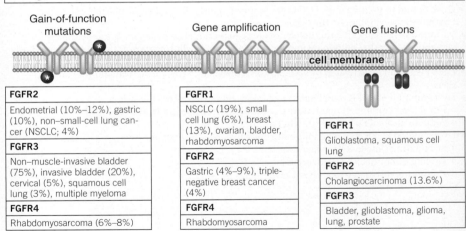

FGFR2
Endometrial (10%–12%), gastric (10%), non–small-cell lung cancer (NSCLC; 4%)

FGFR3
Non–muscle-invasive bladder (75%), invasive bladder (20%), cervical (5%), squamous cell lung (3%), multiple myeloma

FGFR4
Rhabdomyosarcoma (6%–8%)

FGFR1
NSCLC (19%), small cell lung (6%), breast (13%), ovarian, bladder, rhabdomyosarcoma

FGFR2
Gastric (4%–9%), triple-negative breast cancer (4%)

FGFR4
Rhabdomyosarcoma

FGFR1
Glioblastoma, squamous cell lung

FGFR2
Cholangiocarcinoma (13.6%)

FGFR3
Bladder, glioblastoma, glioma, lung, prostate

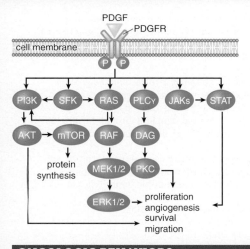

PHYSIOLOGY

- Platelet-derived growth factor (PDGF) A–D are potent mitogens for cells of mesenchymal origin.
- Synthesized, stored, and released by platelets upon activation
- Also produced by smooth muscle cells, activated macrophages, and ECs
- Essential in early development, tissue remodeling, differentiation
- Downstream effector pathways (MAPK, phosphatidylinositol 3-kinase [PI3K], and/or JAK/STAT) are triggered via PDGF receptor (PDGFR)A, B.

ONCOLOGIC BEHAVIORS

- *COL1A1–PDGFB* fusion linked to dermatofibrosarcoma protuberans
- PDGFRA mutations linked to multiple tumor types; germline lesions linked to hereditary gastrointestinal stromal tumors (GIST)
- *PDGFRA* amplification often associated with coalterations in epidermal growth factor receptor (*EGFR*), *KIT*, *KDR*
- Up to 60% of PDGFRA mutant GIST are also D842V, which is associated with primary resistance.

- PDGFs are potent mitogens for cells of mesenchymal origin and are synthesized, stored, and released by platelets upon activation; also produced by smooth muscle cells, activated macrophages, and ECs.
- PDGF signaling network consists of four ligands (PDGFA–D) and two transmembrane tyrosine RTKs (PDGFRα and PDGFRβ).
- These receptors transmit extracellular growth factor signaling to intracellular signaling cascades. Upon binding of the growth factor ligands, the receptors undergo dimerization and autophosphorylation of cytoplasmic kinase domains, activating the receptor.
- Downstream effects of PDGFR activation lead to differential signaling through MAPK, PI3K, and/or JAK/STAT pathways, resulting in cell proliferation, cell differentiation, survival, and migration.
- Dermatofibrosarcoma protuberans is characterized by a chromosomal translocation with formation of COL1A1–PDGFB fusion gene, causing activation of PDGFRβ in tumor cells.
- PDGFRα is encoded by the *PDGFRA* gene, which is altered in multiple tumor types, resulting in constitutive PDGFRα activity.
- Germline mutations in PDGFRA have been described in hereditary GIST.
- PDGFRA amplification has been described in sarcomas and gliomas; however, often it is associated with coalterations in EGFR, KIT, and KDR.
- In about 5% of GIST, somatic PDGFRA mutations in exons 12, 14, and 18 activation loop are the most common and are associated with greater response to PDGFRA-inhibitor imatinib. However, up to 60% of PDGFRA mutant GIST harbors a mutation in exon 18 D842V, which is associated with primary resistance.

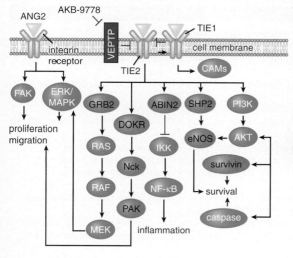

PHYSIOLOGY

- Angiopoietin growth factors (ANG) regulate angiogenesis through activating (ANG1,4) or inhibitory (ANG2,3) effects on TIE1,2.
- ANG-TIE system is critical for cardiac, blood, vascular development and homeostasis.

ASSOCIATED PATHOLOGIC STATES

- inflammation
- metastasis
- tumor angiogenesis
- atherosclerosis
- vascular leakage

ONCOGENIC BEHAVIORS

- Circulating ANG2 predictive of poor prognosis from many cancers
- Low baseline ANG2 predicts better response to anti-VEGF therapy versus colorectal cancer.
- High baseline serum ANG2 predicts poorer outcome from immune checkpoint therapy; potentially immunosuppressive.
- ANG bind to cell surface RTKs with immunoglobulin-like and epithelial growth factor–like domains 1 and 2 (TIE1 and TIE2).
- Four different ANGs have been identified (ANG1, ANG2, ANG3, and ANG4).
- ANG1 and ANG4 are agonists for TIE2, whereas ANG2 and ANG3 are competitive antagonists for TIE1 and TIE2.
- Activation of TIE2 by ANG1 is indispensable for embryonic cardiac development and angiogenesis, and both TIE1 and TIE2 are key regulators of normal formation of blood and lymphatic vessel development as TIE1 and TIE2 are almost exclusively expressed in the endothelium.
- ANG/TIE system is also involved in pathologic processes including inflammation, metastasis, tumor angiogenesis, atherosclerosis, and vascular leakage.
- Upon binding of ANG ligands, TIE2 receptors can form dimers or possibly multimers. Vascular endothelial protein tyrosine phosphatase (VEPTP, encoded by *PTPRB* gene) dephosphorylates active TIE2.
- TIE1 upregulates the cell adhesion molecules (CAMs) VCAM-1, E-selectin, and ICAM-1 through a p38-dependent mechanism.

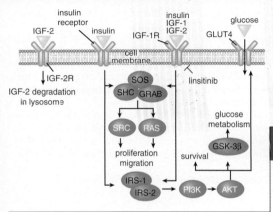

PHYSIOLOGY

- Insulin is a key metabolic regulator and growth factor.
- IGF-*1,2* are structurally similar to insulin.
- IGF-*1R* drives growth.
- IGF-*2R* depletes IGF-2 by endocytosis.

NOTABLE BEHAVIORS IN CANCER

- Hyperinsulinemia due to obesity, diabetes, metabolic syndrome, etc., increases risk of and mortality from cancer
- Glucose transporter (GLUT)4 is overexpressed in pancreatic cancers, possibly linked to castration-resistant phenotype.
- IGF-1R is overexpressed in some cancers, possibly to increase glucose uptake via insulin receptor substrate (IRS)-1-dependent membrane translocation of GLUT.
- IGF levels are prognostic in NSCLC and sarcoma.
- IGF-1R promotes resistance to EGFR drugs by dimerizing with EGFR.
- IGF-1R drugs have limited clinical activity, significant adverse effects, for example, hyperglycemia.

- Insulin-like growth factor family includes two growth factors (IGF-1, IGF-2) and two receptors (IGF-1R, IGF-2R).
- IGF-1 and IGF-2 are polypeptide hormones structurally similar to insulin. IGF-IR, IGF-2R, and insulin receptors are also structurally similar and are able to form heterodimers.
- IGF-1R is activated by IGF-1, IGF-2, and insulin and has a strong growth-promoting effect.
- IGF-2R does not trigger signaling, but regulates extracellular IRS-2 levels through receptor-mediated endocytosis and degradation. Upon phosphorylation, IGF-1R recruits and phosphorylates adaptor proteins IRS-1, IRS-2, and SRC homology 2 domain-containing protein (SHC).
- IRS-1 acts as a second messenger within cell to stimulate transcription of insulin-related genes (e.g., ELK1, glycogen synthase-3 [GSK3]) via PI3K and RAS pathways and also initiates the translocation of GLUT to the cell surface where it facilitates transport of glucose into the cell.
- IRS-2 plays a critical role in cellular motility response, and SHC stimulates activation of MAPK pathway.
- Compared with normal cells, cancer cells have an increased need for glucose, which alters cellular metabolism (i.e., Warburg effect).

- Increased levels of IGF-1R are expressed in certain types of cancer cells (e.g., prostate, pancreatic), which can lead to increased uptake of glucose from blood into tumor. However, IGF-1R expression does not consistently correlate with disease control in heterogeneous groups of patients treated with anti-IGF-1R monoclonal antibodies (mAbs).
- IGF ligand (IGF-1) levels have been shown to have predictive value in NSCLC and sarcoma, but correlation between ligand level and tumor microenvironment has not been established.
- In the presence of epidermal growth factor (EGF) inhibitors, IGF-1R can dimerize with EGFR, allowing pathway signaling to resume, leading to resistance of these inhibitors.
- Although there is compelling preclinical evidence, only limited clinical activity of IGF-1R inhibition has been observed in several tumor types, including NSCLC and breast cancer. More favorable outcomes were observed in patients with sarcoma.
- Furthermore, common adverse effects of IGF-1R inhibition that include hyperglycemia (pituitary feedback loop), nausea, vomiting, fatigue, anorexia, and skin reactions have limited the U.S. Food and Drug Administration (FDA) approval of any IGF-1R pathway inhibitors so far.

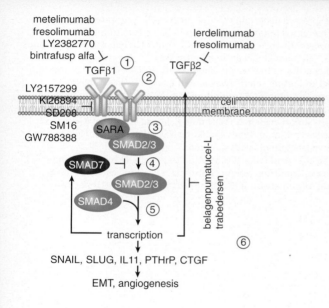

CLASSICAL SIGNALING

1. Activation of transforming growth factor-beta (TGFβ) receptors
2. Oligomerization
3. Phosphorylation of SMAD2/3
4. Translocation of SMADs to nucleus
5. Expression of target genes, for example, cyclin-dependent kinase (CDK) inhibitors
6. Physiologic response, for example, cytoskeletal rearrangement, remodeling of extracellular matrix

NOTABLE BEHAVIORS IN CANCER

- TGFβ is upregulated in some cancers with programmed cell death ligand 1 (PD-L1), inhibits anticancer immunity, and contributes to poor prognosis.
- SMAD4 deletion is common in pancreatic cancers, inactivating mutations in liver, colorectal cancer.
- Germline SMAD4 lesion is linked to hereditary juvenile polyposis.
- TGFβ induces tumor cell migration and boosts epithelial to mesenchymal transition.
- TGFβ is a powerful suppressor of innate and adaptive immunity, promoting immune surveillance by tumor cells.

- TGFβ signaling pathway plays a critical role in cell growth, differentiation, and development. TGFβ stimulates proliferation of mesenchymal cells, but inhibits proliferation of epithelial cells.
- In cancer, TGFβ inhibits immune response against cancer, while stimulating stromal cells to proliferate.
- Signaling is initiated by interaction of the ligand with the receptor and oligomerization of serine/threonine TGFβ receptor kinases and phosphorylation of the cytoplasmic signaling molecules SMAD2 and SMAD3.
- SMAD transcription factors are phosphorylated and translocated to nucleus where they stimulate expression of genes encoding CDK inhibitors or proteins involved in the formation and remodeling of extracellular matrix.
- Activation of pathway is counteracted by inhibitory SMADs (e.g., SMAD7), which are encoded by gene induced by pathway stimulation (feedback mechanism).
- TGFβ/activin and bone morphogenetic protein (BMP) pathways are modulated by MAPK signaling at a number of levels. Moreover, in certain contexts, TGFβ signaling can also affect

SMAD-independent pathways, including ERK, stress-activated protein kinase/c-Jun NH2-terminal kinase (SAPK/JNK), and p38 MAPK pathways.

- Rho GTPase (RhoA) activates downstream target proteins to prompt rearrangement of the cytoskeletal elements associated with cell growth, migration, and invasion.
- A germline mutation in SMAD4 is known to be associated with hereditary juvenile polyposis syndrome.
- Targeting TGFβ can be done by different drugs that include antisense oligonucleotides (AONs), neutralizing antibodies that inhibit ligand–receptor interactions, receptor domain–immunoglobulin fusions that sequester ligands and prevent binding to receptors, and receptor kinase inhibitors.
  - AONs (target TGFβ2): trabedersen (AP12009) and antisense gene-modified allogenic tumor vaccine: Belagenpumatucel-L (Lucanix) are currently in clinical trials.
  - Antibodies: Fresolimumab (GC-1008)—binds TGFβ1 and TGFβ2; IMC-TR1—targets TβRII
  - TGFβ kinase inhibitors/small-molecule inhibitors: LY2157299 (galunisertib); TEW-7197
- Although TGFβ targeting agents, such as galunisertib, have shown dramatic therapeutic effects in animal cancer models and in some cancer patients, it is still not clear how the therapeutic effect in cancer patients is achieved; currently, there is no predictive biomarker for response to drugs targeting the TGFβ pathway.
- TGFβ and PD-L1 are both upregulated in certain types of cancers, and their overexpression is associated with increased evasion of immune surveillance and contributes to poor prognosis.
- Bintrafusp alfa, a bifunctional fusion protein composed of avelumab, an anti-PD-L1 human mAb, bound to the soluble extracellular domain of TGFβRII, has shown to increase natural killer (NK) cell and cytotoxic T-lymphocyte (CTL) activities inhibiting tumor cell proliferation; it is currently being tested in clinical trials.

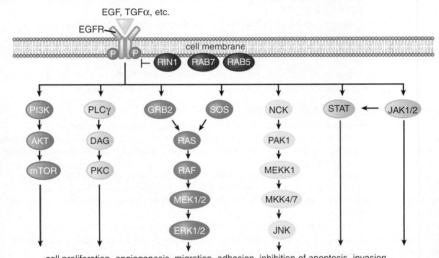

EGF, TGFα, etc.

EGFR

cell membrane

RIN1 RAB7 RAB5

| PI3K | PLCγ | GRB2 SOS | NCK | STAT ← JAK1/2 |

PI3K → AKT → mTOR

PLCγ → DAG → PKC

GRB2, SOS → RAS → RAF → MEK1/2 → ERK1/2

NCK → PAK1 → MEKK1 → MKK4/7 → JNK

cell proliferation, angiogenesis, migration, adhesion, inhibition of apoptosis, invasion

PHYSIOLOGY
- **Family consists of EGFR (ERBB1), HER2 (ERBB2), HER3 (ERBB3), HER4 (ERBB4).**
- **EGFR, HER2, HER4 are active kinases.**

EGF FAMILY OF RECEPTORS

- The EGF family of receptors are transmembrane RTKs that are frequently overexpressed or mutated in a wide variety of epithelial tumors.
- The EGF or ERBB family consists of EGFR (ERBB1), HER2 (ERBB2), HER3 (ERBB3), and HER4 (ERBB4).
- They are characterized by an extracellular ligand-binding domain and an intracellular tyrosine kinase domain except ERBB3, which has a kinase-deficient intracellular domain.

ACTIVATION OF THE RECEPTORS

- The EGF family of receptors is activated by binding to a ligand resulting in homo- or heterodimerization of the receptors and phosphorylation of the receptors at the cytosolic kinase domain. This results in the recruitment of adapter molecules, leading to activation of signaling pathway cascades downstream.
- One of the well-studied pathways acts through the RAS → rapidly accelerated fibrosarcoma (RAF) → ERK cascade. The other major pathway involves the lipid kinase PI3K, AKT, and mammalian target of rapamycin (mTOR). The activation of these pathways leads to cell growth, proliferation, differentiation, and migration.
- The receptor is trafficked through the early and late endosomes and lysosomes, where it is degraded by proteases. This regulation mechanism driven by RAB5, RIN1, and RAB7 ensures downregulation of receptor signaling when not required.

LIGANDS

- EGFR (ERBB1) has seven known ligands: EGF, TGFα, heparin-binding EGF-like growth factor (HBEGF), amphiregulin (AREG), β-cellulin (BTC), epiregulin (EREG), and epigen (EPGN). EGF and TGFα are the most common and most characterized.

- Interestingly, ERBB2 (HER2) does not have a ligand. ERBB2 can heterodimerize with EGFR, ERBB3, and ERBB4, functioning through activation of other receptor family members.
- Neuregulin 1 and 2 bind ERBB3 to activate it, whereas EGF, BTC, and neuregulins (1–4) bind ERBB4.

EGFR SIGNALING IN CANCER

- Dysregulation of EGFR signaling is seen in cancer.
- EGFR kinase domain mutations are commonly seen in lung cancer. These result in constitutive activation of the EGF receptor.
- EGFR overexpression is commonly seen in head and neck squamous cell carcinoma (80%–90%), NSCLC (~60%), triple-negative breast cancer (~60%), colon cancer (>90%), and glioblastoma (~50%). EGFR overexpression can occur by increase in copy number or increase in protein expression.
- Other mechanisms of signaling dysregulation include defective downregulation of the receptor (caused by CBL mutations and seen in EGFRvIII) and cross-talk with other receptors (such as other ERBB family members and G-protein-coupled receptors or GPCRs).

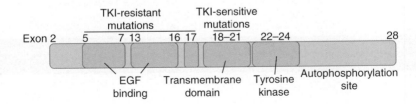

Notable behaviors in cancer	• Overexpressed in head and neck squamous cell carcinoma (80%–90%), NSCLC (~60%), triple-negative breast cancer (~60%), colon cancer (>90%), and glioblastoma (~50%). • Constitutively active mutants common in lung cancer • Normal switch-off mechanisms may be lost • May cross-talk with other receptors	
EGFR-activating mutations	• L858R on exon 21 • in-frame deletion in exon 19	• Account for 90% of activating mutations
	• L861Q (exon 21) • G719X (exon 18) • V765A, T783A (exon 20) • Some in-frame deletion/insertion on exon 20 • T790M: most common lesion that confers resistance to EGFR drugs	
EGFR VIII	• Truncated form after deletion of exons 2–7 by gene rearrangement • Unable to bind ligand, but is constitutively active because of interaction with wild-type EGFR and loss of downregulation mechanism • Preferentially triggers PI3K/AKT, whereas other mutants activate MAPK	

Activating mutations, except exon 20 insertions, hypersensitize cells to EGFR inhibitors. Exon 20 mutations contribute to resistance to EGFR inhibitors.

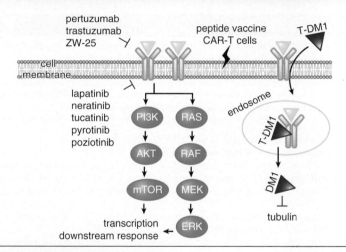

NOTABLE BEHAVIORS IN CANCER

- Overexpression, rather than simple activation, is required for tumorigenic activity.
- Overexpression may alter the repertoire of HER2-containing dimers, resulting in altered signaling.
- Overexpression deregulates cell cycle, polarity, and adhesion.
- Overexpression elicits oncogene addiction, the basis of drug activity.

LESIONS IN CANCER

- Overexpressed/amplified in breast (~30% of tumors), esophageal (~17%), lung (~3%), ovarian (~2%–66%), colorectal (~3%), prostate, salivary gland, bladder cancer
- In-frame A775_G776insYVMA in exon 20 seen in NSCLC
- Activating missense mutations in kinase domain seen in breast, lung, colorectal cancers
- Activating mutations in extracellular domain, for example, S310Y and S310F, are seen in ~1%–2% lung and breast cancers, some colorectal and ovarian cancers.

- HER2 (ERBB2) is the second member of the EGFR family of receptors.
- HER2 heterodimerizes with EGFR as well as ERBB3.
- ERBB2/HER2 is often overexpressed/amplified in various cancer types such as breast (~30% of tumors), esophageal (~17% of tumors), lung (~3%), ovarian (~2%–66%), colorectal cancer (~3%). Amplification is also seen in prostate cancer, salivary gland tumors, and bladder cancers.
- *ERBB2* gene mutations are drivers of several cancer types. In NSCLC, ERBB2 exon 20 in-frame insertion/duplication A775_G776insYVMA is the most prevalent.
- Missense activating mutations in tyrosine kinase domains are seen in breast, lung, and colorectal cancers predominantly.
- Extracellular domain mutations causing enhanced kinase activity such as ERBB2 S310Y and ERBB2 S310F are seen in ~1% to 2% lung and breast cancers, and also a small proportion of colorectal and ovarian cancers.

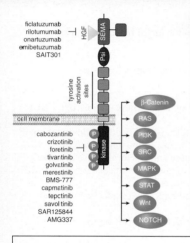

NOTABLE BEHAVIORS IN CANCER

- Deregulation linked to tumor growth, metastasis, poor prognosis
- Hepatocyte growth factor (HGF) lesions linked to kidney, liver, gastric, esophageal, breast, brain, and melanoma
- Cancer stem cells seem to reacquire MET expression, which is normally exclusive to stem and progenitor cells.
- MET activation synergizes with INK4a/ alternate reading frame (ARF) inactivation in rhabdomyosarcoma.
- MET amplification and exon 14 skipping drive NSCLC progression and resistance to EGFR drugs.
- MET amplification linked to aggressive gastric cancer and poor outcome
- Tumor HGF secretion drives MET expression in melanoma.

- Constitutive activation of the HGF promoter is observed in 51% of African-Americans with breast cancer.
- Circulating HGF levels correlated with poorer survival and are potential markers for both presence of cancer and disease stage.

NORMAL BIOLOGY

- c-MET is a proto-oncogene that encodes for hepatocyte growth factor receptor, also known as MET (HGFR), possessing tyrosine kinase activity.
- HGF is the only known ligand of the MET receptor.
- MET induces several biologic responses that collectively give rise to invasive growth.

ROLE IN CANCER

- Abnormal MET activation in cancer correlates with poor prognosis, where uncontrolled MET triggers tumor growth, angiogenesis, and metastasis.
- MET deregulation (MET and HGF amplifications, MET mutations) has been implicated in many types of cancer, including kidney, liver, gastric, esophageal, breast, brain, and melanoma.
- Usually, only stem cells and progenitor cells express MET, which allows for invasive growth; however, cancer stem cells are thought to hijack the ability of normal stem cells to express MET and thus become the cause of cancer persistence and metastasis.
- MET activates multiple signal transduction pathways, including RAS, PI3K, STAT, Wnt, and NOTCH.
- Inactivation of tumor suppressors INK4a/ARF synergizes with MET activation in rhabdomyosarcoma.
- MET expression is driven by HGF secretions in the tumor cell microenvironment in melanoma.
- In NSCLC, c-MET amplification and exon 14 skipping drive progression and resistance to EGFR inhibitors. In gastric cancers, amplification is associated with aggressive disease and poor outcomes.

Physiology	• Receptor for glial cell line–derived neurotropic factors (GDNF) • Activates MAPK and PI3K pathways similar to EGFR.
Notable behaviors in cancer	• Point mutations drive multiple endocrine neoplasia syndromes (MEN2) and familial medullary thyroid cancer. • Fusion with other proteins may cause constitutive activation, potentially via dimerization. • Fusions associated with radiation exposure, seen in NSCLC, Spitz tumors, breast, colon cancers, ~1/3 of papillary thyroid cancers • Fusion partners include KIF5B, CCDC6, GOLGA5, TRIM24, TRIM27, TRIM33, PRKAR1A, MBD1, KTN1, HOOK3, AKAP13, FKBP15, SPECC1L, ERC1, NCOA4, TBL1XR1, RAB6IP2

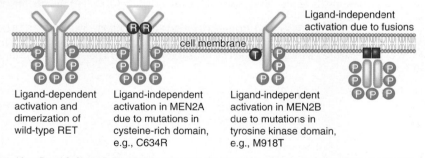

Ligand-dependent activation and dimerization of wild-type RET

Ligand-independent activation in MEN2A due to mutations in cysteine-rich domain, e.g., C634R

Ligand-independent activation in MEN2B due to mutations in tyrosine kinase domain, e.g., M918T

Ligand-independent activation due to fusions

(Adapted from Romei C, Ciampi R, Elisei R. A comprehensive overview of the role of the RET proto-oncogene in thyroid carcinoma. *Nat Rev Endocrinol*. 2016;12(4):192–202.)

- REarranged during Transfection (RET) receptor can activate MAPK and PI3K pathways similar to EGFR.
- RET is a receptor for the GDNF family of extracellular ligands.

ROLE IN CANCER

- Point mutations in RET give rise to MEN2 and familial medullary thyroid cancer.
- Chromosomal rearrangements that create a fusion between RET and other proteins can cause constitutive activation of RET receptor.
- Fusions of RET with other genes have been identified in multiple malignancies.
  - Found in approximately one-third of patients with papillary thyroid cancer. Associated with radiation exposure.
  - RET fusions have also been identified as an oncogenic driver in NSCLC, Spitz tumors, breast, and colon cancers.
  - RET fusion partners include KIF5B, CCDC6, GOLGA5, TRIM24, TRIM27, TRIM33, PRKAR1A, MBD1, KTN1, HOOK3, AKAP13, FKBP15, SPECC1L, ERC1, NCOA4, TBL1XR1, and RAB6IP2. Many of these partners have dimerization motifs, suggesting this as a possible mechanism for RET activation.

Physiology	• Also known as CD246; receptor for insulin • Expressed in brain, testis, small intestine; enhanced expression in developing nervous system; lower expression in adults
Notable behaviors in cancer	• Overactivated following fusion with other genes, typically via constitutive dimerization • Amplification and gene deletions seen in several malignancies, e.g., in 13 of 15 specimens of inflammatory breast cancer • Nonfusion lesions of unknown significance, although mutation and overexpression seen in 40%–100% of neuroblastomas

NOTABLE FUSIONS

Physiology	Partners	Prev. (%)
Lymphoma	NPM, TPM3, TPM4	60
NSCLC	EML4, K1F5B	5
Colorectal	EML4	2
Breast	EML4	2
Renal	EML4, TPM3	2

• **NPM binds ss- and dsDNA; drives DNA repair, stabilizes genome**
• **TPM3 drives muscle contraction**
• **EML4 modifies microtubules**
• **K1F5B required to distribute mitochondria, lysosomes**

ROLE IN CANCER

- Observed mechanisms of oncogenesis involve overactivation of the ALK receptor through fusion gene formation. The most common is the EML4–ALK fusion, occurring in 2% to 7% of NSCLCs.
- ALK fusions were first discovered in lymphoma. In solid tumors, they are found most commonly in lung adenocarcinoma, but have been identified in Spitz tumors, sarcoma, melanoma, breast, colorectal, esophageal, cholangiocarcinoma, thyroid, neuroblastoma, renal cell, renal medullary, and bladder cancers.
- Fusion partner usually has a domain that induces constitutive dimerization with resultant activation.
- In NSCLC, patients with ALK fusions are usually young with minimal or no smoking history.
- ALK amplifications and gene deletions have been identified in several malignancies. At this time, the significance of nonfusion alterations is unclear.
- Crizotinib was the first-generation ALK inhibitor; second-generation inhibitors include ceritinib, alectinib, and brigatinib; lorlatinib is a third-generation inhibitor.

Physiology	• Regulates cell survival, proliferation, differentiation • Expressed as multiple transcript variants encoding isoforms • Strongly expressed by hematopoietic stem cells, multipotent progenitors, common myeloid progenitors, early thymocyte progenitors; lower levels of expression in common lymphoid progenitors, mast cells, melanocytes, interstitial cells of Cajal in digestive tract
Lesions in Cancer	• Activating mutations linked to GIST, testicular seminoma, mast cell disease, melanoma, acute myeloid leukemia • Primary mutations in exon 11 and 9 linked to sensitivity and intrinsic resistance to imatinib, respectively • Secondary mutations in kinase domain (exons 13–18) linked to acquired resistance to imatinib

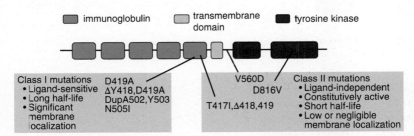

(Adapted from Shi X, Sousa LP, Mandel-Bausch EM, Tome F, Reshetnyak AV, Hadari Y, Schlessinger J, Lax I. Distinct cellular properties of oncogenic KIT receptor tyrosine kinase mutants enable alternative courses of cancer cell inhibition. *Proc Natl Acad Sci U S A*. 2016;113(33):E4784–E4793.)

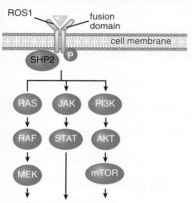

ROS1 / fusion domain
cell membrane
SHP2 / P

RAS → RAF → MEK

JAK → STAT

PI3K → AKT → mTOR

proliferation, transformation, survival

Physiology

- Structurally similar to ALK, but activated by unknown ligand
- Function also unknown, but contains extracellular sequences analogous to cell adhesion proteins, triggers typical RTK pathways
- In normal adults, expression is highest in the kidney, with some expression in stomach, intestines, neural tissue.

Lesions in Cancer

- Fusion with various partners enhances oncogenesis.
- ROS-1 rearrangement relatively rare, seen only in the absence of other known oncogenic driver mutations
- ROS-1 mutation seen in ~2% of NSCLCs

Fusion partners

TPM3	CD74	KDELR2
CEP85L	TFG	ZER
CCDC6	FIG	YWHAE
SLC34A2	SDC4	LRIG3

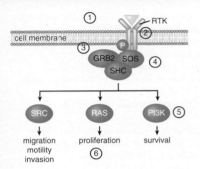

Signaling

1. Activation by growth factors
2. Homo- or heterodimerization
3. Autophosphorylation
4. Recruitment of adaptor proteins
5. Activation of downstream pathways
6. Physiologic response

Oncogenic Mechanisms

- Activating gain-of-function mutations
- Overexpression because of genomic amplification

SRC → migration motility invasion

RAS → proliferation

PI3K → survival

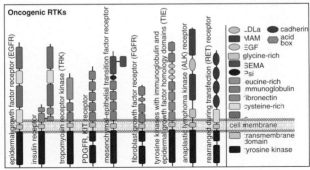

Oncogenic RTKs

- epidermal growth factor receptor (EGFR)
- insulin receptor
- tropomyosin receptor kinase (TRK)
- PDGFR, KIT receptor
- mesenchymal-epithelial transition factor receptor
- fibroblast growth factor receptor (FGFR)
- tyrosine kinases with immunoglobulin and epidermal growth factor homology domains (TIE)
- anaplastic lymphoma kinase (ALK) receptor
- rearranged during transfection (RET) receptor

Legend:
- LDLa
- MAM
- EGF
- glycine-rich
- SEMA
- Psi
- leucine-rich
- immunoglobulin
- fibronectin
- cysteine-rich
- cadherin
- acid box
- cell membrane
- transmembrane domain
- tyrosine kinase

- RTKs are cell surface receptors that function as key regulators of fundamental cellular processes such as proliferation, differentiation, senescence, and migration, among others.
- Binding growth factor ligands to extracellular domain, RTKs induce receptor dimerization (forming either homodimers or heterodimers with other RTKs) followed by their autophosphorylation. This allows for subsequent recruitment of adaptor proteins such as growth factor receptor–bound protein 2 (GRB2), SHC, and Son of Sevenless (SOS) that activate proliferation, survival, and migration pathways (e.g., RAS, PI3K, SRC).
- Tight control of RTK activation is necessary for tissue homeostasis, which is why RTKs constitute one of the biggest classes of oncoproteins.
- Over 20 different classes of RTKs have been identified, including the following that have been previously implicated in cancer initiation and progression: ALK, EGFR, FGFR, IGFR, KIT, MET, PDGFR, RET, TIE, and VEGFR. Each RTK will be discussed in detail in this section.

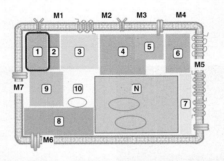

Rapamycin is a naturally occurring "antibiotic" discovered on the Pacific island of Rapa Nui (Easter Island) in the 1970s. This "family" consists of the mTOR complex, PI3K, AKT, phosphatase and tensin homolog (PTEN) and is an important key regulator of the immune system, glucose metabolism, and cell growth.

PI3K activation leads to phosphorylation and activation of AKT, which in turn can activate mTOR. The pathway can be suppressed by tuberous sclerosis (TSC1; hamartin), TSC2 (tuberin), and phosphatidylinositol-3,4,5-trisphosphate 3-phosphatase (PTEN). PI3Ks are divided into three classes according to structural characteristics and substrate specificity. This pathway interacts with IRS to regulate glucose uptake through a series of phosphorylation events. Hyperglycemia and sore mouth are common but manageable side effects in patients taking PI3K inhibitors.

Easter Island is a triangular-shaped Chilean territory in the Pacific Ocean and is known for the remarkable stone head sculptures.

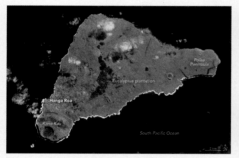

(NASA Earth Observatory image by Jesse Allen, using Landsat data from the U.S. Geological Survey. Available at https://earthobservatory.nasa.gov/images/90027/easter-island)

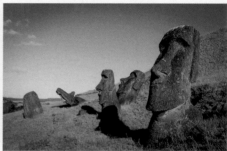

(From Shutterstock.)

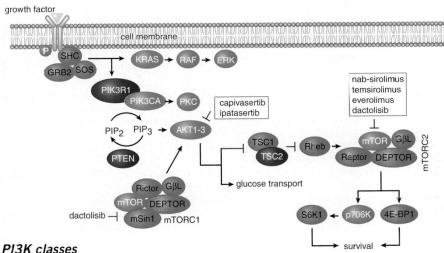

PI3K classes

Class IA	Catalytic	PIK3CA,B,D
	Regulatory	PI3KR1,2,3
Class II	Catalytic	PIK3C2A,2B,2G

Class IB	Catalytic	PIK3CG
	Regulatory	PI3KR5
Class III	Catalytic	PIK3C3

- PI3K/protein kinase B (PKB or AKT)/mTOR pathway is a key regulator of normal cellular processes. Aberrant activation of this pathway leads to survival and proliferation of tumor cells.
- PI3K activation leads to phosphorylation and activation of AKT, which in turn can activate mTOR. The pathway can be suppressed by TSC1 (hamartin), TSC2 (tuberin), and PTEN.
- PI3Ks are divided into three classes according to structural characteristics and substrate specificity:
  - Class I
    - Class IA PI3Ks: heterodimers consisting of a p110 catalytic subunit (isoforms p110α, p110β, and p110δ encoded by the genes *PIK3CA*, *PIK3CB*, and *PIK3CD*, respectively) and a p85 regulatory subunit (isoforms p85α [and slice variants p55α and p50α] encoded by PIK3R1, p85β encoded by PIK3R2, and p85γ encoded by PIK3R3)
    - Class IB PI3Ks: heterodimers consisting of a p110γ (encoded by PIK3CG) and a p101 regulatory subunit (encoded by PIK3R5)
  - Class II: monomers with a single catalytic subunit (isoforms PI3KC2α, PI3KC2β, and PI3KC2γ encoded by PIK3C2A, PIK3C2B, and PIK3C2G, respectively)
  - Class III: single catalytic subunit VPS34 (encoded by *PIK3C3* gene)
- This pathway interacts with the IRS to regulate glucose uptake through a series of phosphorylation events. A common side effect in patients taking PI3Ks inhibitors is hyperglycemia.

Molecule	Notable Behaviors in Cancer
PIK3CA	Activating missense mutations occur throughout, with most in hotspots, e.g., E542K, E545K in exon 9; H1047R in exon 20
PIK3R1	• Substitutions, in-frame insertions, deletions in iSH2 domain that impair inhibitory activity against catalytic subunit • Somatic mutations prevalent in endometrial, glioma, colon cancer • Suppressed in some cancers
PIK3CB	Seen in breast and castration-resistant prostate cancer
PIK3CD PIK3CG	Typically not mutated, but amplified or overexpressed
PIK3R2	• Somatic mutations in endometrial, colorectal cancer, but no hotspot • Overexpression in breast, colon cancer
PIK3C2B	• Like PIK3C2A, expressed in tumor cells • Mutations seen in NSCLC • Amplification in glioblastoma
AKT1	• E17K in melanoma, breast, colorectal, endometrial, ovarian, squamous cell lung cancer; amplification in gastric cancer
AKT2	• Mutations in colorectal cancer; amplification in head and neck, pancreatic, ovarian, breast cancers
AKT3	• Amplification in melanoma, breast, endometrial, ovarian cancer
PTEN	• Germline mutations linked to inherited PTEN hamartoma tumor syndrome (PHTS) that increase the risk of breast, thyroid, endometrial cancer
TSC1/2	• Mutations linked to bladder, kidney cancers

TARGETING AKT MUTATIONS

- AKT (also known as PKB) is a serine–threonine protein kinase expressed as three isoforms AKT1, AKT2, and AKT3 (encoded by the genes *PKBα*, *PKBβ*, and *PKBγ*, respectively).
- Activation through mutation has been reported for all three isoforms (AKT1, AKT2, AKT3) and activation through amplification has been reported for two isoforms only (AKT1, AKT2). They affect survival, proliferation, and apoptosis of cancer cells with additional effects on tumor-induced angiogenesis through activation of other kinases (e.g., BCL-2-associated death promoter [BAD], mouse double minute 2 [MDM2], GSK3β).
  - AKT1 is involved in cell survival and growth.
    - Mutation E17K in AKT1 has been identified in melanoma, breast, colorectal, endometrial, and ovarian cancers.
    - Mutation is most common in breast, colorectal, and squamous cell lung carcinoma cancers; amplification is most common in gastric cancer.
  - AKT2 is involved in invasiveness and insulin responsiveness.
    - Mutation is most common in colorectal cancer; amplification is common in head and neck, pancreatic, ovary, and breast cancers.
  - AKT3 is involved in survival and apoptosis.
    - Amplification is common in a wide variety of cancers, for example, breast, endometrial, ovarian, and melanoma.

TARGETING PTEN AND TSC ALTERATIONS
- PTEN is a lipid phosphatase that removes phosphate on the three positions of PIP3 and converts it back to PIP2.
- Germline mutations in the *PTEN* gene are associated with inherited cancer predisposition syndromes collectively known as PHTS (e.g., Cowden syndrome and Bannayan–Riley–Ruvalcaba syndrome); individuals with PHTS have an increased incidence of breast, thyroid, and endometrial cancers.
- Preclinical data suggest mTOR inhibitors exhibit activity against PTEN alterations.
- TSC1 or hamartin and TSC2 or tuberin proteins are tumor suppressors in the PI3K pathway.
- TSC1–TSC2 (hamartin–tuberin) complex is a critical negative regulator of mTORC1 through its GAP (GTPase-activating protein) activity toward the small G-protein Rheb (Ras homolog enriched in brain).
- Germline TSC1/2 mutations have been linked to bladder and kidney cancers.
- Loss of TSC1/2 function leads to overactivity of mTOR; therefore, mTOR inhibitors may show activity against TSC alterations.

PHYSIOLOGY

- Considered to be class IV PI3Ks
- Activated in response to growth factors and nutrients
- A master regulator of metabolic homeostasis, protein and lipid synthesis, glycolysis, mitochondria biogenesis, lysosome biogenesis, proteasome assembly, and autophagy

NOTABLE BEHAVIORS IN CANCER

- Mutations (potentially hyperactivating, usually rapamycin-sensitive) detected in colorectal, endometrial, lung cancers
- Amplification of other subunits, for example, raptor, has been seen.
- Also activated by oncogenic activation of upstream regulators, for example, RTKs, PI3K
- Mediates metabolic reprogramming to ensure tumor cell survival and proliferation; also responds to upstream metabolic changes, for example, increased glucose or amino acid uptake
- mTORC inhibitors are being tested in combination with other drugs that interfere with cellular metabolism, for example, the diabetes drug metformin.

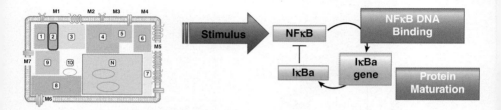

Nuclear factor kappa B (NF-κB) is an ancient protein transcription factor and considered a regulator of innate immunity. The NF-κB signaling pathway links pathogenic signals and cellular danger signals, thus organizing cellular resistance to invading pathogens.

NF-κB is a network hub responsible for complex biologic signaling and is considered a master regulator of evolutionarily conserved biochemical cascades. Other factors are also translocated into the mitochondria and are involved in modulating expression.

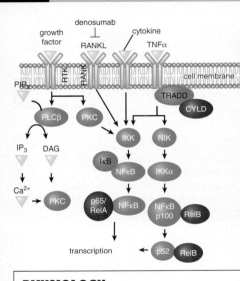

NOTABLE BEHAVIORS IN CANCER

- Osteoclasts, which express RANK, are aberrantly activated in metastatic bone cancer.
- NF-κB links chronic inflammation to cancer.
- NF-κB lesions are typical in lymphoid cancers, rarer in solid cancers.
- NF-κB may be constitutively activated by lesions in upstream regulators or by deregulated secretion of cytokines and other stimuli.
- Constitutive NF-κB activation elicits chemo- and radio-resistance.
- Depending on context, NF-κB can trigger or suppress tumorigenesis.

PHYSIOLOGY

- Cytokine receptors triggered by interferons (e.g., IFNα,β,γ); interleukins (e.g., IL-2)
- RANKL expressed on stromal cells, osteoblasts, T cells
- RANK expressed on osteoclasts, dendritic cells; regulates immune signaling

G-Protein-Coupled Receptors

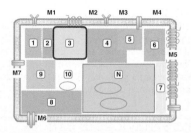

Nobel Prizes in 1994 and 2012

GPCRs are "seven-transmembrane" globular proteins that make up the largest and most diverse group of cell surface receptors. They are named for their binding to guanosine diphosphate (GDP). The conversion of GDP to the triphosphate GTP is the "on/off" switch that positively (+) or negatively (−) affects hundreds of "druggable" enzyme cascades.

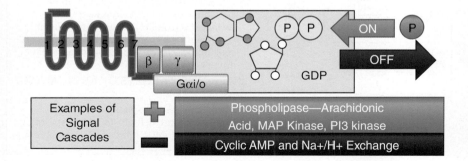

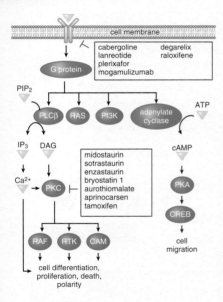

PHYSIOLOGY

- Large family of receptors that regulate multiple signaling pathways
- Activated by diverse ligands, for example, chemokines, hormones, neurotransmitters
- Targeted by the most successful drugs to manage pain, inflammation, neurologic, and metabolic disorders

NOTABLE BEHAVIORS IN CANCER

- Downstream effector PKC frequently dysregulated in cancers
- Deregulated levels of GPCR ligands in the circulation or tumor environment trigger sustained activation, driving tumor growth
- GPCR mutations seen in ~20% of cancers; constitutively active G-protein mutants may drive carcinogenesis.

EMERGING TARGETS OF ANTICANCER DRUGS

- Chemokine, lysophospholipid receptors
- Protease-activated, E-prostanoid receptors
- Smoothened (SMO), Frizzled (FZD) receptors
- GPCRs that regulate Hippo, "transactivate" RTKs

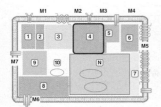

Since the 1980s, the MAP kinases have been an important source of cell signal research. They are specific to the amino acids serine and threonine and control responses to cellular stress: mitogens, heat shock, and inflammatory cytokines. MAPK/ERK regulates cell proliferation, differentiation, mitosis, and apoptosis.

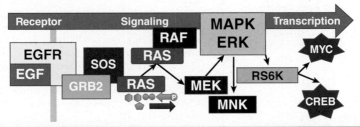

The MAPK "Cascade": Epidermal Growth Factor Receptor (**EGFR**); Growth factor receptor–bound protein 2 (**GRB2**); Son of Sevenless (**SOS**); RAS (RAt Sarcoma virus), a small GTPase that is related to G proteins. Rapidly Accelerated Fibrosarcoma (**RAF**); MEK is the MAP Kinase Kinase that activates MAPK/ERK. MNKs are downstream effector kinases; RS6K is Ribosomal S6 Kinase; MYK is named for MYeloCytomatosis avian virus. CREB is Cyclic AMP Response Element–Binding Protein.

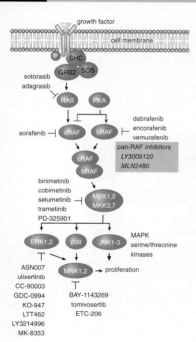

NOTABLE BEHAVIORS IN CANCER

- Sustained pathway signaling following oncogenic activation
- RAS mutations present in up to 30% of cancers
- Constitutively active KRAS (mutated in codons 12, 13, and 61) frequent in pancreatic, colon, lung cancer; KRAS mutations most common Ras lesions (25%–30%)
- HRAS mutations most frequent in bladder cancer, seminoma, Hurthle cell carcinoma
- NRAS mutations common in leukemia, melanoma, thyroid, rectal, follicular cancers
- CRAF overexpressed in lung, liver, prostate, neuroendocrine, myeloid leukemia
- BRAF seen in melanoma (30%–60%), thyroid cancer (30%–50%), colorectal cancer (5%–20%), of which 905 is V600E.
- MEK1/2 mutation and BRAF amplification in V600E cancers may confer resistance to MEK drugs.

- Signaling through the RAS/RAF/MEK/ERK (MAPK) pathway is essential for the proliferation of normal cells as well as for many cancer cells.
- Activation of pathway occurs through growth factor binding to RTKs and also by other extra- and intracellular stimuli.
- MAPK are involved in directing cellular responses to a variety of stimuli and help regulate proliferation, gene expression, and apoptosis, among others.
- In cancer cells, pathway signaling is often heightened as a consequence of oncogenic activation of RTKs, RAS, or RAF. The pathway cascade ultimately leads to ERK activation.
- MAPK kinases activated by MEK1/2 were previously known as ERK1 and ERK2 (extracellular signal–regulated kinases). MAPKs are serine/threonine kinases that include ERK1/2, P38 kinase, ERK5, and c-Jun (JNK1/2/3) kinases.

TARGETING BRAF

- RAF kinase family is serine/threonine-specific protein kinases that mediate signal transduction in MAPK pathway. Raf kinase family consists of three isoforms: RAF-1/CRAF, BRAF, ARAF.
- All Raf proteins share MEK1/2 kinases as a substrate.
- CRAF overexpression is found in a variety of primary human cancers: lung, liver, prostate, neuroendocrine tumors, and myeloid leukemia.
- BRAF mutations are found in melanoma (30%–60%), thyroid cancer (30%–50%), colorectal cancer (5%–20%).
- The most common BRAF mutation, valine (V) is substituted for by glutamate (E) at codon 600 (now referred to as V600E) in the activation segment, which accounts for 90% of BRAF mutations that are seen in human cancers. BRAF V600E mutation indicates poor prognosis in colorectal cancers.

TARGETING KRAS

- Specific KRASG12C inhibitors are now approved or in clinical trials, e.g., sotorasib and adagrasib.
- KRASG12D or pan-RAS inhibitors are upcoming.

TARGETING MEK

- MAP kinase kinases or MAPKK (also known as MEK or MAP2K) is a family of kinase enzymes in the RAS MAPK pathway.
- Inhibitors of MEK1/2 have shown efficacy in BRAF- and KRAS-mutated cancers.
- Mutations in MEK1/2 and BRAF amplification have been identified as potential mechanisms of resistance to MEK inhibitors in cancer cells harboring BRAF V600E mutation.

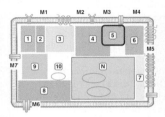

Peyton Rous discovered Rous sarcoma virus (RSV) in the early 1900s working with naturally occurring tumors in chickens. He found that by injecting RSV as a cell filtrate, RSV could induce solid tumors in closely related healthy fowl. He was awarded the Nobel Prize in 1966 for the discovery that viruses could cause tumors and cancer.

The genetic material of RSV—RSV is derived from the more common avian leukosis virus (ALV)—is ribonucleic acid (RNA), which can be transcribed into DNA by reverse transcriptase. Once incorporated into host DNA, proto-oncogene cellular c-Src function increases. Src is a nine-member family of nonreceptor tyrosine kinases. Src triggers downstream phosphorylation signaling and is linked to cancer promotion and carcinogenesis. Bishop and Varmus were awarded the Nobel Prize in 1989 for their work that included the startling discovery that one Src gene is normally present in virtually all animals and is "hijacked" as part of the process of carcinogenesis.

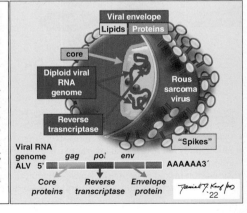

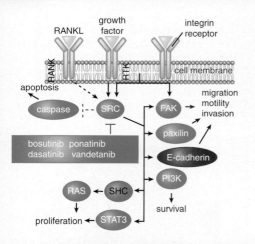

PHYSIOLOGY
- SRC is a nonreceptor tyrosine kinase that triggers phosphorylation cascades.
- Integrins mediate cell–matrix interactions, attachment of actin cytoskeleton at focal adhesion sites.
- May trigger or protect cells from apoptosis
- SRC may also act as direct effector of G proteins, and thus of GPCRs.

NOTABLE BEHAVIORS IN CANCER

- Pathway activated in ~50% of colon, liver, lung, breast, pancreatic tumors
- SRC usually overexpressed/overactive but not mutated, although mutations have been seen in colon cancer
- Activation linked to epithelial–mesenchymal transition, malignant transformation, and, subsequently, heavy migration of and invasion by cancer cells

- E-cadherin mutations seen in gastric, prostate cancers
- Altered integrin expression enables metastasis.
- SRC may also control tumor angiogenesis.
- SRC (short for sarcoma) is a family of nonreceptor protein tyrosine kinases that play an important role in the regulation of cell adhesion, invasion, and motility by phosphorylating specific tyrosine residues in other proteins such as RAS, CAMs (e.g., FAK, focal adhesion protein), and cadherins (e.g., E-cadherins).
- FAK activation by SRC is particularly important for cell adhesion and motility that leads to metastasis.
- SRC activates RAS pathway via SHC.
- SRC also activates E-cadherin, a tumor suppressor that regulates cell invasion.
- Activation of pathway is observed in approximately 50% tumors from colon, liver, lung, breast, and pancreas.
- SRC kinases are usually overexpressed or overactive in cancers, but not mutated, although mutations have been identified (e.g., colon cancer).
  - Activation is often associated with advanced stages of cancer, where cells become highly invasive and migratory.
  - Mutations in E-cadherin have been identified in gastric and prostate cancers.
- SRC is activated by RTK, integrin, VEGFR, and RANK/tumor necrosis factor (TNF)-11.
- Integrin receptors are a family of more than 24 heterodimers that mediate interactions between extracellular matrix and cells and also intracellular signal transduction.
- Altered integrin receptor expression in cancer cells can enable the mobility of metastasizing cells.
- Integrins mediate cell–matrix interactions by binding to extracellular matrix.
- Provide a focus to organize attachment of actin cytoskeleton at focal adhesion contacts

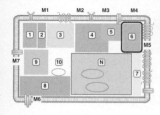

Rolf Kemler et al. (late 1980s) isolated β-catenin and two other molecules, associated with cell adhesion (E-cadherin).

Wnt (**W**ingless fruit fly **Int**egrated) proteins bind to FZD membrane seven-pass receptors. β-Catenin (Axin, Dsh, APC, GSK3, casein kinase-1 [CK1]) is phosphorylated and targeted in the "off state" and for degradation. FZD inhibits phosphorylation and β-catenin accumulates in the nucleus, binds to T-cell factors (TCF), and regulates the cell cycle.

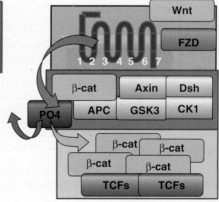

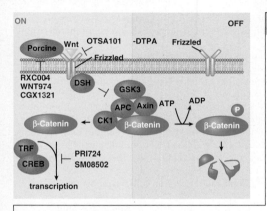

PHYSIOLOGY

- Pivotal in cell proliferation, differentiation, growth, survival, development, regeneration, homeostasis
- Regulates stemness, including of cancer stem cells; can induce dedifferentiation of intestinal epithelial cells into stem cells
- Controls proliferation, maturation, and differentiation of T cells and dendritic cells
- Deregulation drives cancer, metabolic disorders, degenerative diseases

- β-Catenin overexpression, impaired β-catenin degradation, overexpression of Wnt ligands seen in cancer cells
- Persistent signaling because of loss of APC is a key driver of colorectal cancer.
- Wnt signaling activated in 50% of breast cancers and linked to poorer overall survival

- Wnt signaling delays senescence because of $BRAFV^{600E}$ or $NRAS^{Q61K}$, increasing the risk of developing melanoma; mediates phenotypic switching in melanomas between proliferative and invasive states.
- The Wnt signaling pathway is pivotal in cell proliferation, differentiation, growth, survival, development, regeneration, and homeostasis.
- Signaling is initiated by binding of the Wnt proteins to their seven-pass transmembrane receptors called FZD, which then activates β-catenin.
- In the absence of the ligand, the Wnt pathway is in an "off" state with β-catenin phosphorylated and targeted for degradation. In the "on" state, however, FZD is activated by ligand binding, which then inhibits phosphorylation and results in the translocation of β-catenin to the nucleus.
- β-Catenin initiates the transcription of its target gene with a nuclear binding partner, transcription factors of the TCF/lymphoid enhancer factor (Lef) family. These regulate the cell cycle including c-myc and CCND1.
- Porcupine protein (PORCN), located in the endoplasmic reticulum (ER), is important for processing Wnt ligand secretion.
- Deregulation of Wnt signaling contributes to the disease states such as cancer, metabolic diseases, and also degenerative diseases. Thus, inhibitors of this pathway could be used to reverse the pathologic state.
- Dysregulation of the pathway in cancer cells may be associated with mutations in β-catenin that result in overexpression, deficiencies in β-catenin destruction complex, and overexpression of Wnt ligands.
- Small-molecule inhibitors have been used to target the Wnt signaling pathway by targeting cytoplasmic proteins, transcription factors, and/or other coactivators.

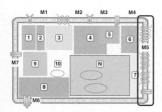

In 1933, Thomas Morgan Hunt received the Nobel Prize for research on *Drosophila melanogaster*—fruit fly genes (FFG). Many of these genes are also fundamental to normal human development because they are mutated and "hijacked" in the process of carcinogenesis. Mutated FFGs are important new drug targets.

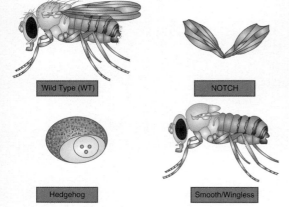

Wild Type (WT)

NOTCH

Hedgehog

Smooth/Wingless

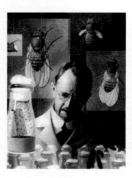

T.M. Hunt

(Courtesy of the Caltech Archives.)

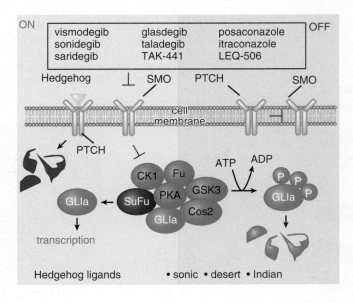

PHYSIOLOGY

- Canonical hedgehog (Hh) signaling occurs mostly in primary cilia (PC), which are immotile but are sensors for mechanical forces, chemicals, light, osmolarity, temperature, gravity.
- Inactive or poorly active in adults except during wound healing, other tissue repair
- Mediates progenitor/stem cell renewal
- Inappropriately activated in basal cell, brain, gastrointestinal, lung, breast, prostate cancer, one-third of malignant tumors
- Activation boosts antiapoptotic genes, angiogenic factors (angiopoietin-1,2), metastatic genes, cyclins D1,B1
- Suppresses apoptotic, cell adhesion, tight junction molecules
- Aberrant activation because of mutations in pathway components or sustained autocrine, paracrine activation
- Paracrine Hh signaling promotes tumorigenesis.
- Sensitive to environmental toxins, for example, piperonyl butoxide, which is common in household and agricultural pesticides

- The Hh pathway can be simplified into four fundamental components: (a) the ligand Hh, (b) the receptor Patched (Patch), (c) the signal transducer Smo, and (d) the effector transcription factor (Gli).
- Canonical Hh signaling occurs predominantly in the PC (Ng and Curran, 2011). PC are tubulin-polymerized immotile cilia that assemble from the centriole at the end of mitosis.
- Components of the Hh pathway concentrate in PC (Ramsbottom and Pownall, 2016; Roy, 2012), and a complex PC trafficking system regulates the interaction of Hh pathway components to enhance, or block, the Hh-initiated signal.

- **OFF State:** In the absence of Hh ligand, the receptor Patch prevents a GPCR-like protein—Smo—from entering the PC, repressing Smo activity.
- This allows the sequential phosphorylation of Gli by several kinases: protein kinase A (PKA), GSK3β, and CK1.
- Phosphorylated Gli is susceptible for ubiquitination by Skp-Cullin-F-box (SCF) protein/β-transducin repeat–containing protein (TrCP), which primes Gli to limited degradation in the proteasome.
- **ON State:** When Hh binds to Patch, it removes Patch from the PC, allowing Smo to enter the PC. The complex Hh–Patch is degraded in vesicles in the cytoplasm. The entry of Smo into the PC allows Smo activation.
- Active Smo abrogates phosphorylation and subsequent degradation of Gli. Full-length Gli translocates to the nucleus where it acts as a transcription factor for several target genes.
- Of note, Shh, Ihh, and Dhh ligands similarly activate the Hh pathway. Gli-1 does not undergo proteasomal degradation, and in the absence of ligand, Gli-2 is preferentially completely degraded in the proteasome, whereas Gli-3 is partially degraded, and hence Gli-1 and Gli-2 act mostly as transcription promoters and Gli-3 can act as a transcription repressor.
- Many human cancers, including brain, gastrointestinal, lung, breast, and prostate cancers, demonstrate inappropriate activation of this pathway.
- Paracrine Hh signaling from the tumor to the surrounding stroma has been shown to promote tumorigenesis.
- Targeted inhibition of Hh signaling may prove effective in the treatment and prevention of many types of human cancers.

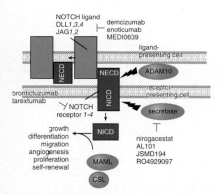

PHYSIOLOGY

- Essential for the development of nervous, cardiovascular, endocrine, respiratory system
- Signaling can be modified by glycosylation and fucosylation of NOTCH receptors, which can affect ligand–receptor interactions.
- Signaling also depends on endocytosis and trafficking of ligands and receptors, which can determine concentrations at cell surface.

CANCER-LINKED LESIONS IN NOTCH RECEPTORS

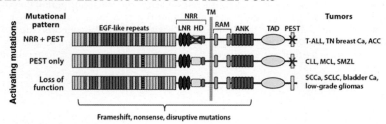

(Republished with permission of Annual Reviews, Inc., from Aster JC, Pear WS, Blacklow SC. The varied roles of Notch in cancer. *Annu Rev Pathol*. 2017 Jan 24;12:245-275.)

- NOTCH is a family of four transmembrane receptors (NOTCH 1–4) that are involved in cell–cell interaction and is found in most multicellular organisms.
- NOTCH signaling is critical to the differentiation and maintenance of several organs that include skin, blood, intestine, liver, and muscle.
- In cancers, mutations in NOTCH can be either activating or inactivating, resulting in oncogenic activity or loss of tumor suppressive function, respectively.
- The NOTCH receptor can be broadly structured into four regions: extracellular domain (NECD), transmembrane domain, intracellular domain (NICD), and the PEST domain located at the C-terminus.
- Two types of NOTCH ligands are known: Delta-like ligands (DLL1, DLL3, DLL4) and Jagged-like ligands (JAG1 and JAG2).
- The binding of the NOTCH ligand to its receptor results in a sequence of two proteolytic events. First, an ADAM family metalloprotease called ADAM10 cleaves the NOTCH protein just outside the plasma membrane. This releases the NECD that will continue to interact with the ligand.
- After the first cleavage, an enzyme called γ-secretase cleaves the remaining part of the NOTCH protein, releasing the NICD from the plasma membrane that translocates to the nucleus.
- In the nucleus, it interacts with DNA where it binds with transcription factors (RBP-J/CSL) and coactivators (Mastermind family, MamL) to induce transcription of target genes, promoting cell proliferation, differentiation, growth, migration, angiogenesis, and self-renewal.

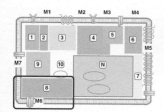

Caspases are activated by DRs and cellular "stress." They work through a network of intermediate molecules to cause cell death: Bid, BCL-2/BCL-Xl, ICAD, IAPS, Smac/Diablo, Omi/HtrA2, cytochrome c, Apaf1, AIF.

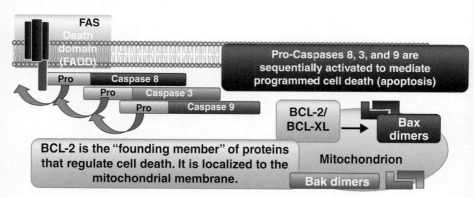

FAS

Death domain (FADD)

Pro | Caspase 8

Pro | Caspase 3

Pro | Caspase 9

Pro-Caspases 8, 3, and 9 are sequentially activated to mediate programmed cell death (apoptosis)

BCL-2/BCL-XL → Bax dimers

Mitochondrion

Bak dimers

BCL-2 is the "founding member" of proteins that regulate cell death. It is localized to the mitochondrial membrane.

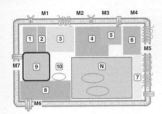

JAK-STAT inhibitors are used in the treatment of autoimmune diseases (rheumatoid arthritis and ulcerative colitis) as well as myeloproliferative disorders (polycythemia vera/essential thrombocytosis).

JAK/STAT has three main components:

1. Receptor is activated by cytokines or other chemical messengers.
2. JAKs (named because of its two nearly identical sequences) attached to the receptor bind phosphates and attract STAT proteins.
3. STATs form dimers and then translocate into nucleus where they bind to promoters, enhancers, and epigenetic regions to control transcription of target genes, microRNAs, and long noncoding RNAs.

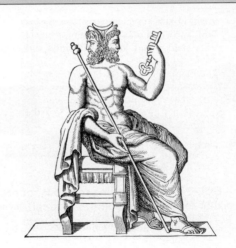

(From Alamy.)

- Among STAT target genes are those encoding SOCS (suppressor of cytokine signaling) factors, which inhibit JAK and contribute to termination of STAT signals.
- STATs can also induce apoptosis mainly by transcriptional activation of genes that encode proteins that trigger cell death process such as BCL-XL (B-cell lymphoma extra-large) and caspases (cysteine-dependent aspartate-directed proteases).
- Signaling through STAT factors in cancers can vary widely because of the many different STATs (e.g., STAT5 in hematologic cancers; STAT3 in breast cancer, head and neck cancer).
- STAT activity is also cross-regulated by protein kinases of MAPK, NF-κB, and PI3K pathways. Dysregulation of pathway may be caused by activating mutations in JAK or inactivation of SOCS.

PHYSIOLOGY
- JAK/STAT signaling mediated by JAK1–4 and STAT1–4,5A,5B,6
- STAT activity cross-regulated by MAPK, NF-κB, PI3K
- Essential in mammary gland, white blood, adipose, neuronal, cardiac, liver, stem cells
- Mediates nearly all immune regulatory processes.

NOTABLE BEHAVIORS IN CANCER
- Deregulation may be due to activating JAK mutations or inactivation of SOCS
- Deregulation may contribute to cancer, immune diseases
- Heterogeneous effects in cancer
- V617F in JAK2 seen in 50% to 95% of classical myeloproliferative neoplasms, polycythemia vera, essential thrombocytosis, primary myelofibrosis
- JAK/STAT activation in head and neck, high-grade ovarian epithelial cancers
- JAK2 amplification in gastric adenocarcinoma
- STAT1,2 drive antitumor immunity; STAT3 linked to cancer cell survival, immune suppression, and sustained inflammation in the tumor microenvironment

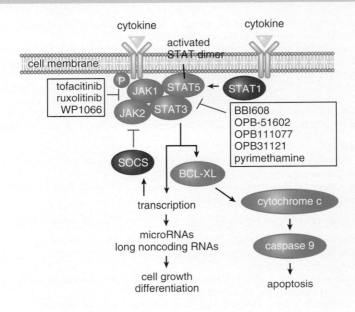

- JAK/STAT pathway transmits information through the cell membrane from chemical signals outside the cell and into genome DNA sites to regulate cell growth and differentiation.
- Many JAK/STAT pathways are important in white blood cells, mammary gland, adipocytes, neuronal cells, cardiomyocytes, hepatocytes, stem cells, and the like, and JAK/STAT deregulations may contribute to development of various diseases including immune diseases and cancers.
- There are four JAK family members (JAK1, JAK2, JAK3, and JAK4 or TYK2) and seven STAT family members (STAT1, STAT2, STAT3, STAT4, STAT5A, STAT5B, and STAT6).
- Receptor is activated by signal from cytokines (e.g., interferon, IL), growth factors, or other chemical messengers.
- After binding of ligand, cytokine receptors recruit JAKs, which phosphorylate each other and the receptor proteins, and create docking sites for STAT proteins, mostly STAT1, STAT3, and STAT5.
- STATs form dimers then translocate into nucleus. They then bind to different DNA sequence promoters, enhancers, and epigenetic regions to control transcription of target genes, microRNAs, and long noncoding RNAs and modify epigenetic markers and chromatin structures.

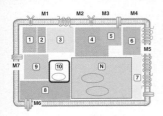

Three pathways promote Programmed Cell Death:

1. Extrinsic—TNF-Related Apoptosis-Inducing Ligand (TNF/TRAIL), FS7-associated surface antigen (FAS)
2. Intrinsic—Mitochondrial-based w/ DNA damage, ROS through BCL-2, BCL-XL, and dimers of Bax/Bak
3. CASPASE-independent pathway

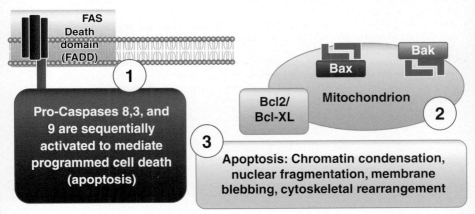

FAS Death domain (FADD)

1

Pro-Caspases 8,3, and 9 are sequentially activated to mediate programmed cell death (apoptosis)

Bax

Bak

Bcl2/ Bcl-XL

Mitochondrion

2

3

Apoptosis: Chromatin condensation, nuclear fragmentation, membrane blebbing, cytoskeletal rearrangement

- DRs include Fas, TNFR, DR3, and DR4/5.
- After binding of ligands (e.g., FasL, TNF-α, AP0-3L/TWEAK, AP0-2L/TRAIL), DRs form dimers or trimers and recruit adaptor proteins that activate the caspase (casp) cascade via the mitochondria, which ultimately leads to apoptosis.
- Fas receptor (also known as apoptosis antigen 1: APO-1 or tumor necrosis factor receptor superfamily member 6 or TNFRSF6) forms the death-inducing signaling complex (DISC) as a result of ligand (FasL) binding.
- DISC is composed of the DR, adaptor protein FADD (Fas-associated protein with death domain), and caspase 8.
- TRAIL receptors 1 and 2 (TRAIL-R1 and -R2, also known as DR4 and DR5) are activated by TRAIL and also form DISC that leads to caspase cascade and apoptosis.
- DISC is inhibited by regulator FLIP (FLICE-like inhibitory protein, also known as caspase 8 and FADD-like apoptosis regulator or CFLAR).
- Other adaptor and regulator proteins mediate apoptotic signaling through different mechanisms, including RIP (receptor-interacting protein), DAXX (Fas death domain–associated xx), and ASK1 (apoptosis signal-regulating kinase 1, also known as MAP3K5).
- RIP activates BID (BH3 interacting-domain death agonist), a member of the proapoptotic BCL-2 (B-cell lymphoma 2) family.
- ASK1 is a member of the MAPKK kinase family and activates JNK (described in RAS pathway).
- Regulator proteins transport into the mitochondria and lead to a cascade of caspase activation that ultimately ends at apoptosis (PD).
- The process of apoptosis is regulated by several other signaling pathways:
  - AKT signaling through the inhibition of BAD
  - Abnormality sensor membrane detection system that responds to changes in pH or cellular damage and triggers cell death through BIM (BCL-2-like protein 11 proapoptotic regulator)
  - TP53 signaling through activation of BAX (BCL-2-like protein 4) proapoptotic regulator

- Proapoptotic factors act through metallothioneins (MTs), a family of proteins localized in the membrane of the Golgi apparatus that bind metals and control oxidative stress.
  - BCL-2 directly inhibits MT.
- In the absence of caspase activation, stimulation of DRs may lead to an alternative pathway of PD called necroptosis.
- Lenalidomide is a thalidomide analog and an FDA-approved inhibitor of TNF-α in multiple myeloma and mantle cell lymphoma.

NOTABLE BEHAVIORS IN CANCER
- Deregulated apoptosis linked to tumor initiation, progression, and chemoresistance
- Ligands of TNF receptors, that is, DRs, are considered as alternative to conventional chemo- or radiotherapy because of apoptotic effects independent of p53, which is often mutated in tumors.
- Some tumors are resistant to TRAIL-induced apoptosis, which is the most tumor cell–selective death mechanism.

PHYSIOLOGY
- Apoptosis is a key (silent/noninflammatory) mechanism maintaining tissue homeostasis.
- Apoptotic cells are swiftly cleared by phagocytosis to prevent release of intracellular components, which may inappropriately trigger signaling.
- DRs include Fas, TNFR, DR3, DR4/5.
- In the absence of caspase activation, DRs may trigger (inflammatory) necroptosis instead of apoptosis.

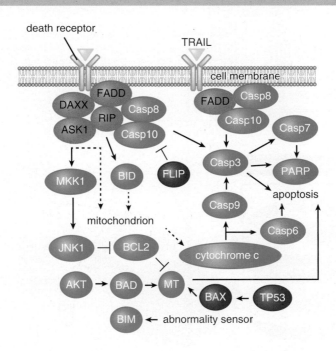

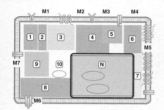

A remarkable number of factors are devoted to transcribing, controlling, and repairing DNA in order to maintain the integrity of the chromosomes, the cell cycle, and the thousands of "apps" present in every cell of the body.

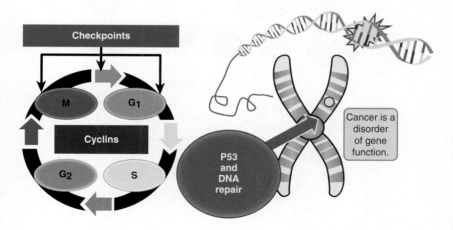

Checkpoints

Cyclins

M

G_1

G_2

S

P53 and DNA repair

Cancer is a disorder of gene function.

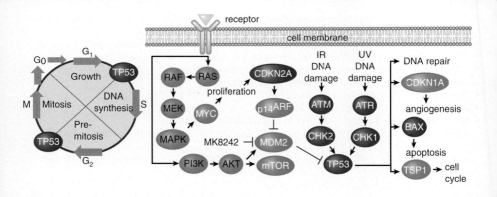

PHYSIOLOGY
- Cell cycle regulation mitigates genomic instability.
- TP53 regulates hundreds of genes and prevents genome damage.

NOTABLE BEHAVIORS IN CANCER
- Rare germline CHK2 mutations predispose to breast, colorectal cancer; somatic mutations seen in small subsets of malignancies.
- TP53 considered the most mutated genes in cancer; mutations can be inherited or somatic.
- TP53 may also be inactivated following loss of p14ARF, loss of upstream activators, loss of downstream effectors.

- *TP53* gene encodes for cellular tumor antigen (TA) or phosphoprotein p53 (name is in reference to apparent molecular mass of 53 kDa).
- Main function of TP53 is prevention of damage to genome, making it a tumor suppressor.
- TP53 acts as a transcriptional activator to several hundred genes.
- TP53 is an important regulator of G1/S and G2/M checkpoints.
- Considered the most frequently mutated gene in cancer
- Mutations may be inherited or sporadic.
- MDM2 is a negative regulator of TP53.
- MDM2 responsible for rapid turnover of TP53 (half-life 10–20 min)
  ○ MDM2 binds to TP53, blocking its transcriptional activity and initiating its transport out of the nucleus.
- MDM2 is activated by the PI3K pathway via AKT, but inhibited by RAS pathway via MYC and p14ARF.
- P14ARF is an ARF product of CDKN2A locus.
- MYC is a transcription factor that promotes proliferation by regulating the expression of specific target genes such as CDKN2A (cyclin-dependent kinase inhibitor 2A).
- Some tumors harbor amplifications of *MDM2* gene, which diminishes TP53 function.
- MDM2 inhibitors (e.g., MK-8242) are not effective against mutated TP53 because they function to silence normal TP53 function.
- Other mechanisms of TP53 inactivation include the following:
  ○ Loss of ARF (p14)
  ○ Loss of function of upstream activators including ATM and ATR, both activated by DNA double-strand breaks (DSBs)
  ○ Loss of function of downstream effectors, including angiogenesis regulator TSP1, apoptosis regulator BAX, and cell cycle regulator CDKN1A (cyclin-dependent kinase inhibitor 1A or p21)

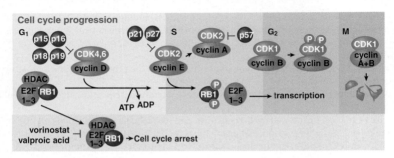

NOTABLE BEHAVIORS IN CANCER

- Loss of RB1 may result in deregulated cell proliferation.
- E2F overactivation may protect against effects of RB1 loss by inducing apoptosis.
- CDK mutation, hypermethylation, deletion are seen in various cancers.
- p15 is often deleted with p16, but may be crucial only in some leukemias.
- p57 inactivation is seen in some cancers.
- p21, p27 rarely mutated, but often downregulated; are good markers of progression and aggression.

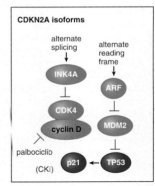

- RB1 controls transition from G1 to S phase of cell cycle by binding to E2F1, E2F2, or E2F3 proteins and thereby repressing promoters of genes needed for the entrance into S phase.
- Phosphorylation performed by CDK4/cyclin D followed by CDK2/cyclin E is needed to inactivate RB1:
  - Activities of CDK4 and CDK2 protein kinases depend on the presence of their regulatory subunits, that is, cyclin D and cyclin E, respectively.
  - Regulatory activities of these subunits fluctuate in a coordinate fashion in the course of the cell cycle.
- Loss of RB1 function upsets cell cycle regulation and may lead to unrestrained cell proliferation.
- Overactivity of E2F factor may protect against loss of RB1 function by inducing apoptosis.
- RB1/E2F complex recruits histone deacetylase (HDAC) protein, which suppresses DNA synthesis.
- HDAC inhibitors valproic acid and vorinostat are FDA-approved neuroleptics currently in clinical trials for cancer.
- Two classes of protein inhibitors of CDKs also control cell cycle:
  - CIP/KIP comprises proteins p21 (*CDKN1A* gene), p27 (*CDKN1B* gene), and p57 (*CDKN1C* gene).
  - INK comprises proteins p15 (*CDKN2B* gene), p16 (*CDKN2A* gene), p18 (*CDKN2C* gene), and p19 (*CDKN2D* gene).
- In a wide range of human cancers, *CDKN2A* gene is inactivated by mutation, hypermethylation, or deletion (regarded as tumor suppressor gene).
- CDKN2B often deleted together with CDKN2A, which may only be crucial in certain leukemia types.
- Inactivation of CDKN1C may be relevant in a small range of cancers.

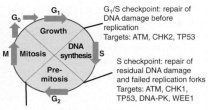

G$_1$/S checkpoint: repair of
DNA damage before
replication
Targets: ATM, CHK2, TP53

S checkpoint: repair of
residual DNA damage
and failed replication forks
Targets: ATM, CHK1,
TP53, DNA-PK, WEE1

G$_2$/M checkpoint: repair
of residual DNA damage
before cell division
Targets: CHK1, MYT, WEE1

BRCA1,2

- Enable repair of DSBs

- Mutations in 5%–10% of all breast cancers; germ-line mutations in hereditary breast, ovarian cancer

- Indirectly targeted

- Therapeutic strategies quickly evolving with knowledge and understanding of DNA damage response (DDR)

DNA DAMAGE REPAIR PATHWAYS
(deficiencies drive carcinogenesis)

Damage	Damaging Agents	Repair Mechanism	Targets
Single-strand breaks	RTx Alkylating agents	Base excision	APE1 PARP
DSBs	RTx, Topo I inhibitors Nucleoside analog	Homologous recombination	ATR ATM
	RTx Topo I inhibitors	Nonhomologous end-joining	ATM DNA-PK
Bulky adducts	UV light Platinum agents	Nucleotide excision + translesion synthesis	ERCC1, XP polymerases
Substitutions insertions deletions	Replication errors Alkylating agents	Mismatch repair (MMR)	MLH, MSH MTH1, etc.

- Human cells are constantly exposed to exogenous and endogenous factors that might damage the genomic integrity and its correct transmission to the next generation.
- To respond to these threats, cells have developed an arsenal of enzymatic tools called DDR.
  - Modified bases and the DNA single-strand breaks (SSBs) are the most common form of DNA damage, and these are repaired by the base excision repair (BER) pathway.
  - For DNA DSBs, there are two major forms of repair: homologous recombination repair (HRR) and nonhomologous end-joining (NHEJ) pathways.
  - The nucleotide excision repair (NER) pathway deals with modified nucleotides that distort the structure of the double helix and it deals with UV-induced or platinum-induced DNA damage.
  - The MMR pathway deals with replication errors, including mismatch base-pairing as well as nucleotide insertions and deletions.
- DDR deficiency causes genetic aberrations that drive carcinogenesis.
- Breast cancer type 1 and type 2 (BRCA1 and BRCA2) are tumor suppressor genes that play an important role in the error-free repair of DNA DSBs, with BRCA1 also having a role in cell cycle checkpoint regulation.
- Cells with loss-of-function BRCA mutations have deficient HRR. Germline mutations in *BRCA1/2* genes are associated with hereditary breast and ovarian cancers. These mutations increase the risk of other cancers, including colon, pancreatic, and prostate. BRCA1/2 mutations account for 5% to 10% of all breast cancer cases.
- Cancer cells that have a reduced capacity to DNA repair pathway (that harbor a BRCA1 or BRCA2 mutation) are solely dependent on another, alternative pathway. This concept of synthetic lethality in cancer treatment is best demonstrated by sensitivity to poly (ADP-ribose) polymerase (PARP) inhibitors that are effective in patients with BRCA1/BRCA2-mutated cancers.

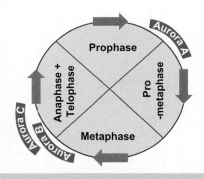

PHYSIOLOGY

- Regulates events in mitosis, including chromosome segregation, spindle checkpoint
- Aurora A required for centrosome function; expression regulated by p53; interacts with BRCA1
- Aurora B required for attachment of mitotic spindle to centromere; phosphorylates histone-H3; function regulated/modified by topoisomerase II, survivin, borealin, INCENP
- In mutually antagonistic relationship with TP53

NOTABLE BEHAVIORS IN CANCER

- Defects in chromosome segregation promote genetic instability, cell cycle progression, deregulated proliferation, tumorigenesis
- Mutated or amplified in cancer cells; diffusely distributed rather than concentrated at specific subcellular structures
- Overexpressed in cancer stem cells
- Stabilize MYC, reinforcing its tumorigenic properties
- Mutations in chromosome 20q13, which spans Aurora A, linked to poor prognosis
- Aurora A overexpression associated with poorer prognosis in specific cancers, predictive of distant metastasis in triple-negative breast cancer, others
- Aurora A variants Phe31/Ile and 91A-169G haplotype predict poor response to cisplatin-based therapy

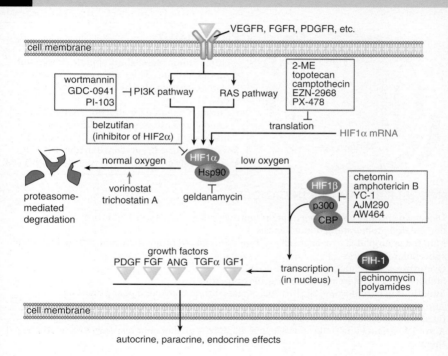

- Angiogenesis is a hallmark of cancer represented by the development of new blood vessels to keep up with the tumor needs, a process that is tightly controlled by pro- and antiangiogenic chemical signals.
- The **angiogenic switch** occurs when, in the hypoxic and inflammatory context of cancer, proangiogenic signals outweigh antiangiogenic signals, leading to tumor neovascularization. The shift in balance toward proangiogenic signals favors the abnormal and rapid growth and proliferation of local blood vessels.
- The sprouting of new blood vessels from the existing vasculature is the most widely investigated mode of new vessel formation in tumors. There are five other mechanisms of new vessel recruitment:
  - Vasculogenesis involves vessel formation by endothelial progenitor cells (EPCs), which are recruited from the bone marrow and/or are resident in vascular walls.
  - Intussusception is the splitting of preexisting vessels to give rise to daughter vessels.
  - Vessel co-option occurs when cancer cells grow around and co-opt the existing vasculature.
  - Vascular mimicry is a process in which cancer cells get incorporated into the blood vessel wall.
  - Tumor stem cell to EC differentiation occurs when cancer stem cell–like cells differentiate into ECs.
- Tumor angiogenesis, which allows for continued tumor growth, is often a deregulated process that results in incomplete, irregular, tortuous, and leaky capillaries. Tumor vessels exhibit bidirectional blood flow, are not constantly perfused, and tend to be larger than normal vessels with an altered surface area-to-volume ratio that results in poor nutrient delivery and waste removal.

Tumor hypoxia and inflammation trigger a proangiogenic switch that overcomes normal antiangiogenic mechanisms.

Angiogenic Switch

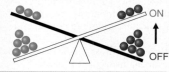

Activators, *e.g.*,	Inhibitors, *e.g.*,
● HIF-1α	● angiostatin
● cytokines (IL-8)	● tumstatin
● growth factors	● endostatin
● inflammation	● TSP-1
	● TP53

(Modified from Hanahan D, Folkman J. Patterns and emerging mechanisms of the angiogenic switch during tumorigenesis. *Cell*. 1996;86:353–364. With permission from Elsevier.)

Angiogenic Effects Of Genetic Lesions

Gain of Function: Oncogenes		
PI3K	↑VEGF	↓TSP-1
HRAS	↑VEGF	
EGFR	↑VEGF, ↑FGF, ↑IL-8	
ERBB2	↑VEGF	
BCL2	↑VEGF	
SRC	↑VEGF	↓TSP-1
FOS	↑VEGF	
Loss of Function: Tumor Suppressors		
TP53	↑VEGF	↓TSP-1
VHL	↑VEGF	
PTEN	↑VEGF	
RB		↓TSP-1

Adapted from Wicki A, Christofori G. The angiogenic switch in tumorigenesis. In: Marmé D, Fusenig N, eds. *Tumor Angiogenesis: Basic Mechanisms and Cancer Therapy*. Springer; 2008:73.

NEW TUMOR VESSELS FORM BY

- Co-opting of existing vessels
- Differentiation of EPCs into new vessels
- Differentiation of cancer stem cell–like cells into ECs
- Incorporation of cancer cells into vessel walls
- Splitting of/sprouting from existing vessels

- Hypoxia or low oxygen tension results from uncontrolled proliferation of cancer cells in the absence of a functional and adequate vascular bed. It is a major driver of tumor angiogenesis.
  - The 2019 Nobel Prize was awarded to William Kaelin Jr., Sir Peter Ratcliffe, and Gregg Semenza for elucidating the importance of hypoxia-induced factors that respond to changes in oxygen levels.
  - Under normoxic conditions, hypoxia-inducible transcription factor-1 alpha (HIF-1α) subunits are subjected to von Hippel–Lindau (VHL)-directed protein degradation. VHL itself is a tumor suppressor, and VHL mutations have been implicated in malignancies such as renal cell carcinoma.
- Hypoxic conditions stabilize HIF-1α, allowing it to translocate to the nucleus and, along with HIF-1β, initiate the transcription of proangiogenic genes such as VEGF. Examples of proangiogenic signals secreted by tumors include the following:
  - Growth factors such as FGF, ANG, PDGF, VEGF
  - Cytokines such as IL-8
- TP53 negatively regulates angiogenesis by downregulating VEGF and other proangiogenic factors while increasing the expression of antiangiogenic signals such as thrombospondin 1 (TSP1). Loss of P53 function promotes VEGF expression and tumor angiogenesis, although the underlying mechanisms remain unclear and controversial.
- Other examples of endogenous inhibitors of angiogenesis include angiostatin, endostatin, tumstatin, and camstatin.

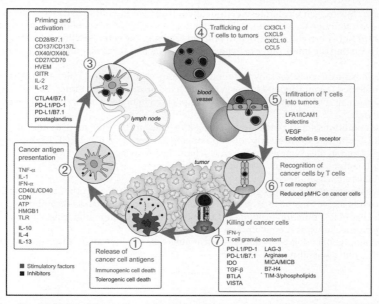

(Reprinted from Chen DS, Mellman I. Oncology meets immunology: the cancer-immunity cycle. *Immunity*. 2013;39(1):1–10. With permission from Elsevier.)

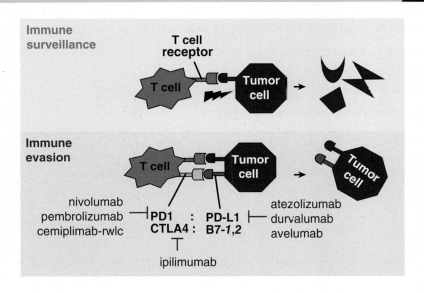

OTHER MODIFIERS OF ANTITUMOR IMMUNITY

Activating receptors (targeted by activators)
- 41BB
- CD28
- GITR
- OX40
- CD27
- HVEM

Inhibitory receptors (targeted by inhibitors)
- VISTA
- TIM-3
- BTLA
- LAG-3

Adoptive Cell Therapy	Chimeric Antigen Receptor T Cells (CAR-T)
Isolation of tumor-infiltrating lymphocytes (TILs)	Isolation of native T cells from patient
↓	↓
Expansion in vitro	Genetic engineering to express CAR
↓	↓
Reinfusion after lymphodepletion	Expansion in vitro
	↓
	Reinfusion

PD-1/PD-L1

- PD-1 is a cell surface protein involved in downregulating T-cell response, preventing autoimmunity under normal conditions.
- PD-1 is typically expressed on T cells and has two ligands, PD-L1 and PD-L2. Interactions between PD-1 and PD-L1 result in T-cell downregulation, impairment, exhaustion, and apoptosis, all of which lead to immune evasion. By hyperexpressing PD-L1, certain cancers can thwart the host immune system.

CTLA-4

- Cytotoxic T-lymphocyte antigen 4 (CTLA-4) is a receptor found exclusively on T cells. Activation of CTLA-4 downregulates T-cell activation and therefore immune response.
- CD80 (B7-1) and CD86 (B7-2) are ligands for CTLA-4, which when bound to each other prevent T-cell activation and immune signaling. Antibodies inhibiting CTLA-4, therefore, promote activation of effector T cells and downregulation of T regulatory cells (Tregs).
- When compared with PD1/PD-L1 blockade, CTLA-4 inhibition generally creates more immune-related toxicities. Where PD1/PD-L1–directed therapies depend on interaction of tumor and T cells, blocking CTLA-4 upregulates the earlier stages of T-cell activation and is independent of tumor interaction.

GITR

- Glucocorticoid-induced TNF receptor (GITR) is a receptor that belongs to the TNF receptor family, like OX-40 and 4-1BB. It is a costimulatory receptor that is highly expressed on Tregs, but is also found on T-effector cells, NK cells, macrophages, and dendritic cells. The ligand for GITR (GITRL) is expressed on antigen-presenting cells.

- Modulation of the GITR and GITRL results in intratumoral Treg inhibition and expansion of cytotoxic and memory CD8+ T cells.
- Antibodies to GITR or GITRL fusion proteins are in the early clinical phases of development and are being evaluated in solid tumors.
- Current clinical trials are evaluating GITR/GITRL modulation in combination with PD-1 or CTLA-4 inhibitors.

4-1BB

- 4-1BB (CD137) is a receptor that belongs to the TNF receptor family, like OX-40 and GITR. It is expressed on multiple immune cells with its downstream effect being activating and upregulating cytotoxic T cells. There is some evidence to suggest that activation of 4-1BB enhances antibody-dependent cell-mediated cytotoxicity (ADCC).
- There are currently two 4-1BB monoclonal antibodies being investigated—urelumab, a fully humanized immunoglobulin G (IgG)4, and utomilumab, a fully humanized IgG2—both of which are being investigated in clinical trials as a single agent and in combination with other immune checkpoint inhibitors.
- Although 4-1BB targeted therapies have a high potential for antitumor effect, there have been severe adverse immune-related events including hematologic toxicity and hepatitis.

OX40

- OX40 (CD134) is a costimulatory receptor that belongs to the TNF receptor family, like 4-1BB and GITR. It is expressed on T cells following their activation and promotes their survival during immune response.

- Modulation of OX40 or its ligand (OX40L) results in expansion and promotion of cytotoxic CD8+ T cells alongside nonregulatory CD4+ T cells.
- Several clinical trials with OX40 agonists are in clinical trials mostly in combination with PD1/PD-L1 and CTLA-4 inhibitors.

LAG3

- Lymphocyte activation gene 3 (*LAG-3*) (CD223) is a surface protein expressed on activated T cells, B cells, NK cells, and dendritic cells. LAG-3 is similar in structure to CD4 and binds to MHC Class II.
- LAG-3 functions as an immune checkpoint, and its interaction with MHC Class II inhibits downstream effects on CD4+ T cells. Increased LAG-3 expression on tumor samples has been identified in colorectal cancer and melanoma. By increasing LAG-3 expression, cancer cells can evade immune recognition and destruction.
- Blockade of LAG-3 leads to activation of T cells and inhibition of Tregs and upregulation of T-cell proliferation.
- LAG-3 antibodies are being investigated alone and in combination with PD-1 inhibitors.

TIM-3

- T-cell immunoglobulin mucin-3 (TIM-3) is a receptor expressed on a variety of cells including T cells, Tregs, NK cells, and dendritic cells. TIM-3+ T cells are considered dysfunctional and exhausted.
- TIM-3 functions as an immune checkpoint similar to, and possibly in conjunction with, PD-1.
- Patients previously failing PD-1 inhibitors have developed immune escape by upregulating TIM-3 as a response.

TIGIT

- T-cell immunoreceptor with Ig and ITIM domains (TIGIT) interacts with CD155 to suppress T cells and NKs, thereby inhibiting immune reactions, for example, antitumor immunity.
- Overexpressed on TA-specific CD8+ T cells and CD8+ TILs from patients with melanoma, breast cancer, non–small-cell lung carcinoma, colon adenocarcinoma, gastric cancer, acute myeloid leukemia, and multiple myeloma
- Dual blockade of TIGIT and PD-1 leads to increased cell proliferation, cytokine production, and degranulation of TA-specific CD8+ T cells and TIL CD8+ T cells.

ADOPTIVE CELL THERAPY

- Cell therapy involves the infusion of autologous or allogeneic immune cells used to target cancer cells.
- TILs were first used in the treatment of melanoma. TILs are essentially host immune cells that are isolated from the patient's own tumor sample. The TILs are expanded in vitro to a prespecified cell count and infused into the same patient after having received lympho-depleting chemotherapy. Patients have attained sustained complete response using TILs, and trials are ongoing.
- CAR-T use genetically altered autologous T cells that target certain antigens. The patient's native T cells are obtained peripherally through lymphopheresis. They are then genetically altered using a variety of different techniques to express a CAR. Once the CAR-T is generated, it is expanded in vitro and eventually infused back into a patient that has received lympho-depleting chemotherapy.
- CAR-T can target a variety of antigens, but the most common in development has been the B-cell antigen CD19.
- The use of CAR-T is being investigated in solid tumors with targets including EGFR, HER2, CEA, MSLN, PSMA, and CA125.

THYROID FUNCTION

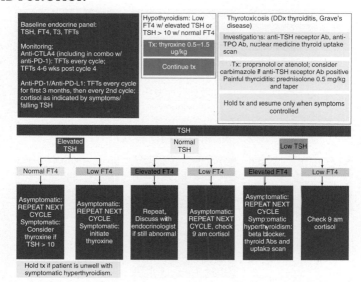

Baseline endocrine panel: TSH, FT4, T3, TFTs

Monitoring:
Anti-CTLA4 (including in combo w/ anti-PD-1): TFTs every cycle; TFTs 4-6 wks post cycle 4

Anti-PD-1/Anti-PD-L1: TFTs every cycle for first 3 months, then every 2nd cycle; cortisol as indicated by symptoms/ falling TSH

Hypothyroidism: Low FT4 w/ elevated TSH or TSH > 10 w/ normal FT4

Tx: thyroxine 0.5–1.5 ug/kg

Continue tx

Thyrotoxicosis (DDx thyroiditis, Grave's disease)

Investigations: anti-TSH receptor Ab, anti-TPO Ab, nuclear medicine thyroid uptake scan

Tx: propranolol or atenolol; consider carbimazole if anti-TSH receptor Ab positive
Painful thyroiditis: prednisolone 0.5 mg/kg and taper

Hold tx and resume only when symptoms controlled

TSH

Elevated TSH

Normal TSH

Low TSH

Normal FT4 | Low FT4 | Elevated FT4 | Low FT4 | Elevated FT4 | Low FT4

Asymptomatic: REPEAT NEXT CYCLE
Symptomatic: Consider thyroxine if TSH > 10

Asymptomatic: REPEAT NEXT CYCLE
Symptomatic: initiate thyroxine

Repeat, Discuss with endocrinologist if still abnormal

Asymptomatic: REPEAT NEXT CYCLE, check 9 am cortisol

Asymptomatic: REPEAT NEXT CYCLE
Symptomatic hyperthyroidism: beta blocker, thyroid Abs and uptake scan

Check 9 am cortisol

Hold tx if patient is unwell with symptomatic hyperthyroidism.

(Data from Haanen J, Carbonnel F, Robert C, et al. Management of toxicities from immunotherapy: ESMO Clinical Practice Guidelines for diagnosis, treatment and follow-up. *Ann Oncol*. 2017;28:iv119–iv142.)

Management of Immune-Related Adverse Events (irAEs) *(continued)*

DIARRHEA AND COLITIS

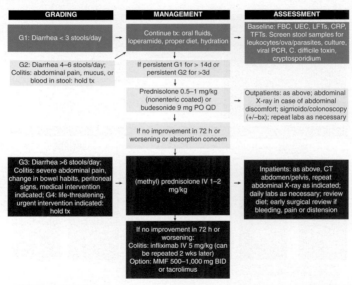

GRADING	MANAGEMENT	ASSESSMENT
G1: Diarrhea < 3 stools/day	Continue tx: oral fluids, loperamide, proper diet, hydration	Baseline: FBC, UEC, LFTs, CRP, TFTs. Screen stool samples for leukocytes/ova/parasites, culture, viral PCR, C. difficile toxin, cryptosporidium
G2: Diarrhea 4–6 stools/day; Colitis: abdominal pain, mucus, or blood in stool: hold tx	If persistent G1 for > 14d or persistent G2 for >3d → Prednisolone 0.5–1 mg/kg (nonenteric coated) or budesonide 9 mg PO QD	Outpatients: as above; abdominal X-ray in case of abdominal discomfort; sigmoido/colonoscopy (+/–bx); repeat labs as necessary
	If no improvement in 72 h or worsening or absorption concern	
G3: Diarrhea >6 stools/day; Colitis: severe abdominal pain, change in bowel habits, peritoneal signs, medical intervention indicated; G4: life-threatening, urgent intervention indicated: hold tx	(methyl) prednisolone IV 1–2 mg/kg	Inpatients: as above, CT abdomen/pelvis, repeat abdominal X-ray as indicated; daily labs as necessary; review diet; early surgical review if bleeding, pain or distension
	If no improvement in 72 h or worsening: Colitis: infliximab IV 5 mg/kg (can be repeated 2 wks later) Option: MMF 500–1,000 mg BID or tacrolimus	

(Data from Haanen J, Carbonnel F, Robert C, et al. Management of toxicities from immunotherapy: ESMO Clinical Practice Guidelines for diagnosis, treatment and follow-up. *Ann Oncol.* 2017;28:iv119–iv142.)

HEPATITIS

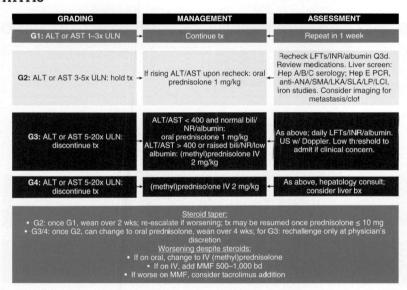

GRADING	MANAGEMENT	ASSESSMENT
G1: ALT or AST 1–3x ULN	Continue tx	Repeat in 1 week
G2: ALT or AST 3-5x ULN: hold tx	If rising ALT/AST upon recheck: oral prednisolone 1 mg/kg	Recheck LFTs/INR/albumin Q3d. Review medications. Liver screen: Hep A/B/C serology; Hep E PCR, anti-ANA/SMA/LKA/SLA/LP/LCI, iron studies. Consider imaging for metastasis/clot
G3: ALT or AST 5-20x ULN: discontinue tx	ALT/AST < 400 and normal bili/INR/albumin: oral prednisolone 1 mg/kg ALT/AST > 400 or raised bili/INR/low albumin: (methyl)prednisolone IV 2 mg/kg	As above; daily LFTs/INR/albumin. US w/ Doppler. Low threshold to admit if clinical concern.
G4: ALT or AST 5-20x ULN: discontinue tx	(methyl)prednisolone IV 2 mg/kg	As above, hepatology consult; consider liver bx

Steroid taper:
- G2: once G1, wean over 2 wks; re-escalate if worsening; tx may be resumed once prednisolone ≤ 10 mg
- G3/4: once G2, can change to oral prednisolone, wean over 4 wks; for G3: rechallenge only at physician's discretion

Worsening despite steroids:
- If on oral, change to IV (methyl)prednisolone
- If on IV, add MMF 500–1,000 bd
- If worse on MMF, consider tacrolimus addition

(Data from Haanen J, Carbonnel F, Robert C, et al. Management of toxicities from immunotherapy: ESMO Clinical Practice Guidelines for diagnosis, treatment and follow-up. *Ann Oncol.* 2017;28:iv119–iv142.)

PERIPHERAL NEUROLOGIC TOXICITY

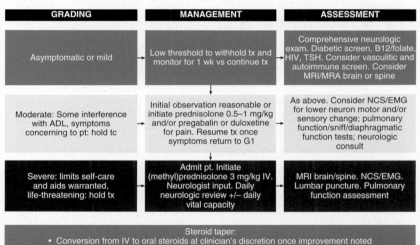

GRADING	MANAGEMENT	ASSESSMENT
Asymptomatic or mild	Low threshold to withhold tx and monitor for 1 wk vs continue tx	Comprehensive neurologic exam. Diabetic screen, B12/folate, HIV, TSH. Consider vasculitic and autoimmune screen. Consider MRI/MRA brain or spine
Moderate: Some interference with ADL, symptoms concerning to pt: hold tc	Initial observation reasonable or initiate prednisolone 0.5–1 mg/kg and/or pregabalin or duloxetine for pain. Resume tx once symptoms return to G1	As above. Consider NCS/EMG for lower neuron motor and/or sensory change; pulmonary function/sniff/diaphragmatic function tests; neurologic consult
Severe: limits self-care and aids warranted, life-threatening: hold tx	Admit pt. Initiate (methyl)prednisolone 3 mg/kg IV. Neurologist input. Daily neurologic review +/– daily vital capacity	MRI brain/spine. NCS/EMG. Lumbar puncture. Pulmonary function assessment

Steroid taper:
- Conversion from IV to oral steroids at clinician's discretion once improvement noted
- Suggested oral prednisolone taper: 4–8 wks
- Consider PJP prophylaxis/vit D if >4 wks duration

(Data from Haanen J, Carbonnel F, Robert C, et al. Management of toxicities from immunotherapy: ESMO Clinical Practice Guidelines for diagnosis, treatment and follow-up. *Ann Oncol.* 2017;28:iv119–iv142.)

PNEUMONITIS

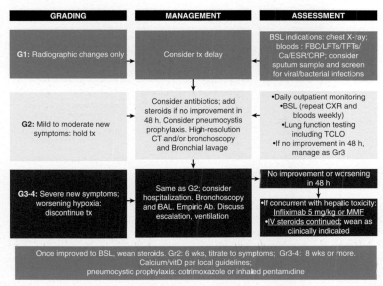

GRADING	MANAGEMENT	ASSESSMENT
G1: Radiographic changes only	Consider tx delay	BSL indications: chest X-ray; bloods : FBC/LFTs/TFTs/Ca/ESR/CRP; consider sputum sample and screen for viral/bacterial infections
G2: Mild to moderate new symptoms: hold tx	Consider antibiotics; add steroids if no improvement in 48 h. Consider pneumocystis prophylaxis. High-resolution CT and/or bronchoscopy and Bronchial lavage	•Daily outpatient monitoring •BSL (repeat CXR and bloods weekly) •Lung function testing including TCLO •If no improvement in 48 h, manage as Gr3
G3-4: Severe new symptoms; worsening hypoxia: discontinue tx	Same as G2; consider hospitalization. Bronchoscopy and BAL. Empiric Ab. Discuss escalation, ventilation	No improvement or worsening in 48 h
		•If concurrent with hepatic toxicity: <u>Infliximab 5 mg/kg or MMF</u> •<u>IV steroids continued</u>; wean as clinically indicated

Once improved to BSL, wean steroids. Gr2: 6 wks, titrate to symptoms; Gr3-4: 8 wks or more. Calcium/vitD per local guidelines; pneumocystic prophylaxis: cotrimoxazole or inhaled pentamidine

(Data from Haanen J, Carbonnel F, Robert C, et al. Management of toxicities from immunotherapy: ESMO Clinical Practice Guidelines for diagnosis, treatment and follow-up. *Ann Oncol.* 2017;28:iv119–iv142.)

NEPHRITIS

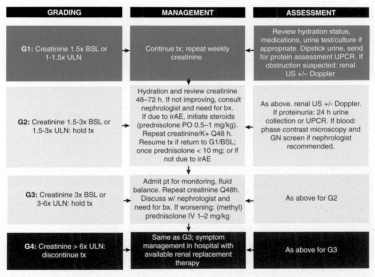

GRADING	MANAGEMENT	ASSESSMENT
G1: Creatinine 1.5x BSL or 1-1.5x ULN	Continue tx; repeat weekly creatinine	Review hydration status, medications, urine test/culture if appropriate. Dipstick urine, send for protein assessment UPCR. If obstruction suspected: renal US +/– Doppler
G2: Creatinine 1.5-3x BSL or 1.5-3x ULN: hold tx	Hydration and review creatinine 48–72 h. If not improving, consult nephrologist and need for bx. If due to irAE, initiate steroids (prednisolone PO 0.5–1 mg/kg). Repeat creatinine/K+ Q48 h. Resume tx if return to G1/BSL; once prednisolone < 10 mg; or if not due to irAE	As above. renal US +/- Doppler. If proteinuria: 24 h urine collection or UPCR. If blood: phase contrast microscopy and GN screen if nephrologist recommended.
G3: Creatinine 3x BSL or 3-6x ULN: hold tx	Admit pt for monitoring, fluid balance. Repeat creatinine Q48h. Discuss w/ nephrologist and need for bx. If worsening: (methyl) prednisolone IV 1–2 mg/kg	As above for G2
G4: Creatinine > 6x ULN: discontinue tx	Same as G3; symptom management in hospital with available renal replacement therapy	As above for G3

(Data from Haanen J, Carbonnel F, Robert C, et al. Management of toxicities from immunotherapy: ESMO Clinical Practice Guidelines for diagnosis, treatment and follow-up. *Ann Oncol.* 2017;28:iv119–iv142.)

SKIN RASH/TOXICITY

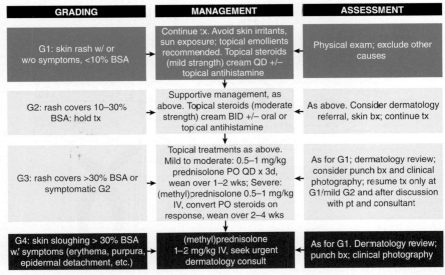

GRADING	MANAGEMENT	ASSESSMENT
G1: skin rash w/ or w/o symptoms, <10% BSA	Continue tx. Avoid skin irritants, sun exposure; topical emollients recommended. Topical steroids (mild strength) cream QD +/– topical antihistamine	Physical exam; exclude other causes
G2: rash covers 10–30% BSA: hold tx	Supportive management, as above. Topical steroids (moderate strength) cream BID +/– oral or topical antihistamine	As above. Consider dermatology referral, skin bx; continue tx
G3: rash covers >30% BSA or symptomatic G2	Topical treatments as above. Mild to moderate: 0.5–1 mg/kg prednisolone PO QD x 3d, wean over 1–2 wks; Severe: (methyl)prednisolone 0.5–1 mg/kg IV, convert PO steroids on response, wean over 2–4 wks	As for G1; dermatology review; consider punch bx and clinical photography; resume tx only at G1/mild G2 and after discussion with pt and consultant
G4: skin sloughing > 30% BSA w/ symptoms (erythema, purpura, epidermal detachment, etc.)	(methyl)prednisolone 1–2 mg/kg IV, seek urgent dermatology consult	As for G1. Dermatology review; punch bx; clinical photography

(Data from Haanen J, Carbonnel F, Robert C, et al. Management of toxicities from immunotherapy: ESMO Clinical Practice Guidelines for diagnosis, treatment and follow-up. *Ann Oncol*. 2017;28:iv119–iv142.)

Epigenetics

HERITABLE GENOMIC CHANGES NOT CAUSED BY CHANGES IN DNA SEQUENCE

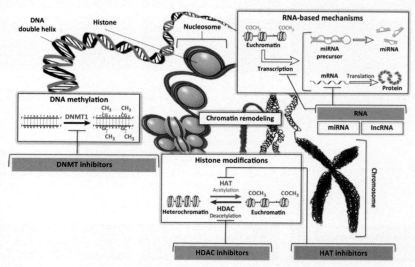

(Reprinted from Schiano C, Vietri MT, Grimaldi V, et al. Epigenetic-related therapeutic challenges in cardiovascular disease. *Trends Pharmacol Sci*. 2015;36:226–235. With permission from Elsevier.)

- **Epigenetics** are defined as heritable changes in the genome that are not caused by alterations in DNA sequence. The DNA exists in the form of chromatin, which is composed of units of nucleosomes. Nucleosome contains an octamer of histone core and the wrapping DNA of 147 bp.
- **Epigenetic mechanisms** include the DNA methylation, histone posttranslational modification, nucleosome restructure, and noncoding RNAs. These mechanisms regulate the switch between the active "euchromatic" and the suppressive "heterochromatic" transcription states.
  - **DNA methylation** involves the covalent transfer of a methyl group to the C-5 position of the cytosine ring of DNA by DNA methyltransferase (DNMT). In cancer cells, DNAs are globally hypomethylated but locally hypermethylated at the promoters of tumor suppressor genes. DNMT is overexpressed in many cancer types including leukemia and lung, breast, gastric, and colorectal cancers.
  - **DNMT inhibitors** azacitidine and decitabine are approved by the FDA for myelodysplastic syndrome. In clinical trials, low doses of DNMT inhibitors are used to sensitize cancer cells to radiation therapy, chemotherapy, and immunotherapies.
- **Histone modifications** are posttranscriptional modifications of the histones in a highly dynamic manner, mainly including histone acetylation, methylation, phosphorylation, ubiquitylation, and sumoylation.
- **Histone modifiers** respond to the upstream signals, recognize and bind (readers) to specific histone regions, and catalytically modify (writers or erasers) histone residues. Many of these modifications are abnormally regulated in cancer.

- **Histone acetylation** occurs on lysine residues on the histone tail and is associated with transcription activation. It is catalyzed by competing enzymes such as histone lysine acetyltransferases (HATs) and HDACs.
- **HDAC inhibitors** induce reexpression of tumor suppressors such as p21, p53, and NF-κB. Vorinostat, belinostat, and romidepsin are FDA-approved HDAC inhibitors for T-cell lymphoma. Panobinostat is another FDA-approved HDAC inhibitor in treating multiple myeloma.
- **Bromodomain and extraterminal protein (BET)** is a subfamily of bromodomains, which are histone acetylation readers. BET is a key player in transcriptional elongation and cell cycle progression. **BET inhibitors** have shown antitumor effects in NUT-midline carcinoma and hematologic malignancies in clinical trials.
- **Histone methylation** occurs on arginine and lysine residues and may either activate or inactivate transcription.
  - **EZH2** is the catalytic subunit of PRC2 complex, which trimethylates H3K27. High activity of EZH2 results in alterations in cell self-renewal and differentiation, cell cycle progression, and DNA repair. **EZH2 inhibitors** show antitumor and synthetic lethal effects with deficiency of SWI/SNF chromatin remodeling complexes.
  - **PRMT5**, a histone methyltransferase, is overexpressed in AML, lymphomas, glioblastomas, and lung and ovarian cancers. **PRMT5 inhibitors** are being tested in treating non-Hodgkin lymphoma and other solid tumors in clinical trials.
  - **Histone lysine demethylase LSD1** demethylates H3K4 and H3K9. **LSD1 inhibitors** induce apoptosis and prodifferentiation in leukemia cells in preclinical studies and are being tested in clinical trials.
- **Chromatin remodeling** uses the energy from ATP hydrolysis to mobilize and exchange histones, and thus allows open chromatin for gene activation. It is regulated by families of SWI/SNF, ISWI, and NuRD/Mi-2/CHD. The components of SWI/SNF family are tumor suppressors, for example, SNF5 loss leads to the development of malignant rhabdoid tumors. SWI/SNF deficiency is combined with other antitumor agents to reach therapeutic synthetic lethality in clinical trials.

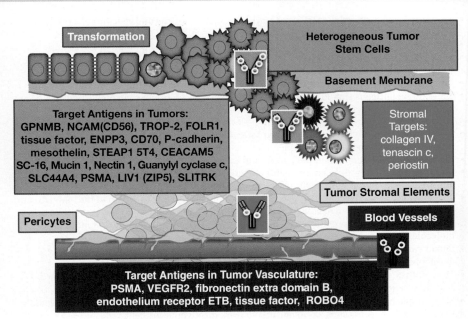

- Antibody–drug conjugates (ADCs) are a hybrid of cytotoxic drug and specific antibody joined by a linker.
- They provide targeted delivery of a cytotoxic agent with a reduced amount of toxicity.
- Their efficacy depends not on a mutation in the genome, but on a suitable marker on the cell surface.
- A successful ADC depends on a firmly attached cell surface antigen for the antibody to bind.
- These target antigens should be expressed at higher levels on tumor than on normal cells. Drug uptake should be via receptor-mediated endocytosis.
- Patients tend to benefit proportionally to the level of antigen expression on tumor cells.
- ADC specificity is limited because of the bystander effect, which causes cell death in adjacent cells that did not internalize the drug.
- Alternatively, ADCs can target the stroma and vasculature rather than the tumor itself.
- Commonly, the antibody portion is a human IgG1, which has the occasional benefit of activating antibody-dependent cellular cytotoxicity.
- The linker is a crucial piece of an ADC because it must not release the toxin in the bloodstream, while also releasing when necessary after endocytosis. The linker usually holds multiple molecules of a toxin to provide adequate cellular kill, with an optimal ratio of four toxin molecules to one antibody.
- Linker can be cleavable or noncleavable, with both approaches successfully used in drug development. (T-DM1 is a noncleavable linker.)
- The cytotoxic payload must be highly potent even at nanomolar concentrations, making traditional chemotherapy ineffective.
- Microtubule inhibitors such as auristatins cause G2/M-cell cycle arrest (brentuximab–vedotin).
- DNA-damaging agents such as calicheamicin work throughout the cell cycle (inotuzumab–ozogamicin).

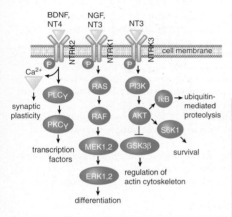

PHYSIOLOGY

- Neurotrophin receptors that regulate neuronal development and function; as well as memory, body weight, appetite, proprioception, pain, thermal regulation

NOTABLE BEHAVIORS IN CANCER

- Activation of downstream pathways drives tumor growth.
- Gene fusions pathognomonic in rare cancers such as congenital fibrosarcoma, secretory breast cancer, mammary analogue secretory carcinoma (MASC) of salivary gland
- Fusion partners include TPR, ETV6, TP53, TFG
- Mutations, splice variants, and overexpression also potentially tumorigenic
- Fusions also seen in papillary thyroid carcinoma (12%–14.5%), lung adenocarcinoma (3.3%), Spitzoid neoplasms (16%), pediatric high-grade glioma (40%)
- Highly responsive to first-generation inhibitors, but eventually acquire resistance, most commonly through solvent front mutations; resistance can be overcome by second-generation inhibitors currently in clinical trials; NGS needed to identify resistance mutations postprogression/nonresponse

- The tropomyosin-related kinases (TRKs) are neurotrophin receptors from the tyrosine kinase family and consist of three members: TRKA, TRKB, and TRKC, which are encoded by *NTRK1*, *NTRK2*, and *NTRK3* genes. The corresponding in vivo ligands are as follows: TRKA—neurotrophic growth factor (NGF) and neurotrophin-3 (NT-3); TRKB—brain-derived neurotrophic factor (BDNF) and neurotrophin-4 (NT-4); TRKC—NT-3 (Amatu et al., 2016).
- The TRK receptor family is involved in neuronal development, including the growth and function of neuronal synapses. In adults, TRK receptors regulate memory, body weight, appetite, proprioception, pain, and thermal regulation.
- Tropomyosin sequences cause activation of the kinase activity of the receptor with downstream activation of MAPK, PI3K, and PLCg pathways, resulting in cell proliferation, increased cell survival, and migration leading to tumor growth.
- Gene fusions involving the NTRK family are pathognomonic in rare cancers such as congenital fibrosarcoma, secretory breast cancer, and MASC of the salivary gland.
- *NTRK* gene fusions have been described across several cancer types with varying frequencies such as the following:
  - Papillary thyroid carcinoma (NTRK1—12%; NTRK3—14.5%)
  - Lung adenocarcinoma (3.3%)
  - Spitzoid neoplasms (16%)
  - Pediatric high-grade glioma (40%)

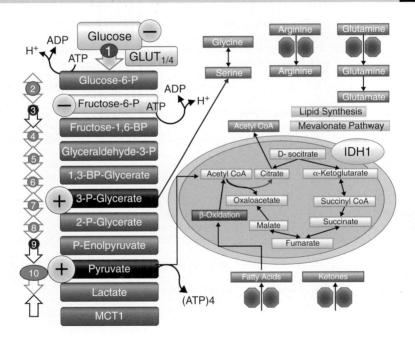

- Tumor cells metabolize glucose, lactate, pyruvate, hydroxybutyrate, acetate, glutamine, arginine, and fatty acids at much higher rates than nontumor tissue.
- These intermediary metabolites are released by catabolic cells, taken up by tumor cells, and used to replenish TCA-cycle intermediates and to fuel oxidative phosphorylation (reverse Warburg effect).
- Enasidenib (formerly AG-221) is a first-in-class inhibitor of mutated isocitrate dehydrogenase 2 (IDH2) and is now FDA-approved to treat acute myeloid leukemia.
- Similarly, ivosidenib, an inhibitor of IDH1, is FDA-approved in cholangiocarcinoma. The IDH enzyme normally metabolizes isocitrate into α-ketoglutarate. When mutated, it also converts α-ketoglutarate into 2-hydroxyglutarate, an oncometabolite that causes cell differentiation defects by impairing histone demethylation.
- Targeting glycolysis, mitochondrial metabolism, and amino acid metabolism with drug combinations holds promise as an antitumor strategy, and the following drugs are in early-phase trials:
  - Drugs inhibiting glycolysis—silibinin (GLUT1 inhibitor) (Ooi and Gomperts, 2015), TLN-232 (inhibits PKM2 dimerization and activity) (Vander Heiden et al., 2010)
  - Drugs inhibiting glutamine metabolism—CB-839 (Gross et al., 2014) and bis-2-(5-phenylacetamido-1,2,4-thiadiazol-2-yl)ethyl sulfide (BPTES) (Xiang et al., 2015) (glutaminase inhibitors)
  - Drugs targeting lactate, pyruvate, and acetyl-CoA production—AZD3965 (MCT1 inhibitor) (Polański et al., 2014)
  - Drugs degrading circulating arginine—ADI-PEG20 (Ascierto et al., 2005)

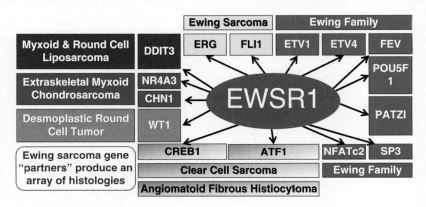

ATF1, cyclic AMP (cAMP)–dependent Transcription Factor 1; CHN1, CHimaerin Nervous system 1 protein gene; CREB1, cAMP Responsive Element–Binding protein 1; DDIT3, DNA Damage Inducible Transcript 3 gene; ERG, Erythroblast transformation factor–Related Gene; ETV1, ETS Variant 1; ETV4, E-Twenty-six Translocation Variant 4; FEV, Fifth Ewing Variant protein (ETS oncogene family); FLI1, Friend Leukemia Integration 1 gene; NFATC2, Nuclear Factor of Activated T Cells 2; NR4A3, Nuclear (hormone) Receptor member 4A3; PATZ1, POZ/BTB and AT Hook–Containing Zinc Finger 1; POU5F1, Protein coding POU class 5 homeobox 1 gene; SP3, GT/GC box promoter transcription factor gene; WT1, Wilms Tumor protein coding gene 1.

SECTION 4

Targeted and Immunotherapy Agents

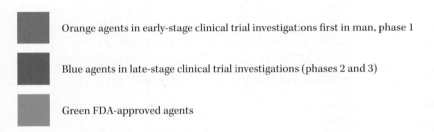

Orange agents in early-stage clinical trial investigations first in man, phase 1

Blue agents in late-stage clinical trial investigations (phases 2 and 3)

Green FDA-approved agents

- 17-AAG: 17-allylaminogeldanamycin
- 2HG: 2-hydroxyglutarate
- 5FU: 5-fluorouracil
- ADCC: antibody-dependent cell-mediated cytotoxicity
- AICARFT: aminoimidazole carboxamide ribonucleotide formyltransferase
- ALK: anaplastic lymphoma kinase
- ALT: alanine transaminase
- AML: acute myelogenous leukemia
- AR: androgen receptor
- AST: aspartate aminotransferase
- ATM: ataxia telangiectasia mutated
- AURKA: Aurora A kinase
- AURKB: Aurora B kinase
- BCRP: breast cancer resistance protein
- BNP: brain natriuretic peptide
- BRCA: BReast CAncer susceptibility gene
- BTK: Bruton's tyrosine kinase
- CAR: chimeric antigen receptor
- CBP: CREB-binding protein
- CCR4: CC chemokine receptor 4
- CD: cytosine deaminase
- CDK: cyclin-dependent kinase
- CLL: chronic lymphocytic leukemia
- CMV: cytomegalovirus
- CPK: creatine phosphokinase

- CREB: cAMP response element-binding protein
- CTCL: cutaneous T-cell lymphoma
- CTLA4: cytotoxic T-lymphocyte–associated antigen 4
- DHFR: dihydrofolate reductase
- DOE: dyspnea on exertion
- DPD: dihydropyrimidine dehydrogenase
- DVT: deep vein thrombosis
- EF: ejection fraction
- EGFR: epidermal growth factor receptor
- EKG: electrocardiogram
- ERK2: extracellular signal–related kinase 2
- Fc: fragment crystallizable
- FGFR: fibroblast growth factor receptor
- FKBP-12: FK506-binding protein-12
- FLT3: FMS-related tyrosine kinase receptor-3
- FOLFIRI: folinic acid/fluorouracil/irinotecan
- FOLR1: folate receptor 1
- FPGS: folylpolyglutamate synthetase
- GARFT: glycinamide ribonucleotide formyltransferase
- GE: gastroesophageal
- GERD: gastroesophageal reflux disease
- GGT: γ-glutamyl transferase
- GI: gastrointestinal
- GM-CSF: granulocyte-macrophage colony-stimulating factor
- HCC: hepatocellular carcinoma

- HDAC: histone deacetylase
- HER2: human epidermal growth factor receptor 2
- HSV: herpes simplex virus
- IDH: isocitrate dehydrogenase
- Ig: immunoglobulin
- IGF-1R: insulin-like growth factor-1 receptor
- ITD: internal tandem duplication
- ITP: immune thrombocytopenic purpura
- JAK: Janus kinase
- KDR: kinase insert domain receptor
- KLF4: Kruppel-like factor 4
- KRAS: Kirsten rat sarcoma
- LD: lactate dehydrogenase
- LVEF: left ventricular ejection fraction
- mAb: monoclonal antibody
- MAPK: mitogen-activated protein kinase
- MCL: mantle cell lymphoma
- mCRC: metastatic colorectal cancer
- MDS: myelodysplastic syndrome
- MEK1: mitogen-activated protein kinase kinase 1
- MET: mesenchymal–epithelial transition
- MM: multiple myeloma
- MTC: medullary thyroid carcinoma
- MTF-1: metal-regulatory transcription factor 1
- mTOR: mammalian target of rapamycin

- MWF: Monday, Wednesday, Friday
- NHL: non-Hodgkin lymphoma
- NRAS: neuroblastoma RAS viral oncogene homolog
- NSCLC: non–small-cell lung cancer
- NTRK: neurotrophic tropomyosin receptor kinase
- PAP: prostatic-acid phosphatase
- PARP: poly (ADP-ribose) polymerase
- PDGFR: platelet-derived growth factor receptor
- PD-L1: programmed death ligand 1
- PEG: polyethylene glycol
- PFS: progression-free survival
- PI3K: phosphatidylinositol 3-kinase
- PIP3: phosphatidylinositol-3,4,5-trisphosphate
- PKC: protein kinase C
- pNET: pancreatic neuroendocrine tumor
- PTCH: patched
- PTCL: peripheral T-cell lymphoma
- RANKL: receptor activator of nuclear factor-κB ligand
- RAS: rat sarcoma virus
- RET: rearranged during transfection
- RFC-1: reduced folate carrier
- RTKs: receptor tyrosine kinases
- SAPK: stress-activated protein kinase
- SCCHN: squamous cell carcinoma of the head and neck
- scFv: single-chain variable fragment

- SCLC: small-cell lung cancer
- SMO: small-molecule smoothened
- STAT3: signal transducer and activator of transcription 3
- STS: soft-tissue sarcoma
- SYK: spleen tyrosine kinase
- TAA: tumor-associated antigen
- TCR: T-cell receptor
- TEN: toxic epidermal necrolysis
- TGF: transforming growth factor
- TLS: tumor lysis syndrome
- TRK: tropomyosin receptor kinase
- TS: thymidylate synthase
- URI: upper respiratory infection
- VEGF: vascular endothelial growth factor
- VEGFR: vascular endothelial growth factor receptor
- XRT: radiotherapy

Abemaciclib

- **Alias:** LY2835219
- **Brand Name:** Verzenio
- **Type Mechanism:** CDK4/6 inhibitor blocks early G1 retinoblastoma (Rb) protein phosphorylation and G1-S cell-cycle transition.
- **Drug Class:** Cyclin-dependent kinase inhibitor
- **Mechanism of Action:** CDK4/6 inhibitor
- **FDA Approval Date:** September 28, 2017
- **Indications:** Advanced or metastatic breast cancer with hormone receptor (HR) (+) and HER2(−)
- **Dose:** 150 to 200 mg twice daily (BID)
- **Half-life:** 18.3 hours
- **Metabolism:** Major CYP3A4 substrate
- **Side Effects:** Diarrhea, neutropenia and leukopenia, nausea, abdominal pain, infections, fatigue, anemia, alopecia, decreased appetite, vomiting, transaminitis, headache
- **Clinical Pearls:** Need premedication with 5HT3 antagonist before each dose. Considered as moderate-to-high emetogenic potential.

Abiraterone Acetate

- **Alias:** CB7630
- **Brand Name:** Zytiga; Yonsa (micronized formulation)
- **Type Mechanism:** Selectively and irreversibly inhibits 17-α-hydroxylase/C17,20-lyase (CYP17), an enzyme required for testosterone synthesis. The inhibition of CYP17 results in increased mineralocorticoid production by the adrenals and suppression of testosterone production by both the testes and the adrenals.
- **Drug Class:** Androgen inhibitor
- **Mechanism of Action:** CYP17 inhibitor
- **FDA Approval Date:** April 28, 2011
- **Indications:** 2011 approved for late-stage prostate cancer; 2018 approval for the treatment of earlier form of metastatic prostate cancer with prednisone
- **Dose:** 1,000 mg orally (PO) daily with prednisone. Give on a fasting stomach 1 hour before and 2 hours after meal.
- **Half-life:** 14.4 to 16.5 hours
- **Metabolism:** Major CYP3A4 substrate
- **Side Effects:** Peripheral edema, fatigue, hypertension (HTN), hyperglycemia/hypertriglyceridemia, lymphopenia, transaminitis, arthralgias/myalgias, diarrhea

- **Clinical Pearls:** Yonza™ (micronized formulation) may be taken regardless of meals; patient should also be receiving gonadotropin-releasing hormone (GnRH) analog concurrently or have had a bilateral orchiectomy.

Acalabrutinib

- **Alias:** ACP-196
- **Brand Name:** Calquence
- **Type Mechanism:** An orally available inhibitor of BTK with potential antineoplastic activity. Upon administration, acalabrutinib inhibits the activity of BTK and prevents the activation of the B-cell antigen receptor (BCR) signaling pathway. This prevents both B-cell activation and BTK-mediated activation of downstream survival pathways. This leads to an inhibition of the growth of malignant B cells that overexpress BTK. BTK, a member of the src-related BTK/Tec family of cytoplasmic tyrosine kinases, is overexpressed in B-cell malignancies; it plays an important role in B lymphocyte development, activation, signaling, proliferation, and survival.
- **Drug Class:** Tyrosine kinase inhibitor (TKI)
- **Mechanism of Action:** A selective and irreversible second-generation BTK inhibitor. BTK inhibition results in decreased malignant B-cell proliferation and tumor growth.
- **FDA Approval Date:** October 31, 2017
- **Indications:** Previously treated MCL; CLL or small lymphocytic lymphoma (SLL) in adults
- **Dose:** 100 mg PO Q 12 hours regardless of meals
- **Half-life:** 1 hour; ACP-5862 (active metabolite) 3.5 hours
- **Metabolism:** Major CYP3A4 substrates. May dose-adjust with moderate inhibitors of CYP3A4
- **Side Effects:** Headache, fatigue, skin rash, diarrhea, bruise, neutropenia, myalgias, anemia, rare increase in serum creatinine (SCr), increased uric acid, abdominal pain, transaminitis, hyperbilirubinemia
- **Clinical Pearls:** Avoid use with proton-pump inhibitors; take 2 hours before H2 antagonist; separate from antacids by 2 hours.

Acalisib

- **Alias:** GS-9820
- **Type Mechanism:** A second-generation inhibitor of the β and δ isoforms of the 110-kDa catalytic subunit of class IA PI3K that inhibits the activity of PI3K, thereby preventing the production of the second

messenger PIP3, which decreases tumor cell proliferation and induces cell death
- **Drug Class:** PI3K inhibitor
- **Phase:** Phase 1/2
- **Indications:** Relapsed/refractory lymphoid malignancies (CLL and B-cell lymphomas)
- **Dose:** 200 to 400 mg PO BID
- **Side Effects:** Diarrhea, rash, weight loss, ALT/AST elevations, dysgeusia, fever, nausea, neutropenia, anemia, increased SCr, pneumonia

(Kater et al., 2018)

Adavosertib

- **Alias:** AZD1775; MK-1775
- **Type Mechanism:** It selectively targets and inhibits WEE1, a tyrosine kinase that phosphorylates cyclin-dependent kinase 1 (CDK1, CDC2) to inactivate the CDC2/cyclin B complex. Inhibition of WEE1 activity prevents the phosphorylation of CDC2 and impairs the G2 DNA damage checkpoint.
- **Drug Class:** Cell-cycle inhibitor
- **Mechanism of Action:** WEE1 inhibitor
- **Phase:** Phase 2
- **Indications:** Phase 2 combination with olaparib in recurrent ovarian, primary peritoneal, or fallopian tube cancer; phase 2 studies in advanced solid tumors that have SETD2 mutation; phase 2 in recurrent uterine serous carcinoma or uterine carcinosarcoma
- **Dose:** Intermittent dosing daily to BID for 5 days on, 2 days off, or Q other week 5 days on, 2 days off with dose ranging from 200 to 300 mg on empty stomach with or without chemotherapy/biotherapy
- **Half-life:** 18.3 hours
- **Metabolism:** Major substrate of CYP3A4
- **Side Effects:** Nausea, vomiting—can be controlled by using 5HT3 + steroids as premedications; fatigue, diarrhea, anemia, thrombocytopenia, and leukopenia/neutropenia; loss of appetite
- **Clinical Pearls:** High-fat meal was shown not to have clinically relevant effect on exposure of adavosertib, suggesting that it can be dosed regardless of meals.

(Kato et al., 2020; Nagard et al., 2020)

Ado-Trastuzumab Emtansine

- **Alias:** T-DM1; trastuzumab-DM1; trastuzumab-MCC-DM1
- **Brand Name:** Kadcyla
- **Type Mechanism:** A HER2 antibody–drug conjugate (ADC) that incorporates the HER2-targeted actions of trastuzumab with the microtubule inhibitor DM1 (a maitansine

derivative). The conjugate, which is linked via a stable thioether linker, allows for selective delivery into HER2 overexpressing cells, resulting in cell-cycle arrest and apoptosis.

- **Drug Class:** ADC
- **Mechanism of Action:** HER2 ADC
- **FDA Approval Date:** February 22, 2013
- **Indications:** HER2-positive metastatic breast cancer patients who have previously had trastuzumab-based treatment with taxanes
- **Dose:** 3.6 mg/kg intravenous (IV) Q 3 weeks over 90 minutes with the first dose, then may decrease to 30 minutes if tolerated
- **Half-life:** 4 days
- **Metabolism:** Major CYP3A4 substrate
- **Side Effects:** Fatigue, headache, neuropathy, skin rash, nausea, stomatitis, abdominal pain, muscle pain, arthralgias, cough, fever, thrombocytopenia, anemia

Afatinib Dimaleate

- **Brand Name:** Gilotrif
- **Type Mechanism:** A dimaleate salt form of afatinib, an orally bioavailable anilinoquinazoline derivative and inhibitor of the RTK EGFR (ErbB).

Upon administration, afatinib selectively and irreversibly binds to and inhibits the epidermal growth factor receptors 1 (ErbB1; EGFR), 2 (ErbB2; HER2), and 4 (ErbB4; HER4), and certain EGFR mutants, including those caused by EGFR exon 19 deletion mutations or exon 21 (L858R) mutations. In addition, afatinib inhibits the EGFR T790M gatekeeper mutation, which is resistant to the treatment with the first-generation EGFR inhibitors. EGFR, HER2, and HER4 are RTKs that belong to the EGFR superfamily.

- **Drug Class:** EGFR inhibitor
- **Mechanism of Action:** A TKI that covalently binds to EGFR (ErbB1), HER2 (ErbB2), and HER4 (ErbB4) to irreversibly inhibit tyrosine kinase autophosphorylation and downregulate ErbB signaling
- **FDA Approval Date:** July 12, 2013
- **Indications:** Metastatic EGFR mutation–positive NSCLC and metastatic squamous cell lung cancer
- **Dose:** 40 mg PO daily. Administer ≥1 hour before or 2 hours after a meal.
- **Half-life:** 37 hours
- **Metabolism:** P-glycoprotein/ABCB1 major substrate
- **Side Effects:** Acneiform eruption, skin rash, paronychia, xeroderma, pruritis,

cheilitis, diarrhea, stomatitis, nausea, vomiting, lymphocytopenia, transaminitis, hyperbilirubinemia, hypokalemia
- **Clinical Pearls:** Binding to T790M can lead to longer time to resistance.

Afuresertib

- **Alias:** GSK2110183
- **Type Mechanism:** Inhibitor of the serine/threonine protein kinase Akt (protein kinase B) with potential antineoplastic activity. Afuresertib binds to and inhibits the activity of Akt, which may result in inhibition of the PI3K/Akt signaling pathway and tumor cell proliferation and the induction of tumor cell apoptosis.
- **Drug Class:** AKT inhibitor
- **Mechanism of Action:** Inhibitor of protein kinase B (AKT)/PI3K pathway
- **Phase:** Phase 1/2
- **Indications:** Undergoing trials in platinum-resistant ovarian cancer, MCRPC, and relapsed/refractory MM
- **Dose:** 125 mg PO daily in combination with paclitaxel and carboplatin
- **Half-life:** 1.7 days
- **Side Effects:** Nausea, diarrhea, dyspepsia, fatigue, gastrointestinal (GI) reflux, rash, neutropenia, odynophagia, asthenia

- **Clinical Pearls:** Most useful in tumors with PTEN deficiency and PIK3 mutations

(Nitulescu et al., 2016; Spencer et al., 2014)

Alectinib

- **Alias:** AF802; CH5424802; RG7853; RO5424802
- **Brand Name:** Alecensa
- **Type Mechanism:** A tyrosine kinase receptor inhibitor that inhibits ALK and RET, resulting in decreased tumor cell viability. Alectinib is more potent than crizotinib against ALK and can inhibit most of the clinically observed acquired ALK resistance mutations to crizotinib.
- **Drug Class:** Tyrosine kinase receptor inhibitor
- **Mechanism of Action:** ALK and RET inhibitors
- **FDA Approval Date:** December 11, 2015
- **Indications:** Metastatic NSCLC with ALK-positive mutation
- **Dose:** 600 mg BID with food
- **Half-life:** 33 hours ; M4-active metabolite 31 hours
- **Metabolism:** Minor CYP3A4 substrate
- **Side Effects:** Edema, bradycardia, fatigue, headache, rash, hyperglycemia,

hypophosphatemia, transaminitis, hyperbilirubinemia, muscle pain, increased CPK, increased SCr, constipation

- **Clinical Pearls:** Dose adjustment needed for both grade 2 transaminitis and hyperbilirubinemia.

Alemtuzumab (Campath-1H)

- **Alias:** mAb CD52; anti-CD52 mAb; humanized IgG1 anti-CD52 mAb
- **Brand Name:** Lemtrada
- **Type Mechanism:** Binds to CD52, a nonmodulating antigen present on the surface of B and T lymphocytes, a majority of monocytes, macrophages, natural killer (NK) cells, and a subpopulation of granulocytes. After binding to $CD52^+$ cells, an antibody-dependent lysis of malignant cells occurs.
- **Drug Class:** Anti-CD52 mAb
- **FDA Approval Date:** As of September 4, 2012, alemtuzumab (Campath) is no longer commercially available in the United States (or Europe).
  - In February 2014, alemtuzumab was launched under a different trade name of Lemtrada for use in multiple sclerosis with lower doses.

- **Indications:** Campath remains accessible (free of charge) through the Campath Distribution Program for the treatment of B-cell CLL and select unlabeled uses.
- **Dose:** 3 mg IV on day 1; if no reaction, increase to 10 mg IV on day 3; again if no reaction, increase to full dose at 30 mg IV three times a week (TIW) for a total of 12 doses
- **Half-life:** 11 hours (following first 30-mg dose); 6 days (following last 30-mg dose)
- **Side Effects:** Black box warning: potentially life-threatening cytopenias, opportunistic infections, infusion reactions, hypotension/HTN, fevers, chills, lymphopenia, rash
- **Clinical Pearls:** Premedications needed with diphenhydramine and acetaminophen. Moderate emetogenic potential. If given as IV, need to infuse over 4 hours.

Alisertib

- **Alias:** MLN8237
- **Type Mechanism:** Second-generation, orally bioavailable, selective binding to and inhibiting Aurora A kinase in cells. Inhibition of Aurora A results in delayed mitotic entry and progression through mitosis, leading to

an accumulation of cells with a tetraploid DNA content. This results in a process called *mitotic slippage*, causing apoptosis, senescence, or reenter the cell cycle.

- **Drug Class:** Mitotic inhibitor
- **Mechanism of Action:** Aurora kinase inhibitor
- **Phase:** Phase 2/3
- **Indications:** Phase 2 in relapsed/refractory neuroblastoma; phase 3 relapsed/refractory PTCL; phase 2 SCLC, CRPC, and neuroendocrine prostate cancer; phase 2 high-risk AML
- **Dose:** 50 mg BID for 7 consecutive days of the 21-day cycle (10 mg enteric coated tablet). Fast 2 hours before and 1 hour after dosing
- **Half-life:** 19 to 23 hours
- **Metabolism:** Excreted primarily unchanged
- **Side Effects:** Fatigue, neutropenia, nausea, stomatitis, HTN

(DuBois et al., 2018; O'Connor et al., 2019)

All-Trans Retinoic Acid (ATRA)

- **Type Mechanism:** Binds one or more nuclear receptors and decreases proliferation and induces differentiation of acute promyelocytic leukemia (APL) cells; initially produces maturation of primitive promyelocytes and repopulates the marrow and peripheral blood with normal hematopoietic cells

- **Drug Class:** Retinoic acid derivative
- **Mechanism of Action:** Induces maturation of promyelocytic cells
- **FDA Approval Date:** November 2, 1995
- **Indications:** APL
- **Dose:** 45 mg/m^2/day in 2 divided doses until complete response (CR)
- **Half-life:** 0.5 to 2 hours
- **Metabolism:** Minor substrates of CYP2B6, CYP2C8, CYP2C9, and CYP2A6; weak inducer of CYPE1
- **Side Effects:** Peripheral edema, cardiac arrhythmia, flushing, headache, skin rash, xeroderma, hypercholesterolemia, transaminitis, APL differentiation syndrome
- **Clinical Pearls:** Steroids should be given in conjunction with ATRA if present with high white blood cell count (WBC) >5,000 due to APL differentiation syndrome.

Alpelisib

- **Alias:** BYL719
- **Brand Name:** Piqray
- **Type Mechanism:** An orally bioavailable PI3K inhibitor that specifically inhibits PIK3 in the PI3K/AKT kinase (or protein kinase B)

signaling pathway, thereby inhibiting the activation of the PI3K signaling pathway. This may result in inhibition of tumor cell growth and survival in susceptible tumor cell populations; inhibits the PI3K-α isoform and much less strongly the β, δ, and γ isoforms.

- **Mechanism of Action:** PI3 kinase inhibitor
- **FDA Approval Date:** May 24, 2019
- **Indications:** Breast cancer, advanced or metastatic (HR positive, HER2 negative, PIK3CA mutated)
- **Dose:** 300 mg PO once daily
- **Half-life:** 8 to 9 hours
- **Metabolism:** Minor CYP3A4 substrate; BCRP/ABCG2 substrate
- **Side Effects:** Hyperglycemia, erythematous rash, xeroderma, edema, stomatitis, nausea/vomiting, diarrhea, fatigue, anorexia, increased lipase, lymphopenia, thrombocytopenia, prolonged partial thromboplastin time (PTT), elevated ALT, increased SCr

Alrizomadlin

- **Alias:** APG 115
- **Type Mechanism:** Activates the p53/p21 pathway to restore p53 function by inhibiting the MDM2, a mouse double minute 2 homolog. This results in potent antiproliferative and apoptogenic activities and induces cell-cycle arrest in p53 wild type (WT).
- **Drug Class:** MDM2 antagonist
- **Phase:** Phase 2
- **Indications:** p53 WT salivary gland carcinoma, relapsed/refractory unresectable or metastatic melanoma, NSCLC, malignant peripheral nerve sheath tumor, liposarcoma, ATM-mutant solid tumors, and urothelial carcinoma
- **Dose:** 100 mg PO every other day (QOD) for 2 weeks on, 1 week off (in combination with pembrolizumab)
- **Side Effects:** Nausea, thrombocytopenia, vomiting, fatigue, loss of appetite, diarrhea, neutropenia, pain in extremity, anemia
- **Clinical Pearls:** It has been granted a fast track designation by the FDA for the treatment of relapsed/refractory unresectable or metastatic melanoma who are relapsed or refractory to prior immune-oncologic agents.

(Rasco et al., 2019)

Altiratinib

- **Alias:** DC-2701; DP-5164
- **Type Mechanism:** Inhibitor of c-Met/hepatocyte growth factor receptor (HGFR), VEGFR2, Tie2 RTK (TIE2), and TRK

- **Drug Class:** Multitargeted TKI
- **Mechanism of Action:** MET/TIE2/VEFGR2/TRK (A, B, C) kinase inhibitor
- **Phase:** Phase 1
- **Indications:** Solid tumors
- **Dose:** PO BID for a 28-day cycle

AMG337

- **Type Mechanism:** A small molecule that inhibit the enzymatic activity of the c-Met tyrosine kinase
- **Drug Class:** c-MET inhibitor
- **Mechanism of Action:** c-Met inhibitor selectively binds to c-Met, thereby disrupting c-Met signal transduction pathways. This may induce cell death in tumor cells overexpressing c-Met protein or expressing constitutively activated c-Met protein.
- **Phase:** Phase 2
- **Indications:** MET-amplified GE junction (GEJ) cancer, gastric cancer, and esophageal cancer
- **Dose:** RP2D: 300 mg PO daily
- **Half-life:** 5.9 to 7 hours
- **Side Effects:** Headache, nausea/vomiting, fatigue, constipation, abdominal pain, peripheral edema, rash

(Kwak et al., 2015)

Amivantamab-vmjw

- **Alias:** JNJ-61186372; 2171511-58-1
- **Brand Name:** Rybrevant
- **Type Mechanism:** A human bispecific antibody (bsAb) targeting both EGFR and HGFR (c-Met) that simultaneously targets and binds to WT or certain mutant forms of both EGFR and c-Met expressed on cancer cells, thereby preventing receptor phosphorylation. This prevents activation of both EGFR- and c-MET–mediated signaling pathways.
- **Drug Class:** EGFR and c-MET inhibitor
- **FDA Approval Date:** May 21, 2021
- **Indications:** Locally advanced or metastatic NSCLC with EGFR exon 20 insertion mutations after failing platinum-based therapy
- **Dose:** Patient <80 kg: week 1–350 mg IV on day 1 and 700 mg IV on day 2; weeks 2 to 4: 1,050 mg IV once weekly; subsequent dosing Q 2 weeks starting from week 5
  - Patient ≥80 kg: week 1–350 mg IV on day 1 and 1,050 mg IV on day 2
- **Half-life:** 11.3 days
- **Side Effects:** Edema; paronychia; skin rash; xeroderma; decreased serum albumin; decreased serum phosphate, magnesium, and sodium; hyperglycemia; nausea; stomatitis; lymphocytopenia; transaminitis; fatigue; peripheral neuropathy

- **Clinical Pearls:** Recommendation for premedications with acetaminophen 650 to 1,000 mg and diphenhydramine 30 minutes before each dose of amivantamab; administer 60 minutes prior with dexamethasone 10 mg or methylprednisolone 40 mg before week 1 on days 1 and 2.

Anastrozole

- **Alias:** ICI-D1033; ZD1033
- **Brand Name:** Arimidex
- **Type Mechanism:** A potent and selective nonsteroidal aromatase inhibitor. By inhibiting aromatase, the conversion of androstenedione to estrone, and testosterone to estradiol, is prevented, thereby decreasing tumor mass or delaying progression in patients with tumors responsive to hormones. Anastrozole can cause an 85% decrease in estrone sulfate levels.
- **Drug Class:** Aromatase inhibitor
- **Mechanism of Action:** A potent and selective nonsteroidal aromatase inhibitor
- **FDA Approval Date:** December 27, 1995
- **Indications:** HR-positive breast cancer; off-label endometrial and uterine carcinoma; off-label recurrent ovarian cancer
- **Dose:** 1 mg PO daily regardless of meals

- **Half-life:** ~50 hours
- **Side Effects:** Hot flash, nausea, GI distress, skin rash, depression, fatigue, headache, mood disorder, pharyngitis, arthralgia, arthritis, hypercholesterolemia, transaminitis, osteoporosis

Andecaliximab (GS-5745)

- **Alias:** GS-5745
- **Type Mechanism:** A mAb that inhibits matrix metalloproteinase 9 (MMP9), an extracellular enzyme involved in matrix remodeling, tumor growth, and metastasis. Increased MMP9 expression is associated with poor prognosis across many malignancies, including gastric cancer.
- **Drug Class:** MMP9 mAb inhibitor
- **Mechanism of Action:** A mAb inhibitor of the MMP9
- **Phase:** Phase 2
- **Indications:** Advanced pancreatic adenocarcinoma, NSCLC, HER2 (−) GEJ adenocarcinoma, and gastric cancer
- **Dose:** 800 mg IV on days 1 and 15 of the 28-day cycle
- **Half-life:** 2.4 to 8.3 days
- **Side Effects:** Neutropenia, diarrhea, fatigue, nausea

(Shah et al., 2018)

Anetumab Ravtansine

- **Alias:** BAY94-9343
- **Type Mechanism:** An ADC that is a fully human anti-mesothelin antibody (MF-T) coupled via a reducible disulfide linker to a microtubule-targeting toxophore DM4, binds to mesothelin with high affinity and delivers the microtubule inhibitor DM4 to mesothelin-positive tumor cells
- **Drug Class:** ADC
- **Mechanism of Action:** Anti-mesothelin ADC
- **Phase:** Phase 2 in mesothelin-expressing solid tumors
- **Indications:** Ovarian cancer, pancreatic cancer, NSCLC; indication for mesothelioma did not meet PFS—clinical trial stopped in July 2017 for mesothelioma
- **Dose:** 6.5 mg/kg IV once Q 3 weeks; 1.8 to 2.2 mg/kg IV Q week
- **Half-life:** 4 to 5 days
- **Side Effects:** Fatigue, weakness, neuropathy, nausea, vomiting, anorexia, keratitis/keratopathy

(Chokshi & Hochster, 2018)

Anlotinib

- **Alias:** ALTN HCl
- **Type Mechanism:** Targets multiple RTKs, including VEGFR2 and VEGFR3

- **Drug Class:** VEGF inhibitor
- **Mechanism of Action:** Receptor TKI of VEGFR2/3; can also inhibit both tumor angiogenesis and tumor cell proliferation.
- **Phase:** Phase 3
- **Indications:** Alveolar soft-part sarcoma, leiomyosarcoma, synovial sarcoma
- **Dose:** 12 mg PO daily for 14 days on, 7 days off
- **Half-life:** 116 hours
- **Side Effects:** HTN, fatigue, thyroid-stimulating hormone (TSH) elevation, anorexia, hypertriglyceridemia, hand-foot syndrome, hypercholesterolemia, GGT elevation

(Han et al., 2018; Shen et al., 2018)

Apalutamide

- **Alias:** ARN-509; JNJ-56021927
- **Brand Name:** Erleada
- **Type Mechanism:** Binds directly to the AR ligand-binding domain to prevent AR translocation, DNA binding, and receptor-mediated transcription. AR inhibition results in decreased proliferation of tumor cells and increased apoptosis, leading to a decrease in tumor volume.
- **Drug Class:** A nonsteroidal AR inhibitor
- **Mechanism of Action:** AR inhibitor

- **FDA Approval Date:** February 14, 2018
- **Indications:** Metastatic castrate-sensitive prostate cancer; non-metastatic castrate-resistant prostate cancer (MCRPC)
- **Dose:** 240 mg PO daily (in combination with androgen deprivation therapy)
- **Half-life:** ~3 days
- **Metabolism:** Major CYP2C8 substrate; potent inducer of CYP2C19, CYP3A4, and P-glycoprotein
- **Side Effects:** HTN, peripheral edema, rash, pruritis, hot flash, hypercholesterolemia, hyperglycemia, hypertriglyceridemia, nausea, anemia, lymphopenia, fatigue, arthralgia

Apatinib

- **Alias:** YN968D1; rivoceranib (international nonproprietary name)
- **Type Mechanism:** Orally bioavailable VEGFR2 (KDR) inhibitor; also mildly inhibits RET, KIT, and SRC
- **Drug Class:** Antiangiogenic TKI
- **Mechanism of Action:** Selectively inhibits VEGFR2
- **Phase:** Phase 3 gastric cancer and HCC; FDA granted orphan status in adenoid cystic carcinoma; phase 2 in CRC
- **FDA Approval Date:** Orphan status for adenoid cystic carcinoma
- **Indications:** Gastric cancer, CRC, adenoid cystic carcinoma, HCC
- **Dose:** 850 mg daily in 2 divided doses; optimum dose seen is 500 mg daily.
- **Half-life:** 9 hours
- **Metabolism:** Extensively by CYP3A4/5
- **Side Effects:** HTN, hand-foot syndrome, diarrhea, anemia, thrombocytopenia, neutropenia, proteinuria, fatigue
- **Clinical Pearls:** UGT1A4 and UT2B7 deficiency may affect metabolism of apatinib.

(Du et al., 2020)

Atezolizumab

- **Alias:** MPDL3280A; RO5541267
- **Brand Name:** Tecentriq
- **Type Mechanism:** A humanized mAb inhibiting PD-L1
- **Drug Class:** A humanized mAb immune checkpoint inhibitor
- **Mechanism of Action:** Binds to PD-L1 to selectively prevent the interaction between the programmed cell death-1 (PD-1) and B7.1. PD-L1 is an immune checkpoint protein expressed on tumor cells and tumor-infiltrating cells and downregulates antitumor T-cell function by binding to PD-1

and B7.1; blocking PD-1 and B7.1 interactions restores antitumor T-cell function.

- **FDA Approval Date:** May 18, 2016
- **Indications:** PD-L1–positive triple-negative breast cancer (TNBC); urothelial cancer ineligible for platinum-containing chemotherapy; metastatic NSCLC; SCLC; metastatic HCC; metastatic melanoma
- **Dose:** 840 mg IV Q 2 weeks; 1,200 mg IV Q 3 weeks; or 1,680 mg IV Q 4 weeks
- **Half-life:** 27 days
- **Side Effects:** Peripheral edema, fatigue, skin rash, hyponatremia, decreased appetite, transaminitis, hyperbilirubinemia, infection
- **Clinical Pearls:** When combining with chemotherapy, administer atezolizumab first

---

Avapritinib

- **Alias:** BLU-285
- **Brand Name:** Ayvakit™
- **Type Mechanism:** A potent TKI that blocks PDGFRα
- **Drug Class:** PDGFRα TKI
- **Mechanism of Action:** Targets PDGFRα and PDGFR D842 mutants, as well as KIT exon 11, 11/17, and 17 mutants. It also inhibits autophosphorylation of KIT D816V and PDGFRα D842V, which are mutants associated with resistance to approved kinase inhibitors.
- **FDA Approval Date:** January 9, 2020
- **Indications:** Metastatic gastrointestinal stromal tumor (GIST) with a PDGFRα exon 18 mutation
- **Dose:** 300 mg PO daily
- **Half-life:** 32 to 57 hours
- **Metabolism:** Major CYP3A4 substrate
- **Side Effects:** Edema, hair discoloration, skin rash, dyspepsia, decreased serum albumin, constipation, decreased appetite, diarrhea, neutropenia, transaminitis, cognitive dysfunction, dizziness, fatigue, headache, sleep disorder
- **Clinical Pearls:** Need antiemetics owing to moderate or high emetogenicity

---

Avelumab

- **Alias:** MSB0010718C
- **Brand Name:** Bavencio
- **Type Mechanism:** Fully human mAb that binds to PD-L1 to selectively prevent the interaction between PD-1 and 7.1 receptors, resulting in the restoration of antitumor T-cell function
- **Drug Class:** Anti–PD-L1 mAb
- **FDA Approval Date:** March 23, 2017

- **Indications:** Metastatic Merkel cell carcinoma; locally, advanced, or metastatic urothelial carcinoma following platinum therapy; advanced renal cell carcinoma (RCC)
- **Dose:** 10 mg/kg IV over 60 minutes Q 2 weeks (for gestational trophoblastic neoplasia chemotherapy resistant) or 800 mg (FLAT dose) IV Q 2 weeks; should premedicate with acetaminophen and diphenhydramine for the first four infusions
- **Half-life:** 6.1 days
- **Side Effects:** Peripheral edema, HTN, fatigue, dizziness, skin rash, nausea, diarrhea, hyponatremia, decreased appetite, abdominal pain, transaminitis, arthralgia, infusion-related reaction with chills, fevers

---

Axicabtagene Ciloleucel

- **Alias:** KTE-C19 CAR; axicel
- **Brand Name:** Yescarta
- **Type Mechanism:** A CD19-directed genetically modified autologous T-cell immunotherapy in which a patient's T cells are reprogrammed with a transgene encoding a CAR to identify and eliminate CD19-expressing malignant and normal cells
- **Drug Class:** CAR T-cell immunotherapy
- **Mechanism of Action:** A preparation of autologous peripheral blood T lymphocytes that have been transduced with a γ-retroviral vector expressing a CAR consisting of an anti-CD19 scFv coupled to the costimulatory signaling domain CD28 and the ζ chain of the TCR/CD3 complex (CD3-ζ), resulting in immunostimulation
- **FDA Approval Date:** October 18, 2017
- **Indications:** Relapsed/refractory follicular lymphoma (FL); relapsed/refractory large B-cell lymphoma
- **Dose:** A treatment course consists of lymphodepleting chemotherapy with fludarabine and cyclophosphamide on the fifth, fourth, and third day before axicabtagene ciloleucel infusion (confirm the availability of autologous axicabtagene ciloleucel before initiating).
- **Half-life:** Duration: Anti-CD19 CAR T cells displayed an initial rapid expansion followed by a decline to near baseline levels by 3 months after axicabtagene ciloleucel infusion. Peak level of anti-CD19 CAR T cells occurred within the 7 to 14 days after infusion.
- **Side Effects:** Cytokine release syndrome (CRS), tachycardia; neurologic toxicities, such as cerebral edema, ataxia, blurred vision, headaches; hypotension;

hypogammaglobulinemia; fatigue; nausea; abdominal pain

- **Clinical Pearls:** Premedications with acetaminophen and diphenhydramine before infusion; tocilizumab should be on standby before infusion and after. No prophylactic steroids allowed owing to possible interference with axicabtagene ciloleucel.

Axitinib

- **Alias:** AG-013736
- **Brand Name:** Inlyta
- **Type Mechanism:** Selective second-generation, orally bioavailable inhibitor of VEGFRs (VEGFR-1, VEGFR-2, and VEGFR-3), PDGFR, and KIT
- **Drug Class:** VEGF TKI
- **FDA Approval Date:** January 27, 2012
- **Indications:** Advanced RCC; off-label use for differentiated thyroid cancer
- **Dose:** Optimum dose is 10 mg PO BID; recommend to dose escalate Q 2 weeks starting at 5 mg.
- **Half-life:** 2 to 6 hours
- **Metabolism:** Major CYP3A4 substrate and UGT1A1 substrate
- **Side Effects:** Diarrhea, HTN, fatigue, decreased appetite, palmar–plantar erythrodysesthesia, skin rash, stomatitis,

hypothyroidism, transaminitis, increased SCr, nausea/vomiting

- **Clinical Pearls:** Dysphonia (hoarseness) may occur while taking. Advise patients to avoid irritants and to drink plenty of fluids.

Belagenpumatucel-L

- **Brand Name:** Lucanix
- **Type Mechanism:** A therapeutic, gene-modified, allogeneic cell vaccine composing of four NSCLC cell lines (two adenocarcinoma, one large cell carcinoma, and one squamous cell carcinoma [SCC]), transfected by a TGF-β2 antisense plasmid, and then expanded, irradiated with 100 Gy and frozen. The vaccine promotes the suppression of NSCLC cells by the activation of a cytotoxic T lymphocyte (CTL) response and enhancing the immune response due to the suppression of TGF-β2 messenger RNA (mRNA) produced by tumor cells.
- **Drug Class:** Allogeneic cancer vaccine
- **Mechanism of Action:** Belagenpumatucel-L may elicit a CTL response against host NSCLC cells, resulting in decreased tumor cell proliferation; vaccine immunogenicity may be potentiated by suppression of tumor TGF-β2 production by antisense RNA

expressed by the vaccine plasmid TGF-β2 antisense transgene.

- **Phase:** Phase 3 in NSCLC
- **Indications:** Advanced NSCLC (adenocarcinoma, SCC, and large cell carcinoma)
- **Dose:** 1.25, 2.5, or 5×10^7 cells given as intradermal injection once a month or once Q other month for total maximum injection of 16
- **Side Effects:** Local injection site reaction such as erythema and induration, rash

(Decoster et al., 2012; Giaccone et al., 2015)

Belantamab Mafodotin

- **Alias:** GSK2857916; J6M0-mcMMAF
- **Brand Name:** Blenrep
- **Type Mechanism:** An afucosylated, humanized ADC directed against B-cell maturation antigen (BCMA); BCMA is expressed on MM cells but is mostly absent on naive and memory B cells. The antibody is conjugated by a protease-resistant maleimidocaproyl linker to microtubule-disrupting monomethyl auristatin F (MMAF).
- **Drug Class:** ADC
- **FDA Approval Date:** August 5, 2020
- **Indications:** Relapsed/refractory MM
- **Dose:** 2.5 mg/kg IV Q 3 weeks
- **Half-life:** 14 days
- **Side Effects:** Hypoalbuminemia, hypokalemia, hyponatremia, increased GGT, hyperglycemia, anemia, lymphocytopenia, thrombocytopenia, increased AST, increased alkaline phosphatase (ALP), fatigue, arthralgias, asthenia, blurred vision, epithelial keratopathy

Belinostat

- **Alias:** PXD101
- **Brand Name:** Beleodaq
- **Type Mechanism:** A novel hydroxamic acid–type HDAC inhibitor that targets HDAC enzymes, thereby inhibiting tumor cell proliferation, inducing apoptosis, promoting cellular differentiation, and inhibiting angiogenesis
- **Drug Class:** HDAC inhibitor
- **Mechanism of Action:** An HDAC inhibitor that catalyzes acetyl group removal from protein lysine residues (of histone and some nonhistone proteins). Inhibition of HDAC results in accumulation of acetyl groups, leading to cell-cycle arrest and apoptosis. Belinostat has preferential cytotoxicity toward tumor cells versus normal cells.
- **FDA Approval Date:** July 3, 2014

- **Indications:** Relapsed/refractory PTCL
- **Dose:** 1,000 mg/m^2 IV on days 1 to 5 Q 21 days
- **Half-life:** 1.1 hours
- **Metabolism:** Weak substrates of CYP2C9, CYP3A4, P-glycoprotein/ABCB1, and UGT1A1
- **Side Effects:** Peripheral edema, prolonged QT, fatigue, chills, headache, rash, pruritus, hypokalemia, anemia, thrombocytopenia, dyspnea, fevers, hypotension, elevated SCr
- **Clinical Pearls:** Dose only if absolute neutrophil count (ANC) is ≥1,000/mm^3 and platelets ≥50,000/mm^3. NOTE: If the patient is homozygous for UGT1A1*28 allele, reduce the initial dose to 750 mg/m^2.

Belizatinib

- **Alias:** TSR-011; UN2-Z8A6022P3J
- **Type Mechanism:** Dual, potent inhibitor of ALK and TRKA, TRKB, and TRKC, including crizotinib-resistant ALK mutations
- **Drug Class:** ALK inhibitor
- **Phase:** Phase 2
- **Indications:** ALK-positive NSCLC
- **Dose:** RP2D: 40 mg PO Q 8 hours
- **Half-life:** 7 to 27 hours
- **Metabolism:** CYP3A4 and CYP2D6 inhibitors

- **Side Effects:** QT prolongation, constipation, decreased appetite, vomiting, fatigue

(Weiss et al., 2014)

Bemarituzumab

- **Alias:** FPA144
- **Type Mechanism:** A glycoengineered, humanized mAb directed against the FGFR2b that specifically binds to and inhibits FGFR2b on tumor cell surfaces, which prevents FGFR2 from binding to its ligands, FGFR2b activation, and the activation of FGFR2b-mediated signal transduction pathways. The binding of bemarituzumab to FGFR2b protein also induces ADCC against FGFR2b-expressing tumor cells.
- **Phase:** Phase 2/3
- **Indications:** GE adenocarcinoma or gastric carcinoma with FGFR2b overexpression
- **Dose:** 15 mg/kg IV Q 2 weeks in combination with mFOLFOX
- **Half-life:** 12.8 days
- **Side Effects:** Fatigue, nausea, dry eyes, anemia, neutropenia, increased AST, vomiting, infusion reaction

(Catenacci et al., 2020)

Bempegaldesleukin

- **Type Mechanism:** A PEGylated interleukin-2 (IL-2) acting as a CD122-preferential IL-2 pathway agonist designed to activate and proliferate CD8$^+$ T cells and NK cells
- **Phase:** Phase 3
- **Indications:** Metastatic melanoma
- **Dose:** 0.006 mg/kg IV Q 3 weeks
- **Half-life:** 20 hours
- **Side Effects:** Flulike symptoms, rash, fatigue, hypotension

(Khushalani et al., 2020)

Berzosertib

- **Alias:** VX-970; M6620
- **Type Mechanism:** An inhibitor of ataxia telangiectasia and rad3-related (ATR) kinase, a DNA damage response kinase that selectively binds to and inhibits ATR kinase activity and prevents ATR-mediated signaling in the ATR-checkpoint kinase 1 (CHK1) signaling pathway. This prevents DNA damage checkpoint activation, disrupts DNA damage repair, and induces tumor cell apoptosis.
- **Drug Class:** ATR inhibitor
- **Phase:** Phase 2
- **Indications:** mCRC, small-cell neuroendocrine cancers, platinum-resistant SCLC, and platinum-resistant serous ovarian cancer harboring molecular aberrations, including ATM loss and an ARID1A mutation
- **Dose:** 240 mg/m^2 IV once weekly or twice weekly as monotherapy or 90 mg/m^2 IV weekly (combined with carboplatin AUC5)
- **Half-life:** 18.5 hours for once weekly dosing; 12.8 hours for twice weekly dosing; 14.3 hours for combination therapy
- **Side Effects:** Flushing, nausea, pruritus, headache, infusion-related side effects, such as flushing, fatigue, thrombocytopenia, neutropenia, and anemia

(Yap et al., 2020)

Bevacizumab

- **Brand Name:** Avastin
- **Type Mechanism:** A recombinant humanized mAb directed against the VEGF, a proangiogenic cytokine
  - Binds to VEGF and inhibits receptor binding, thereby preventing the growth and maintenance of tumor blood vessels
- **Drug Class:** VEGF inhibitor
- **FDA Approval Date:** February 26, 2004
- **Indications:** Colon, lung, and renal carcinomas and glioblastoma multiforme
- **Dose:** 5 to 10 mg/kg IV Q 2 weeks or 15 mg/kg IV Q 3 weeks
- **Half-life:** 20 days

- **Side Effects:** HTN, severe or fatal hemorrhage (GI bleed, hemoptysis, central nervous system [CNS] bleed), bowel perforation, fistulas/abscess formation, proteinuria
- **Clinical Pearls:** Have patients monitor blood pressure and bring the log to appointments. Avoid use in patients with severe hypertension requiring multiple antihypertensive medications for control.

BI 811283

- **Type Mechanism:** Binds to and inhibits Aurora kinases, resulting in disruption of the assembly of the mitotic spindle apparatus, disruption of chromosome segregation, and inhibition of cell proliferation
- **Drug Class:** AURKB inhibitor
- **Mechanism of Action:** A small-molecule inhibitor of the serine/threonine protein kinase Aurora kinase
- **Phase:** Phase 1
- **Dose:** 230 mg as 24-hour continuous infusion on day 1 of a 21-day cycle
- **Half-life:** 12 to 26 hours
- **Side Effects:** Neutropenia, leukopenia, febrile neutropenia, fatigue, alopecia, diarrhea, decreased appetite

(Mross et al., 2016)

Bicalutamide

- **Alias:** CDX; ICI-176334
- **Brand Name:** Casodex
- **Type Mechanism:** A pure nonsteroidal AR inhibitor, specifically a competitive inhibitor for the binding of dihydrotestosterone and testosterone
- **Drug Class:** Antiandrogen
- **FDA Approval Date:** October 4, 1995
- **Indications:** Metastatic prostate cancer
- **Dose:** 50 mg PO daily
- **Half-life:** 6 days
- **Metabolism:** Substrate of CYP3A4
- **Side Effects:** AST and ALT increase, hyperbilirubinemia, ALP increase, nausea, pain (bone, back, pelvis), anorexia, fatigue, diarrhea, hot flashes, limb edema
- **Clinical Pearls:** Use in combination with luteinizing hormone–releasing hormone (LHRH) analog such as leuprolide.

Binimetinib

- **Alias:** ARRY-162; MEK162; ARRY-43162
- **Type Mechanism:** An orally available inhibitor of MEK1/2 prevents the activation of MEK1/2-dependent effector proteins and transcription factors, which may result in the inhibition of growth factor–mediated cell

signaling. This may eventually lead to an inhibition of tumor cell proliferation and an inhibition in the production of various inflammatory cytokines, including IL-1, IL-6, and tumor necrosis factor (TNF).

- **Drug Class:** MEK1/2 inhibitor
- **FDA Approval Date:** June 27, 2018
- **Indications:** Unresectable or metastatic melanoma; off-label use for metastatic, refractory, RAS WT, and BRAF V600E–mutant CRC
- **Dose:** 45 mg PO Q 12 hours
- **Half-life:** 3.5 hours
- **Metabolism:** BCRP/ABCG2 substrate; UGT1A1 substrate
- **Side Effects:** Skin rash, fatigue, dermatitis acneiform, peripheral edema, diarrhea, nausea, elevated CPK, anemia, increased GGT, transaminitis
- **Clinical Pearls:** Use in combination with encorafenib in melanoma.

Bintrafusp Alfa

- **Alias:** M7824; MSB0011359C
- **Type Mechanism:** A first-in-class bifunctional fusion protein composed of the extracellular domain of TGF-β receptor 2 (a TGF-β "trap") fused to a human IgG1 antibody blocking PD-L1
- **Drug Class:** TGF-β/PD-L1 inhibitor
- **Phase:** Phase 1/2
- **Indications:** NSCLC; biliary tract cancer including ampullary cancer, intrahepatic and extrahepatic cholangiocarcinoma
- **Dose:** RP2D: 1,200 mg IV Q 2 weeks
- **Side Effects:** Rash, fever, maculopapular rash, increased lipase, pruritis

(Vugmeyster et al., 2020)

Blinatumomab

- **Alias:** MEDI-538; MT-103; AMG-103
- **Brand Name:** Blincyto
- **Type Mechanism:** A recombinant, single-chain, anti-CD19/anti-CD3 bispecific mAb that possesses two antigen-recognition sites, one for the CD3 complex, a group of T-cell surface glycoproteins that complex with the TCR, and one for CD19, a TAA overexpressed on the surface of B cells
- **Mechanism of Action:** It activates endogenous T cells by connecting CD3 in the TCR complex with CD19 on B cells (malignant and benign), thus forming a cytolytic synapse between a cytotoxic T cell and the cancer target B cell. It mediates the production of cytolytic proteins, release of inflammatory cytokines, and proliferation of T cells, which result in a lysis of CD19-positive cells.

- **FDA Approval Date:** December 4, 2014
- **Indications:** Relapsed/refractory acute lymphoblastic leukemia with CD19$^+$ disease
- **Dose:** Patients ≥45 kg: cycles 1 to 4: 28 mcg IV continuous infusion on days 1 to 28 of a 6-week cycle. Patients <45 kg: cycles 1 to 4: 15 mcg/m^2/day (max 28 mcg/day) IV continuous infusion on days 1 to 28 of a 6-week cycle
- **Half-life:** 2 hours
- **Side Effects:** Edema, HTN, cardiac arrhythmia, headache, rash, headache, pyrexia, tremors, fatigue, lymphopenia, CRS, infusion-related side effects, fever
- **Clinical Pearls:** Premedications with IV equivalent of 100 mg prednisone 1 hour before first dose of each cycle.

BMS-936559

- **Alias:** MDX1105
- **Type Mechanism:** High-affinity, fully humanized PD-L1–specific IgG4 mAb that inhibits the binding of PD-L1 to both PD-1 and CD80
- **Phase:** No active clinical trials for cancer in the United States; previous studies in melanoma and hematologic malignancies were withdrawn.
- **Indications:** Advanced solid tumors, especially melanoma, RCC, NSCLC, and ovarian cancer

- **Dose:** 0.3 to 10 mg/kg as 60-minute infusion Q 2 weeks
- **Half-life:** 15 days
- **Side Effects:** Rash, pruritis, hypothyroidism related to hypophysitis, hepatitis, diarrhea
- **Clinical Pearls:** May require antihistamines and antipyretics as premedications

(Brahmer et al., 2012; Gay et al., 2017)

Bortezomib

- **Alias:** PS-341; MLN341
- **Brand Name:** Velcade
- **Type Mechanism:** Reversibly inhibits the 26S proteasome, a large protease complex that degrades ubiquitinated protein with an unusual boron "backbone"
  - Inhibits nuclear factor NFκB, a protein that is constitutively activated in some cancers, thereby interfering with NFκB-mediated cell survival, tumor growth, and angiogenesis
- **Drug Class:** Proteasome inhibitor
- **FDA Approval Date:** May 13, 2003
- **Indications:** MCL; MM: Off label for mycosis fungoides, relapsed/refractory FL, relapsed/refractory PTCL, systemic light-chain amyloidosis, and Waldenström macroglobulinemia
- **Dose:** 1.3 mg/m^2 IV or subcutaneous (SC) twice weekly (Days 1, 4, 8, 11, 22, 25, 29, and

32 of a 42-day cycle for 4 cycles, then 1.3 mg/m^2 IV on days 1, 8, 22, and 29 of a 42-day cycle for 5 cycles)
- **Half-life:** 76 to 108 hours
- **Metabolism:** Major substrate of CYP3A4
- **Side Effects:** Peripheral neuropathy, neutropenia, thrombocytopenia, neuralgia, paresthesia, skin rash, diarrhea, nausea/vomiting, anorexia, anemia, herpes zoster reactivation
- **Clinical Pearls:** Consider using SC route if patient has high risk for peripheral neuropathy; NOTE: Reconstituted concentrations for IV and SC administration are different.

Bosutinib

- **Alias:** SKI-606
- **Brand Name:** Bosulif
- **Type Mechanism:** BCR-ABL inhibitor with activities against SRC family (including SRC, LYN, and HCK); very minimal activity in KIT and PDGFR
  - Activity in 16 of 18 imatinib-resistant BCR-ABL mutations, with exception being the T315I and V299L mutants
- **Drug Class:** BCR-ABL TKI
- **FDA Approval Date:** September 4, 2012
- **Indications:** Ph+ chronic myelogenous leukemia (CML)
- **Dose:** 400 mg PO daily for newly diagnosed Ph+ CML; 500 mg PO daily for Ph+ CML resistant or intolerant to prior therapy
- **Half-life:** 22 to 27 hours
- **Metabolism:** Major CYP3A4 substrate
- **Side Effects:** Nausea/vomiting (moderate-to-high emetogenicity), diarrhea, edema, myelosuppression, skin rash, abdominal pain, pyrexia, transaminitis, chest pain, anemia, neutropenia, thrombocytopenia, fatigue, arthralgia

Brentuximab Vedotin

- **Alias:** SGN-35
- **Brand Name:** Adcetris
- **Type Mechanism:** An ADC directed at CD30 consisting of three components: (1) a CD30-specific chimeric IgG1 antibody cAC10; (2) a microtubule-disrupting agent, MMAE; and (3) a protease-cleavable dipeptide linker (which covalently conjugates MMAE to cAC10). The conjugate binds to cells that express CD30 and forms a complex that is internalized within the cell and releases MMAE. MMAE binds to the tubules and disrupts the cellular microtubule network, inducing cell-cycle arrest (G2/M phase) and apoptosis.

- **Drug Class:** ADC
- **FDA Approval Date:** August 19, 2011
- **Indications:** Anaplastic large cell lymphoma (ALCL) (relapsed primary cutaneous, untreated), CD30-expressing mycosis fungoides and PTCL, or Hodgkin lymphoma (previously untreated, relapsed/refractory, consolidation post-transplant)
- **Dose:** 1.8 mg/kg (cap at max weight of 100 kg) as IV infusion Q 3 weeks; 1.2 mg/kg for mild hepatic impairment or advanced, previously untreated Hodgkin lymphoma
- **Half-life:** 4 to 6 hours for ADC; 3 to 4 hours for the MMAE payload
- **Metabolism:** Minor CYP3A4 and P-glycoprotein substrates
- **Side Effects:** Myelosuppression, fatigue, infusion-related side effects, nausea/vomiting, diarrhea, peripheral sensory/motor neuropathy, pyrexia, pruritus, maculopapular rash
- **Clinical Pearls:** Peripheral neuropathy is generally cumulative. Dose interruption, reduction, or discontinuation may be recommended.

Brexucabtagene Autoleucel

- **Alias:** KTE-X19
- **Brand Name:** Tecartus

- **Type Mechanism:** A CD19-directed genetically modified autologous T-cell immunotherapy in which a patient's T cells are reprogrammed with a transgene encoding a CAR to identify and eliminate CD19-expressing malignant and normal cells. The CAR is composed of a murine single-chain antibody fragment that recognizes CD19 and is fused to CD28 and CD3-ζ. CD3-ζ is a critical component for initiating T-cell activation and antitumor activity. After binding to CD19-expressing cells, the CD28 and CD3-ζ costimulatory domains activate downstream signaling cascades, which results in T-cell activation, proliferation, acquisition of effector functions, and secretion of inflammatory cytokines and chemokines, leading to destruction of CD19-expressing cells.
- **Drug Class:** CAR T-cell immunotherapy
- **FDA Approval Date:** July 24, 2021
- **Indications:** Relapsed/refractory MCL
- **Dose:** Target dose: 2×10^6 CAR-positive viable T cells per kg body weight (BW); maximum dose: 2×10^8 CAR-positive viable T cells
- **Half-life:** 3 months post cell infusion
- **Side Effects:** Edema, HTN, hypotension, thrombosis, skin rash,

hypocalcemia, hyponatremia, hypophosphatemia, increased uric acid, transaminitis, constipation or diarrhea, nausea, anemia, hypogammaglobulinemia, leukopenia, neutropenia, thrombocytopenia, CRS, musculoskeletal pain, fever
- **Clinical Pearls:** Prophylaxis with antibiotic until ANC is >1,000 or 1 month post cell infusion; *Pneumocystis jiroveci* pneumonia (PJP) and antiviral prophylaxis for 1 year post cell infusion

Brigatinib

- **Alias:** AP26113
- **Brand Name:** Alunbrig
- **Type Mechanism:** A broad-spectrum multikinase inhibitor with activity against ALK, ROS1, IGF-1R, and FLT-3, as well as EGFR deletion and point mutations. ALK autophosphorylation and ALK-mediated phosphorylation of downstream signaling proteins STAT3, AKT, ERK1/2, and S6 are inhibited by brigatinib.
- **Mechanism of Action:** ALK and EGFR kinase inhibitor. ALK is a member of the insulin receptor superfamily.
- **FDA Approval Date:** April 28, 2017
- **Indications:** ALK(+), metastatic NSCLC

- **Dose:** 90 mg PO daily for 7 days. If tolerated, may continue to full dose at 180 mg PO daily
- **Half-life:** 25 hours
- **Metabolism:** Major CYP3A4 substrate; BCRP/ABCG2 substrate
- **Side Effects:** HTN, fatigue, headache, peripheral neuropathy, skin rash including palmar–plantar erythrodysesthesia, hyperglycemia, transaminitis, constipation or diarrhea, nausea, anemia, lymphocytopenia, cough, prolonged PTT, neutropenia, bradycardia, angioedema, pruritus

Brivanib Alaninate

- **Alias:** BMS-582664
- **Type Mechanism:** The alaninate salt of a VEGFR2 inhibitor that strongly binds to and inhibits VEGFR2 and FGFR tyrosine kinases
- **Mechanism of Action:** VEGFR2 and FGFR dual inhibitor
- **Phase:** Phase 2
- **Indications:** Cervical cancer, endometrial cancer, STS, ovarian cancer, HCC
- **Dose:** 800 mg PO daily
- **Half-life:** 13.8 hours
- **Side Effects:** Nausea/vomiting, diarrhea, constipation, fatigue, transaminitis, HTN, thrombocytopenia

(Jonker et al., 2007)

Bryostatin 1

- **Alias:** B705008K112
- **Type Mechanism:** A macrocyclic lactone isolated from the bryozoan *Bugula neritina* that binds to and inhibits the cell signaling enzyme PKC, resulting in the inhibition of tumor cell proliferation, promotion of tumor cell differentiation, and induction of tumor cell apoptosis. This agent may act synergistically with other chemotherapeutic agents.
- **Mechanism of Action:** Protein kinase C inhibitor
- **Indications:** Metastatic breast cancer, cervical cancer, pancreatic cancer
- **Dose:** RP2D: 24 mcg/m^2 IV over 5 days, 16 mcg/m^2 IV over 6 days, and 8 mcg/m^2 IV over 14 days
- **Side Effects:** Myalgias, nausea, vomiting, fatigue, myelosuppression, ALT/AST elevation

(El-Rayes et al., 2006)

Buparlisib

- **Alias:** BKM120
- **Type Mechanism:** Inhibits class I PIK3 in the PI3K/AKT kinase (or protein kinase B) signaling pathway in an adenosine triphosphate (ATP)-competitive manner, thereby inhibiting the production of the secondary messenger PIP3 and activation of the PI3K signaling pathway. This may result in inhibition of tumor cell growth and survival in susceptible tumor cell populations.
- **Mechanism of Action:** Pan-PI3K inhibitor
- **Phase:** Phase 2/3
- **Indications:** HER2—advanced, metastatic breast cancer; platinum-pretreated recurrent or metastatic SCCHN
- **Dose:** 100 mg PO daily in combination with fulvestrant. Take dose 1 hour after breakfast and fast for 2 hours after dosing.
- **Half-life:** 40 hours
- **Metabolism:** Moderate/reversible inhibitor of CYP3A4
- **Side Effects:** Rash, anorexia, mood alteration, diarrhea, hyperglycemia, elevated ALT, fatigue, pyrexia, pneumonitis
- **Clinical Pearls:** Studies in advanced breast cancer in combination with paclitaxel did not show improvement in PFS. Trial was stopped at the end of phase 2.

(Martín et al., 2017)

Cabozantinib

- **Alias:** XL-184

- **Brand Name:** Cometriq (for MTC); Cabometyx (for HCC and RCC)
- **Type Mechanism:** Potent inhibitor of RTKs, including AXL, FLT-3, KIT, MET, RET, TIE-2, TRKB, and VEGFR-1, VEGFR-2, and VEGFR-3. It induces apoptosis of cancer cells and suppresses tumor growth, metastasis, and angiogenesis.
- **Drug Class:** Multikinase inhibitor
- **Mechanism of Action:** Multikinase inhibitor
- **FDA Approval Date:** November 29, 2012
- **Indications:** Advanced HCC and RCC; metastatic MTC
- **Dose:** HCC dosing: 60 mg PO daily; RCC dosing: 40 mg PO daily with nivolumab or 60 mg PO daily (monotherapy); MTC dosing: 140 mg PO daily
- **Half-life:** Cometriq = ~55 hours; Cabometyx = ~99 hours
- **Metabolism:** Major CYP3A4 substrate
- **Side Effects:** Hemorrhage, perforation/fistula (U.S. box warning), HTN, stomatitis, palmar–plantar erythrodysesthesia, decreased appetite, weight loss, nausea/vomiting, diarrhea, tiredness and weakness, change in hair color, liver dysfunction (hyperbilirubinemia, transaminitis, increases alkaline phosphatase)
- **Clinical Pearls:** May affect the rate of wound healing; patients should notify doctor before surgery or dental work; moderate-to-high emetogenicity.

Camrelizumab

- **Alias:** SHR-1211
- **Type Mechanism:** An mAb directed against PD-1 (PCD-1) that binds to and blocks the binding of PD-1, expressed on activated T lymphocytes, B cells, and NK cells, to its ligands PD-L1, overexpressed on certain cancer cells, and PD-L2, which is primarily expressed on antigen-presenting cells (APCs). This prevents the activation of PD-1 and its downstream signaling pathways. Activation of CTLs and cell-mediated immune responses against tumor cells or pathogens.
- **Drug Class:** Checkpoint inhibitor
- **Mechanism of Action:** Monoclonal PD-1 inhibitor
- **Phase:** Phase 2/3
- **Indications:** Advanced SCC, NSCLC, HCC, advanced cervical cancer, and Hodgkin lymphoma
- **Dose:** 200 mg IV Q 2 weeks
- **Half-life:** 3 to 11 days
- **Side Effects:** Hyperbilirubinemia, stomatitis, anemia, diarrhea, increased ALT/AST, leukopenia, thrombocytopenia, rash, hyponatremia, hypochloremia

(Jackson et al., 2018)

Capivasertib

- **Alias:** AZD5363
- **Type Mechanism:** A novel pyrrolopyrimidine derivative and an inhibitor of the serine/threonine protein kinase AKT (protein kinase B) that binds to and inhibits all AKT isoforms. Inhibition of AKT prevents the phosphorylation of AKT substrates that mediate cellular processes, such as cell division, apoptosis, and glucose and fatty acid metabolism.
- **Drug Class:** Oral AKT inhibitor
- **Phase:** Phase 3 in combination with fulvestrant in metastatic ER+/Her2− breast cancer; advanced/metastatic TNBC; phase 3 meningioma
- **Indications:** TNBC; ER+/HER2− metastatic breast cancer
- **Dose:** RP2D: 480 mg PO BID for 4 days on, 3 days off for 21 days
- **Half-life:** 10 hours (range 7–15 hours)
- **Side Effects:** Maculopapular rash, hyperglycemia, diarrhea, nausea, neutropenia, fatigue

(Smyth et al., 2020)

Capmatinib

- **Alias:** INCB028060; INC280
- **Brand Name:** Tabrecta
- **Type Mechanism:** A potent and highly selective inhibitor of MET, including the mutant variant produced by exon 14 skipping. MET exon 14 skipping results in increased downstream MET signaling. It also decreases cancer cell growth and inhibits MET phosphorylation triggered by binding of c-MET (also known as hepatocyte growth factor or HGF) or by MET amplification, as well as MET-mediated phosphorylation of downstream signaling proteins.
- **Drug Class:** MET inhibitor
- **FDA Approval Date:** May 6, 2020
- **Indications:** Metastatic NSCLC with mutation that leads to MET exon 14 skipping
- **Dose:** 400 mg PO BID
- **Half-life:** 6.5 hours
- **Metabolism:** Major CYP3A4 substrate; moderate CYP1A2 inhibitor; P-glycoprotein/ABCB1 inhibitor
- **Side Effects:** Pneumonitis, peripheral leg swelling, nausea, fatigue, vomiting, amylase/lipase elevation, anemia, lymphocytopenia, transaminitis, dyspnea, decreased appetite

Carfilzomib

- **Alias:** PR-171
- **Brand Name:** Kyprolis

- **Type Mechanism:** It inhibits proteasomes, which are responsible for intracellular protein homeostasis. It is a potent, selective, and irreversible inhibitor of chymotrypsin-like activity of the 20S proteasome, leading to cell-cycle arrest and apoptosis.
- **Drug Class:** Proteasome inhibitor
- **FDA Approval Date:** July 20, 2012
- **Indications:** Relapsed/refractory MM
- **Dose:** Cycle 1: 20 mg/m^2 IV on days 1 and 2, then increase to 27 mg/m^2 IV on Days 8, 9, 15, and 16 of 28 days; cycles 2 to 12: 27 mg/m^2 on days 1, 2, 8, 9, 15, and 16 of 28 days; cycle 13+: 27 mg/m^2 IV on days 1, 2, 15, and 16 of 28 days
- **Half-life:** <1 hour on cycle 1 day 1 dose. Proteasome inhibition effect can last up to 48 hours.
- **Metabolism:** Mainly extrahepatic elimination, insignificant CYP metabolism
- **Side Effects:** Fatigue, myelosuppression, nausea/vomiting, diarrhea, pyrexia, increased creatinine, back pain, URI (cough, pneumonia, DOE)
- **Clinical Pearls:** Need premedication with dexamethasone before each dose in cycle 1, then as needed. Maintain adequate hydration and prophylaxis against TLS.

Cediranib Maleate

- **Alias:** AZD 2171
- **Brand Name:** Recentin (tentative trade name)
- **Type Mechanism:** A potent VEGF RTK inhibitor of all three VEGF receptors (VEGFR-1, VEGFR-2, and VEGFR-3). Inhibition of VEGF signaling leads to the inhibition of angiogenesis, lymphangiogenesis, neovascular survival, and vascular permeability. Cediranib also inhibits c-Kit tyrosine kinase.
- **Drug Class:** VEGFR inhibitor
- **Phase:** Phase 2/3; phase 3 monotherapy versus lomustine combination did not show PFS benefit.
- **Indications:** Advanced ovarian cancer with platinum resistance, fallopian tube cancer, and peritoneal cancer; mCRC
- **Dose:** 30 or 45 mg PO daily (20 mg when combined with cytotoxic chemotherapy)
- **Half-life:** 12 to 35 hours
- **Side Effects:** Fatigue, diarrhea, nausea, dysphonia, HTN (proteinuria), neutropenia

(Batchelor et al., 2013)

Cemiplimab

- **Alias:** REGN2810
- **Brand Name:** Libtayo™

- **Type Mechanism:** A recombinant human IgG4 mAb that inhibits PD-1 activity by binding to PD-1 and blocking the interactions with the ligands PD-L1 and PD-L2, releasing PD-1 pathway–mediated inhibition of immune response, including antitumor response
- **Drug Class:** Anti–PD-1 mAb
- **FDA Approval Date:** September 28, 2018
- **Indications:** Locally advanced, metastatic basal cell carcinoma or cutaneous SCC; metastatic NSCLC with high PD-L1 expressions
- **Dose:** 350 mg IV day 1 of Q 3 weeks
- **Half-life:** ~20 days
- **Side Effects:** HTN, pruritus, skin rash, diarrhea, nausea, anemia, fatigue, arthralgia, muscle pain, cough, pneumonia versus pneumonitis

Ceritinib

- **Alias:** LDK378
- **Brand Name:** Zykadia
- **Type Mechanism:** An orally available inhibitor of the RTK activity of ALK that binds to and inhibits WT ALK, ALK fusion proteins, and ALK point mutation variants. Inhibition of ALK leads to both the disruption of ALK-mediated signaling and the inhibition of cell growth in ALK-overexpressing tumor cells.
- **Drug Class:** ALK inhibitor
- **FDA Approval Date:** April 29, 2014
- **Indications:** Metastatic NSCLC with ALK-positive mutation
- **Dose:** 450 mg PO daily with food
- **Half-life:** 41 hours
- **Metabolism:** Major CYP3A4 substrate and major CYP3A4 inhibitor
- **Side Effects:** QT prolongation, nausea/vomiting, abdominal pain, diarrhea, neuropathy, fatigue, skin rash, hyperglycemia, increased lipase, transaminitis, hyperbilirubinemia, visual impairment

Cetuximab

- **Alias:** C225; IMC-C225
- **Brand Name:** Erbitux
- **Type Mechanism:** A recombinant human/mouse chimeric mAb that binds specifically to EGFR (HER1, c-ErbB-1) and competitively inhibits the binding of EGF and other ligands
- **Drug Class:** EGFR inhibitor
- **FDA Approval Date:** February 12, 2004
- **Indications:** KRAS WT CRC; SCCHN; off label for RAS WT, BRAF V600E–mutated CRC, SCC of the penis, and SCC of the skin

- **Dose:** Weekly dose: 400 mg/m^2 as 120-minute IV infusion as an initial dose, followed by 250 mg/m^2 infused over 30 minutes weekly. Biweekly dose: 500 mg/m^2 IV over 120 minutes once Q 2 weeks
- **Half-life:** ~112 hours
- **Side Effects:** Infusion reactions (U.S. box warning), nausea/vomiting, diarrhea, skin problems (acneiform rash, pruritus), hypomagnesemia, stomatitis, lung disease (dyspnea, cough), fatigue, neutropenia, transaminitis, palmar–plantar erythrodysesthesia, xeroderma
- **Clinical Pearls:** Severity of acneiform rash can be minimized with the use of topical steroid cream, topical antibiotic gel, and doxycycline.

Cevostamab

- **Alias:** BFCR4350A
- **Type Mechanism:** A humanized IgG-based T-cell–engaging bsAb targeting the most membrane proximal domain of FcRH5 on myeloma cells and CD3 on T cells. Dual binding facilitates efficient immunologic synapse formation, resulting in T-cell activation and potent killing of myeloma cells
- **Mechanism of Action:** A bispecific T-cell engager (BiTE) antibody. It targets both the TAA Fc receptor–like protein 5 (FCRH5, CD307, FCRL5, IRTA2, BXMAS1) and the CD3 antigen found on T lymphocytes.
- **Phase:** Phase 1/2
- **Indications:** Relapsed/refractory MM
- **Dose:** 3.6 mg IV as first dose, then escalate to target dose of 20 mg IV Q 3 weeks
- **Side Effects:** Lymphopenia, transaminitis, CRS, anemia, thrombocytopenia, neutropenia

(Cohen et al., 2020)

Ciltacabtagene Autoleucel

- **Alias:** Cilta-cel; JNJ-4528; LCAR-B38M CAR-T
- **Type Mechanism:** A second-generation CAR T-cell therapy consisting of a CD3-ζ signaling domain, a 4-1BB costimulatory domain, and two BCMA-binding domains.
- **Phase:** Phase 2/3
- **FDA Approval Date:** FDA granted priority review for the treatment of relapsed/refractory MM. Prescription Drug User Fee Act (PDUFA) target date will be November 29, 2021.
- **Indications:** Relapsed/refractory MM
- **Dose:** Lymphodepletion with fludarabine 30 mg/m^2 for 3 days and cyclophosphamide 300 mg/m^2 IV for 3 days. CAR T-cell target dose is 0.75×10^6 viable CAR-positive T cells/kg.
- **Side Effects:** CRS, neurotoxicity, neutropenia, anemia, thrombocytopenia

(Madduri et al., 2020)

Cixutumumab

- **Alias:** IMC-A12; CIX
- **Type Mechanism:** A fully human IgG1/λ mAb directed at the IGF-IR
  - Has a dual action of inhibiting the binding of IGF-1 and IGF-2 ligands to the IGF-1R and inducing the rapid internalization of the receptor
- **Drug Class:** IGF-1R inhibitor
- **Phase:** Phase 2
- **Indications:** Breast cancer, rhabdomyosarcoma, Ewing sarcoma, NSCLC, pancreatic carcinoma, adrenocortical carcinoma, metastatic prostate cancer, and HCC
- **Dose:** 6 to 10 mg/kg IV Q 1 to 2 weeks
- **Half-life:** 148 to 209 hours
- **Side Effects:** Hyperglycemia, rash, pruritis, fatigue, nephrotoxicity, diarrhea, mucositis, lymphopenia, hypophosphatemia, anemia, neutropenia, hyperlipidemia

(Higano et al., 2007)

Cobimetinib Fumarate

- **Alias:** GDC-0973; XL518
- **Brand Name:** Cotellic
- **Type Mechanism:** An orally bioavailable small-molecule inhibitor of MAP2K1 or MEK1 that specifically binds to and inhibits the catalytic activity of MEK1, resulting in the inhibition of ERK2 phosphorylation and activation and reduced tumor cell proliferation
- **Drug Class:** MEK inhibitor
- **FDA Approval Date:** March 28, 2016
- **Indications:** Unresectable or metastatic melanoma with BRAF V600E or V600K mutation in combination with vemurafenib
- **Dose:** 60 mg daily for 21 days of the 28-day cycle
- **Half-life:** Average 44 hours (range 23–70 hours)
- **Metabolism:** Major CYP3A4 substrate
- **Side Effects:** Decreased LVEF; HTN; photosensitivity; ocular toxicities such as serous retinopathy, chorioretinopathy, and retinal detachment; acneiform eruption; hypophosphatemia; increased GGT; nausea/vomiting; diarrhea; anemia; transaminitis; visual impairment; increased SCr

Copanlisib

- **Alias:** BAY 80-6946
- **Brand Name:** Aliqopa
- **Type Mechanism:** Inhibits PI3K, primarily the P13K-α and P13K-δ isoforms that are expressed in malignant B cells. It induces tumor cell death through apoptosis and inhibition of proliferation of primary malignant B-cell lines. It also inhibits several signaling pathways,

including BCR signaling, CXCR12-mediated chemotaxis of malignant B cells, and NFκB signaling in lymphoma cell lines.

- **FDA Approval Date:** September 14, 2017
- **Indications:** Relapsed FL
- **Dose:** 60 mg IV on days 1, 8, and 15 of a 28-day cycle
- **Half-life:** 39.1 hours (range 14.6–82.4 hours)
- **Metabolism:** Major CYP3A4 substrate; if potent CYP3A4 inhibitors cannot be avoided, may decrease dose of copanlisib to 45 mg
- **Side Effects:** Hyperglycemia, nausea/diarrhea, mucositis, fatigue, HTN, skin rash, hypertriglyceridemia, hypophosphatemia

Crenolanib Besylate

- **Type Mechanism:** A highly selective and potent FLT3 TKI with activity against FLT3/ITD mutants and the FLT3/D835 point mutants. It also has inhibitory effects against PDGFRα and PDGFRβ.
- **Drug Class:** A benzimidazole FLT3 inhibitor
- **Phase:** Phase 2/3
- **Indications:** Newly diagnosed FLT3-mutated AML
- **Dose:** 100 mg PO three times daily (TID), starting 24 hours after chemotherapy until 72 hours before consolidation cycles

- **Side Effects:** Nausea/vomiting, transaminitis, fluid retention

(Wang et al., 2019)

Crizotinib

- **Brand Name:** Xalkori
- **Type Mechanism:** A tyrosine kinase receptor inhibitor that inhibits ALK, HGFR (c-MET), ROS1 (c-ros), and recepteur d'origine nantais (RON). It induces apoptosis and inhibits proliferation and ALK-mediated signaling in ALCL-derived cell lines.
- **FDA Approval Date:** August 26, 2011
- **Indications:** Locally advanced or metastatic ALK-positive NSCLC
- **Dose:** 250 mg PO BID
- **Half-life:** 42 hours
- **Metabolism:** Major CYP3A4 substrate and P-glycoprotein; moderate CYP3A4 inhibitor
- **Side Effects:** Edema, vision problems (diplopia, blurred vision), nausea/vomiting, diarrhea, dysphagia, GERD, reflux esophagitis, skin rash, swelling of hands or feet, fatigue, dizziness, transaminitis
- **Clinical Pearls:** Advise patients to exercise caution when driving or operating machinery because of the risk of developing visual changes such as floaters, blurred vision, light sensitivity, or flashes of light.

Dabrafenib

- **Alias:** GSK2118436
- **Brand Name:** Tafinlar
- **Type Mechanism:** Selectively binds to and inhibits the activity of B-raf, which may inhibit the proliferation of tumor cells that contain a mutated *BRAF* gene
- **FDA Approval Date:** March 29, 2013
- **Indications:** Melanoma with BRAF V600E or V600K; metastatic NSCLC with BRAF V600E; metastatic, anaplastic thyroid cancer with BRAF V600E in combination with trametinib
- **Dose:** 150 mg PO BID on fasting stomach at least 1 hour before or 2 hours after meals
- **Half-life:** Parent drug 8 hours; hydroxy-dabrafenib (active metabolite) 10 hours; desmethyl-dabrafenib (active metabolite) 21 to 22 hours
- **Metabolism:** Major CYP2C8 and CYP3A4 substrates; moderate CYP3A4 inducer
- **Side Effects:** Keratoacanthoma and SCC, fatigue, arthralgias, pyrexia, papilloma, hyperglycemia, hyperkeratosis, palmar–plantar erythrodysesthesia, skin rash, hypophosphatemia
- **Clinical Pearls:** Corticosteroids may be used as an effective fever prophylaxis when fever occurs.

Dacomitinib

- **Alias:** PF-00299804
- **Brand Name:** Vizimpro
- **Type Mechanism:** Second-generation small-molecule inhibitor of the pan-EGFR family of tyrosine kinases (ErbB family) that binds to and inhibits human EGFR subtypes, resulting in inhibition of proliferation and induction of apoptosis in EGFR-expressing tumor cells
- **FDA Approval Date:** September 27, 2018
- **Indications:** First-line EGFR exon 19 del, or exon 21 L858 substitution mutation–positive NSCLC
- **Dose:** 45 mg PO once daily with or without food
- **Half-life:** 70 hours
- **Metabolism:** Major CYP2D6 inhibitor; weak CYP2D6 substrate
- **Side Effects:** Diarrhea, dermatitis acneiform (dry skin), stomatitis, paronychia, liver dysfunction (increased bilirubin, ALT/AST), palmar–plantar erythrodysesthesia, pruritus, skin rash, anemia, limb pain

Dactolisib

- **Alias:** BEZ235; NVP-BEZ235
- **Type Mechanism:** An imidazoquinoline that acts as a dual ATP-competitive PI3K and

mTOR inhibitor for p110α/γ/δ/β and mTOR(p70S6K)

- **Drug Class:** PI3K/mTOR inhibitor
- **Phase:** Phase 1b
- **Indications:** pNETs
- **Dose:** 400 to 800 mg PO daily (in combination with everolimus). Taken with food/breakfast. No Seville orange juice or grapefruit juice
- **Half-life:** 15 to 43 hours
- **Metabolism:** Time-dependent CYP3A4 inhibitor
- **Side Effects:** Nausea/vomiting, fatigue, asthenia, anemia, anorexia, diarrhea, mucositis, myelosuppression, transaminitis

(Wise-Draper et al., 2017)

Danvatirsen

- **Alias:** AZD9150; IONIS-STAT3-2.5; ISIS 481464
- **Type Mechanism:** An antisense oligonucleotide targeting STAT3, leading to apoptosis and reduced tumor cell growth
- **Mechanism of Action:** Generation 2.5 antisense therapy targeting STAT3
- **Phase:** Phase 2 in NSCLC, bladder cancer, head and neck (H&N) cancer, diffuse large B-cell lymphoma (DLBCL), and AML
- **Indications:** SCCHN, NSCLC, bladder cancer, and relapsed/refractory DLBCL

- **Dose:** RP2D: 200 mg (flat dose) IV Q week
- **Half-life:** 20 days
- **Side Effects:** Thrombocytopenia, transaminitis

(Xu et al., 2019)

Daratumumab

- **Alias:** JNJ-54767414
- **Brand Name:** Darzalex
- **Type Mechanism:** An IgG1κ human mAb directed against CD38. It inhibits the growth of CD38-expressing tumor cells by inducing apoptosis directly through Fc-mediated cross-linking as well as by immune-mediated tumor cell lysis through complement-dependent cytotoxicity, antibody-dependent cell-mediated cytotoxicity, and antibody-dependent cellular phagocytosis.
- **FDA Approval Date:** November 16, 2015
- **Indications:** Newly diagnosed or relapsed/refractory MM; off label for relapsed light-chain amyloidosis
- **Dose:** 16 mg/kg (diluted) IV once Q week for 6 to 8 doses, then once Q 2 to 3 weeks for 8 to 16 doses, then once Q 4 weeks
- **Half-life:** 18 ± 9 days
- **Side Effects:** Fatigue, headache, nausea, diarrhea, lymphocytopenia, neutropenia, thrombocytopenia, back pain, arthralgias,

anemia, cough, upper respiratory tract infections, HTN

- **Clinical Pearls:** Need premedications with corticosteroids, oral antipyretic, and oral/IV antihistamine. Post infusion, need oral corticosteroids to reduce the risk of delayed infusion reactions; initiate antiviral prophylaxis 1 week after starting daratumumab and continue until 3 months after completion of treatment; may divide the first dose into half to administer over 2 days.

Darolutamide

- **Alias:** ODM-201; BAY-1841788
- **Brand Name:** Nubeqa
- **Type Mechanism:** An AR antagonist that can also inhibit the transcriptional activity of several AR mutant variants (F877L, F877L/T878A, and H875Y/T878A), which are enzalutamide resistant. It inhibits androgen-induced receptor activation, thus facilitating the formation of inactive complexes that cannot translocate to the nucleus. This prevents binding to and transcription of AR-responsive genes that regulate prostate cancer cell proliferation.
- **Drug Class:** AR antagonist
- **FDA Approval Date:** July 30, 2019
- **Indications:** Non-MCRPC

- **Dose:** 600 mg PO BID (usually in combination with GnRH analog)
- **Half-life:** ~20 hours
- **Metabolism:** Weak CYP3A4 substrate; UGT1A1 and UGT1A9 substrate; BCRP/ABCG2 inhibitor, OATP1B1/1B3 inhibitor
- **Side Effects:** Fatigue, neutropenia, AST elevation, hyperbilirubinemia, asthenia, skin rash

Darovasertib

- **Alias:** IDE196; LXS196
- **Type Mechanism:** A PKC inhibitor that binds to and inhibits PKC, which prevents the activation of PKC-mediated signaling pathways. This may lead to the induction of cell-cycle arrest and apoptosis in susceptible tumor cells.
- **Drug Class:** PKC inhibitor
- **Phase:** Phase 2 basket trial for solid tumors harboring GNAQ, GNA11 mutations, or PRKC fusions, including uveal melanoma, cutaneous melanoma, and CRC
- **Indications:** Metastatic uveal melanoma (MUM), non-MUM tumors harboring GNAQ or GNA11 mutations or PRKC fusions
- **Dose:** 200 to 400 mg PO BID for 28 days
- **Side Effects:** Nausea, vomiting, diarrhea, rash, edema, ALT/AST

elevations, CK elevations, edema, loss of appetite, syncope (associated with transient hypotension)

(NCT02601378 Trial, ongoing)

Dasatinib

- **Alias:** BMS-354825
- **Brand Name:** Sprycel
- **Type Mechanism:** A BCR-ABL TKI that targets most imatinib-resistant BCR-ABL mutations (except the T315I and F317V mutants) by distinctly binding to active and inactive ABL kinase. Kinase inhibition halts proliferation of leukemia cells. It also inhibits SRC family (including SRC, LKC, YES, FYN), c-KIT, EPHA2, and PDGFRβ.
- **Drug Class:** BCR-ABL TKI
- **FDA Approval Date:** June 28, 2006
- **Indications:** Chronic-, accelerated-, or blastic-phase Ph+ CML with new diagnosis or with resistance or intolerance to prior therapy; acute lymphoblastic leukemia (ALL) with Ph+ in adults and in pediatric patients with newly diagnosed ALL Ph+ ≥1 year old; off-label indication for GIST
- **Dose:** 100 mg PO daily for chronic-phase Ph+ CML; 140 mg PO daily for ALL Ph+ or accelerated/blastic-phase CML Ph+

- **Half-life:** 3 to 5 hours
- **Metabolism:** Major CYP3A4 substrate
- **Side Effects:** Myelosuppression, fluid retention (edema, pleural effusion), nausea/vomiting, diarrhea, headache, facial edema, fever, musculoskeletal pain, rash, fatigue
- **Clinical Pearls:** Do not take with proton-pump inhibitors or H2 antagonists. May use antacids spaced by 2 hours before and after dosing.

Debio-1347

- **Type Mechanism:** An orally bioavailable inhibitor of the FGFR1/2/3 that binds to and inhibits FGFR-1, FGFR-2, and FGFR-3, which result in the inhibition of FGFR-mediated signal transduction pathways. This leads to the inhibition of both tumor cell proliferation and angiogenesis and causes cell death in FGFR-overexpressing tumor cells.
- **Drug Class:** FGFR inhibitor
- **Phase:** Phase 1/2
- **Indications:** All solid tumors harboring *FGFR1-3* gene fusion
- **Dose:** P2RD: 80 mg PO daily
- **Half-life:** 11.5 hours
- **Side Effects:** Fatigue, hyperphosphatemia, anemia, alopecia, nausea/vomiting, constipation, palmar–plantar

erythrodysesthesia syndrome, minor blurred vision (dry eyes), xerostomia, hyperbilirubinemia, stomatitis

(Cleary et al., 2020)

Demcizumab

- **Alias:** OMP-21M18
- **Type Mechanism:** A humanized mAb directed against the N-terminal epitope of Notch ligand DLL4 (δ-like 4) that binds to the membrane-binding portion of DLL4 and prevents its interaction with Notch-1 and Notch-4 receptors, thereby inhibiting Notch-mediated signaling and gene transcription, which may impede tumor angiogenesis.
- **Drug Class:** Notch inhibitor
- **Phase:** Phase 1b
- **Indications:** Platinum-resistant epithelial ovarian cancer, primary peritoneal, and fallopian tube cancer; metastatic nonsquamous NSCLC. NOTE: Demcizumab failed phase 2 in pancreatic cancer.
- **Dose:** RP2D: 5 mg/kg IV Q 3 weeks for 4 cycles used in combination with chemotherapy
- **Side Effects:** Diarrhea, fatigue, peripheral edema, nausea, pulmonary HTN, increased BNP

(Coleman et al., 2020)

Dostarlimab

- **Alias:** TSR-042; ANB011
- **Brand Name:** Jemperli
- **Type Mechanism:** An anti–PD-1 humanized IgG4 mAb that inhibits PD-1 activity by binding to the PD-1 receptor on T cells to block PD-1 ligands (PD-L1 and PD-L2) from binding
- **Drug Class:** Anti–PD-1 mAb
- **FDA Approval Date:** April 22, 2021
- **Indications:** Recurrent or advanced endometrial cancer with the presence of deficient mismatch repair (dMMR) in tumor specimen
- **Dose:** 500 mg IV Q 3 weeks for 4 doses, then 1,000 mg IV Q 6 weeks for 5 doses or more. Dose #5 should begin 3 weeks after dose #4.
- **Half-life:** 25.4 days
- **Side Effects:** Pruritus, hypercalcemia, diarrhea, nausea/vomiting, anemia, leukopenia, transaminitis, fatigue, myalgias, asthenia, increased SCr

Double Antiangiogenic Protein

- **Type Mechanism:** A chimeric decoy receptor, namely, double antiangiogenic

protein (DAAP), which can simultaneously bind VEGF-A and angiopoietins (ANGs), blocking their actions
- **Phase:** Preclinical; animal studies

(Koh et al., 2010)

Dovitinib

- **Alias:** TKI258; CHIR-258
- **Type Mechanism:** A benzimidazole–quinoline compound strongly binds to FGFR3 and inhibits its phosphorylation, which may result in the inhibition of tumor cell proliferation and the induction of tumor cell death. It also inhibits other members of the RTK superfamily, including the VEGFR, FGFR1, PDGFR type 3, FMS-like tyrosine kinase 3 (FLT3), stem cell factor receptor (SCFR) (c-KIT), and colony-stimulating factor receptor 1 (CSF1R).
- **Drug Class:** Multitargeted RTK inhibitor
- **Phase:** Phase 2
- **Indications:** Metastatic RCC, HR+, HER2− breast cancer, metastatic adenoid cystic carcinoma, GIST, and advanced/metastatic thyroid cancer
- **Dose:** 500 mg PO once daily (5 days on/2 days off)
- **Half-life:** 13 hours
- **Metabolism:** CYP1A2 inducer

- **Side Effects:** Fatigue, diarrhea, nausea/vomiting, decreased appetite, asthenia, headache, acneiform rash, hypertriglyceridemia, neutropenia, thrombocytopenia

(Escudier et al., 2014)

Durvalumab

- **Alias:** MEDI4736
- **Brand Name:** Imfinzi
- **Type Mechanism:** A human IgG1κ mAb that blocks PD-L1 binding to PD-1 and CD80 (B7.1); PD-L1 blockade leads to increased T-cell activation, allowing T cells to kill tumor cells. PD-L1 is an immune checkpoint protein expressed on tumor cells and tumor-infiltrating cells and downregulates antitumor T-cell function by binding to PD-1 and B7.1; blocking PD-1 and B7.1 interactions restores antitumor T-cell function.
- **Drug Class:** Anti–PD-L1 mAb
- **FDA Approval Date:** May 1, 2017
- **Indications:** Unresectable NSCLC and extensive stage SCLC; locally advanced or metastatic urothelial carcinoma
- **Dose:** 10 mg/kg IV Q 2 weeks; may use flat dosing of 1,500 mg IV Q 3 to 4 weeks for patients ≥30 kg
- **Half-life:** ~18 days

- **Side Effects:** Fatigue, skin rash, muscle pain, peripheral edema, abdominal pain, lymphocytopenia, constipation, immune-mediated pneumonitis

---

Duvelisib

- **Alias:** IPI-145; INK-1197
- **Brand Name:** Copiktra
- **Type Mechanism:** A PI3K inhibitor with dual-inhibitory activity primarily against PI3K-δ and PI3K-γ, which are expressed in hematologic malignancies. Inhibition of PI3K-δ reduced tumor cell proliferation and reduces differentiation and migration of tumor microenvironment support cells. It also inhibits BCR signaling pathways and CXCR12-mediated chemotaxis of malignant B cells as well as CXCL12-induced T-cell migration and M-CSF and IL-4–driven M2 macrophage polarization.
- **Drug Class:** PI3K inhibitor
- **FDA Approval Date:** September 24, 2018
- **Indications:** Relapsed/refractory CLL or SLL with at least two prior therapies; relapsed/refractory FL after at least two prior therapies
- **Dose:** 25 mg PO BID
- **Half-life:** 4.7 hours
- **Metabolism:** Major CYP3A4 substrate

- **Side Effects:** Diarrhea, colitis, neutropenia, rash, fatigue, fevers, nausea, anemia, myalgia, edema, headache, increased serum amylase and lipase, neutropenia, lymphocytosis, thrombocytopenia, lymphocytopenia, transaminitis

---

Elotuzumab

- **Alias:** HuLuc63; BMS-901608; PDL-063
- **Brand Name:** Empliciti
- **Type Mechanism:** A humanized IgG1 immunostimulatory mAb directed against signaling lymphocytic activation molecule family member 7 (SLAMF7, also called CS1 [cell-surface glycoprotein CD2 subset 1]). SLAMF7 is expressed on most myeloma and NK cells, but not on normal tissues. It directly activates NK cells through both the SLAMF7 pathway and Fc receptors. It also targets SLAMF7 on myeloma cells and mediates ADCC through the CD16 pathway. This immunostimulatory activity, through the increased activation of NK cells, increases antitumor activity.
- **FDA Approval Date:** November 30, 2015
- **Indications:** Relapsed/refractory MM (in combination with lenalidomide and

dexamethasone) in patients who have received one to three prior therapies

- **Dose:** Cycles 1 and 2: 10 mg/kg IV weekly on days 1, 8, 15, and 22; cycle 3 and beyond: 10 mg/kg IV Q 2 weeks on days 1 and 15. Both in combination with lenalidomide and dexamethasone
- **Half-life:** 78 to 82.4 days
- **Side Effects:** Constipation, diarrhea, loss of appetite, asthenia, upper respiratory tract infections, nasopharyngitis, lymphocytopenia, thrombocytopenia, peripheral neuropathy, bradycardia <60 bpm, tachycardia >100 bpm, peripheral edema, fatigue, hyperglycemia, peripheral neuropathy, ostealgia
- **Clinical Pearls:** Premedications recommended with dexamethasone, an H1 antagonist, an H2 antagonist, and an antipyretic (acetaminophen) 60 minutes before infusion.

Enasidenib Mesylate

- **Alias:** AG-221; CC-90007
- **Brand Name:** Idhifa
- **Type Mechanism:** A small-molecule inhibitor of the enzyme isocitrate dehydrogenase 2 (IDH2) that targets the mutant IDH2 variants R140Q, R172S, and R172K. Mutant IDH2 inhibition results in decreased 2HG levels, reduced abnormal histone hypermethylation, and restored myeloid differentiation. It also reduces blast counts and increases percentages of mature myeloid cells.
- **Drug Class:** IDH2 inhibitor
- **FDA Approval Date:** August 1, 2017
- **Indications:** Relapsed/refractory ALL with IDH2 mutation
- **Dose:** 100 mg PO daily until disease progression (PD)
- **Half-life:** 7.9 days
- **Metabolism:** Minor CYP1A2, CYP2B6, CYP2C19, CYP2C8, CYP2D6, CYP3A4, UGT1A1, UGT1A3, UGT1A4 substrates; BCRP/ABCG2 inhibitor; OATP1B1/1B3 inhibitor
- **Side Effects:** Hypocalcemia, hypokalemia, nausea, diarrhea, decreased appetite, dysgeusia, hyperbilirubinemia, CRS, TLS

Encorafenib

- **Alias:** LGX818
- **Brand Name:** Braftovi
- **Type Mechanism:** An ATP-competitive inhibitor of protein kinase B-raf (BRAF) that suppresses the MAPK pathway and targets

BRAF V600E, V600 D, and V600 K. It has a longer dissociation half-life than other BRAF inhibitors, allowing for sustained inhibition. BRAF V600 mutations result in constitutive activation of the BRAF pathway (which may stimulate tumor growth); BRAF inhibition inhibits tumor cell growth.

- **Drug Class:** BRAF inhibitor
- **FDA Approval Date:** April 8, 2020
- **Indications:** Metastatic, BRAF V600E–mutant CRC and unresectable/metastatic BRAF V600E– or V600K-mutated melanoma
- **Dose:** CRC: 300 mg PO daily with cetuximab; melanoma: 450 mg PO daily with binimetinib
- **Half-life:** 3.5 hours
- **Metabolism:** Major CYP3A4 substrate
- **Side Effects:** Anemia, hyperglycemia, fever, increased lipase, HTN, fatigue, nausea, arthralgia, palmar–plantar erythrodysesthesia, acneiform eruption, alopecia, hyperkeratosis, xeroderma, arthralgia, increased SCr

Enfortumab Vedotin

- **Alias:** ASG-22CE; anti–Nectin-4 ADC ASG-22CE
- **Brand Name:** Padcev

- **Type Mechanism:** An ADC directed at Nectin-4 (an adhesion protein located on cell surfaces). It contains an IgG1 anti–Nectin-4 antibody conjugated to a microtubule-disrupting agent, MMAE. MMAE is attached to the antibody via a protease-cleavable linker. The ADC binds to Nectin-4-expressing cells to form a complex that is internalized within the cell. Released MMAE binds to the tubules and disrupts the cellular microtubule network, inducing cell-cycle arrest and apoptosis of Nectin-4-expressing cells.
- **Drug Class:** ADC
- **FDA Approval Date:** December 18, 2019
- **Indications:** Advanced/metastatic urothelial cancer
- **Dose:** 1.25 mg/kg IV on days 1, 8, and 15 Q 28 days. NOTE: Dose capped for max weight of 100 kg.
- **Half-life:** ADC = 3.4 days; MMAE = 2.4 days
- **Metabolism:** Minor CYP3A4 substrate; minor P-glycoprotein/ABCB1 substrate
- **Side Effects:** Alopecia, maculopapular rash, pruritus, skin rash, xeroderma, decreased appetite, diarrhea, dysgeusia, nausea/vomiting, anemia, neutropenia, lymphocytopenia, peripheral neuropathy, fatigue, blurred vision, ocular toxicity, elevated SCr

Ensartinib

- **Alias:** X-396
- **Type Mechanism:** A small-molecule second-generation inhibitor of the RTK ALK that binds to and inhibits ALK, ALK fusion proteins, and ALK point mutation variants. Inhibition of ALK leads to the disruption of ALK-mediated signaling and eventually inhibits tumor cell growth in ALK-expressing tumor cells.
- **Drug Class:** ALK inhibitor
- **Phase:** Phase 2/3
- **Indications:** ALK-positive NSCLC who progressed on crizotinib, pediatric patients with relapsed/refractory advanced solid tumors, NHL, or histiocytic disorder
- **Dose:** 225 mg PO daily
- **Half-life:** 27.2 hours
- **Side Effects:** Skin rash, nausea, pruritus, vomiting, fatigue
- **Clinical Pearls:** Take with food will lessen nausea effect.

(Horn et al., 2018)

Entrectinib

- **Alias:** RXDX-101
- **Brand Name:** Rozlytrek
- **Type Mechanism:** Inhibits TRK receptors such as TRKA, TRKB, and TRKC. TRKA, TRKB, and TRKC are encoded by NTRK genes *NTRK1*, *NTRK2*, and *NTRK3*, respectively. It also inhibits proto-oncogenic tyrosine protein kinase ROS1 and ALK. M5 (the major active entrectinib metabolite) demonstrated similar activity (in vitro) against TRK, ROS1, and ALK. Fusion proteins that include TRK, ROS1, or ALK domains act as oncogenic drivers to promote hyperactivation of downstream signaling pathways, resulting in unchecked cell proliferation.
- **Drug Class:** TRK inhibitor
- **FDA Approval Date:** August 15, 2019
- **Indications:** Metastatic NSCLC with ROS1 positive; all metastatic, unresectable solid tumors with *NTRK* gene fusion
- **Dose:** 600 mg PO daily
- **Half-life:** Entrectinib = 20 hours
  - M5 active metabolite = 40 hours
- **Metabolism:** Major CYP3A4 substrate
- **Side Effects:** Edema, hypotension, fatigue, cognitive dysfunction, sleep disorder, myasthenia, hyperuricemia, dysgeusia, constipation, diarrhea, increased lipase, anemia, lymphocytopenia, neutropenia myalgia, arthralgia, visual disturbance, elevated SCr, cough, fever
- **Clinical Pearls:** Avoid grapefruit or grapefruit juice as it may increase the levels of entrectinib.

Enzalutamide

- **Alias:** MDV-3100
- **Brand Name:** Xtandi
- **Type Mechanism:** A pure AR signaling inhibitor with no known agonistic properties. It inhibits AR nuclear translocation, DNA binding, and coactivator mobilization, leading to cellular apoptosis and decreased prostate tumor volume.
- **Drug Class:** AR signaling inhibitor
- **FDA Approval Date:** August 31, 2012
- **Indications:** MCRPC
- **Dose:** 160 mg PO daily
- **Half-life:** Parent drug = 5.8 days
  - *N*-Desmethyl enzalutamide = 7.8 to 8.6 days
- **Metabolism:** Major CYP2C8 and CYP3A4 substrates; moderate CYP2C19 and CYP2C9 inducers; major CYP3A4 inducer
- **Side Effects:** Peripheral edema, HTN, fatigue, hot flashes, back pain/arthralgia, URI, neutropenia, hyperglycemia, nausea, neutropenia, dyspnea

Enzastaurin

- **Alias:** LY317615
- **Type Mechanism:** A synthetic macrocyclic bisindolemaleimide that binds to the ATP-binding site and selectively inhibits PKCβ, an enzyme involved in the induction of VEGF-stimulated neoangiogenesis. This agent may decrease tumor blood supply and so tumor burden.
- **Phase:** Phase 1/2
- **Indications:** Recurrent high-grade glioma, relapsed/refractory DLBCL
- **Dose:** 500 mg PO daily for a 42-day cycle
- **Half-life:** 12 to 40 hours
- **Metabolism:** Major CYP3A4 substrate
- **Side Effects:** Thrombocytopenia, thrombosis, elevated ALT/AST, hyperbilirubinemia, diarrhea, prolonged QTc

(Kreisl et al., 2010)

Epratuzumab

- **Alias:** AMG 412; mAb LL2
- **Type Mechanism:** A recombinant, humanized mAb directed against CD22, a cell-surface glycoprotein present on mature B cells and on many types of malignant B cells. Its antitumor activity appears to be mediated through ADCC.
- **Phase:** Phase 1b; phase 3 for systemic lupus erythematosus
- **Indications:** NHL in combination with rituximab

- **Dose:** A range of 360 mg/m^2 Q 2 weeks IV over 30 to 60 minutes for 4 doses
- **Half-life:** 23 days
- **Side Effects:** Infusion-related side effects (chills, fevers, rigors), infections, fatigue, arthralgia, back pain, flushing, hypotension, tachycardia

(Strauss et al., 2006)

Erdafitinib

- **Alias:** JNJ-42756493
- **Brand Name:** Balversa
- **Type Mechanism:** A pan-FGFR kinase inhibitor that binds to and inhibits FGFR1, FGFR2, FGFR3, and FGFR4 enzyme activity. Erdafitinib also binds to RET, CSF1R, PDGFRα, PDGFRβ, FLT4, KIT, and VEGFR2. FGFR inhibition results in decreased FGFR-related signaling and decreased cell viability in cell lines expressing FGFR genetic alterations, including point mutations, amplifications, and fusions.
- **Drug Class:** FGFR inhibitor
- **FDA Approval Date:** April 14, 2019
- **Indications:** Advanced/metastatic urothelial carcinoma with susceptible FGFR genetic alteration

- **Dose:** 8 mg PO daily for 14 days; if serum phosphate ≤5.5 mg/dL, and no ocular toxicity ≥ grade 2 common terminology criteria for adverse events (CTCAEs), then increase dose 9 mg PO daily.
- **Half-life:** 59 hours
- **Metabolism:** Major CYP2C9 and CYP3A4 substrates
- **Side Effects:** Fatigue, onycholysis, xeroderma, alopecia, palmar–plantar erythrodysesthesia, paronychia, nail discoloration, hyperphosphatemia, hyponatremia, stomatitis, diarrhea, xerostomia, dysgeusia, anemia, thrombocytopenia, leukopenia, transaminitis, dry eyes syndrome, central serous retinopathy, blurred vision, elevated SCr, myalgia

Erlotinib

- **Alias:** OSI-774; CP 358774
- **Brand Name:** Tarceva
- **Type Mechanism:** Reversibly binds to the intracellular catalytic domain of EGFR and inhibits overall HER1/EGFR tyrosine kinase. Active competitive inhibition of ATP inhibits downstream signal transduction of ligand-dependent HER1/EGFR activation.
- **Drug Class:** EGFR inhibitor

- **FDA Approval Date:** November 18, 2004
- **Indications:** Metastatic NSCLC with EGFR exon 19 deletions or exon 21 substitution mutations; locally advanced, unresectable, or metastatic pancreatic cancer (in combination with gemcitabine); off-label use for advanced papillary RCC
- **Dose:** 150 mg once daily (NSCLC) and 100 mg once daily (pancreatic cancer) on empty stomach 1 hour before or 2 hours after meals
- **Half-life:** 36 hours
- **Metabolism:** Major CYP3A4 and CYP1A2 substrates
- **Side Effects:** Rash (acne vulgaris, pruritus), diarrhea, paronychia (hair and nail changes), fatigue, weakness, back pain, cough, dyspnea, conjunctivitis, chest pain, xeroderma, anorexia, nausea, mucositis, dry eyes syndrome, increased ALT and GGT
- **Clinical Pearls:** Severity of acne-form rash can be minimized with the use of topical steroid cream, topical antibiotic gel, and doxycycline; encourage smoking cessation before start because smoking can make the drug less effective.

Everolimus

- **Alias:** RAD001
- **Brand Name:** Afinitor
- **Type Mechanism:** An mTOR inhibitor that has antiproliferative and antiangiogenic properties. Reduces protein synthesis and cell proliferation by binding to the FKBP-12, an intracellular protein, to form a complex that inhibits activation of mTOR serine-threonine kinase activity. Also reduces angiogenesis by inhibiting VEGF and hypoxia-inducible factor (HIF-1) expression.
- **Drug Class:** mTOR inhibitor
- **FDA Approval Date:** March 30, 2009
- **Indications:** Advanced RCC, neuroendocrine carcinomas (GI, lung, or pancreatic origin), and advanced, HR+, HER2− breast cancer in combination with exemestane; off-label use in advanced carcinoid tumors, relapsed/refractory Hodgkin lymphoma, advanced/refractory thymoma and thymic carcinoma
- **Dose:** 10 mg once daily with or without food. Dosing with 5 mg if combined with lenvatinib for RCC
- **Half-life:** 30 hours
- **Metabolism:** Major CYP3A4 substrate and P-glycoprotein substrate
- **Side Effects:** Mouth ulcers, rash (acneiform), delayed wound healing,

nausea/vomiting, fatigue, anorexia (decreased appetite), cough, shortness of breath, thrombocytopenia, diarrhea or constipation, hypercholesterolemia, HTN, hyperglycemia, anemia, leukopenia

- **Clinical Pearls:** Monitor fasting triglycerides and cholesterol. Levels may increase while on treatment despite the patient's dietary habits. Initiate oral care early on (soft toothbrush, salt, and soda swish).

Farletuzumab

- **Alias:** MORAb-003
- **Type Mechanism:** An mAb to folate receptor α that leads to cell-mediated cytotoxicity, complement-dependent killing, and inhibition of growth under limited folate conditions
- **Drug Class:** Folate receptor α inhibitor
- **Phase:** Phase 2/3
- **Indications:** Platinum-sensitive ovarian cancer
- **Dose:** 1.25 or 2.5 mg/kg IV Q week in combination with chemotherapy
- **Half-life:** 56 to 260 hours (increased with dose and multiple infusions)
- **Side Effects:** Fatigue, nausea, drug hypersensitivity, headache, cough, exertional dyspnea

(Konner et al., 2010)

Ficlatuzumab

- **Alias:** AV-299; SCH 900105
- **Type Mechanism:** An mAb directed against human HGF that binds to the soluble ligand HGF, preventing the binding of HGF to its receptor c-Met and activation of the HGF/c-Met signaling pathway, which may result in cell death in c-Met–expressing tumor cells
- **Drug Class:** HGF inhibitor
- **Phase:** Phase 1
- **Indications:** Cetuximab resistant, recurrent/metastatic H&N cancer, and NSCLC
- **Dose:** RP2D: 20 mg/kg IV Q 2 weeks (in combination with cetuximab)
- **Side Effects:** Peripheral edema, flulike symptoms, acneiform rash, hyponatremia, hypoalbuminemia, thromboembolism

(Bauman et al., 2020)

Figitumumab

- **Alias:** CP-751871
- **Type Mechanism:** A human mAb directed against the IGF-1R. Selectively binds to IGF-1R to prevent IGF1 from binding to the receptor and subsequent receptor autophosphorylation
- **Mechanism of Action:** Phase 3 trial for advanced NSCLC failed to show any benefits.

- **Phase:** Currently, no active clinical trials in the United States. Failed to meet the end point of phase 3 trial
- **Dose:** 20 mg/kg IV (day 1 of a 21-day cycle)
- **Half-life:** 3 weeks
- **Side Effects:** Hyperglycemia, nausea/vomiting, muscle cramps, fatigue, anorexia, increased GGT

(Langer et al., 2014)

Foretinib

- **Alias:** GSK1363089; XL880
- **Type Mechanism:** Binds to and selectively inhibits MET and VEGFR2
- **Mechanism of Action:** Phase 2 clinical trials discontinued on October 2015
- **Phase:** Currently under investigation in phase 2 clinical trial for SCCHN, metastatic gastric cancer, papillary RCC, and nonsarcomatous GEJ adenocarcinoma
- **Indications:** SCCHN, metastatic gastric cancer, papillary RCC, and nonsarcomatous GEJ adenocarcinoma
- **Dose:** 240 mg PO daily for 5 days Q 14 days
- **Half-life:** 40 hours
- **Side Effects:** Fatigue, nausea/vomiting, diarrhea, HTN, proteinuria, increased lipase, increased AST

(Choueiri et al., 2013)

Fostamatinib Disodium

- **Alias:** R788; tamatinib fosdium; R935788 sodium
- **Brand Name:** Tavalisse
- **Type Mechanism:** A small-molecule SYK inhibitor. SYK affects cellular proliferation, differentiation, survival, and immune regulation via IgG Fc receptor signaling and is also linked to BCR signaling and autoantibody production (Bussel et al., 2018). The major active metabolite of fostamatinib, R406, inhibits signal transduction of Fc-activating receptors and BCR and reduces antibody-mediated destruction of platelets.
- **Drug Class:** Spleen kinase inhibitor
- **FDA Approval Date:** April 17, 2018
- **Indications:** Chronic or refractory immune thrombocytopenia purpura
- **Dose:** 100 mg PO BID; if platelets does not increase to at least 50,000/mm^3, then increase dose to 150 mg PO BID.
- **Half-life:** Active metabolite R406 = 15 hours
- **Metabolism:** Major CYP3A4 and UGT1A9 substrates; BCRP/ABCG2 inhibitor, P-glycoprotein/ABCB1 inhibitor
- **Side Effects:** Fatigue, dizziness, nausea/vomiting/diarrhea, thrombocytopenia, HTN, neutropenia, increased ALT

Fulvestrant

- **Alias:** ICI-182,780; ZD9238
- **Brand Name:** Faslodex
- **Type Mechanism:** An estrogen receptor antagonist; competitively binds to estrogen receptors on tumors and other tissue targets, producing a nuclear complex that causes a dose-related downregulation of estrogen receptors and inhibits tumor growth
- **Drug Class:** Estrogen receptor antagonist
- **FDA Approval Date:** April 25, 2002
- **Indications:** HR-positive and/or HER2-negative breast cancer as monotherapy or combination therapy (e.g., CDK inhibitors)
- **Dose:** 500 mg intramuscularly (IM) on days 1, 15, and 29 with 500 mg IM monthly maintenance
- **Half-life:** ~40 days
- **Metabolism:** Minor CYP3A4
- **Side Effects:** Decreased serum glucose, hot flash, GGT elevation, transaminitis with ALT/AST elevations, diarrhea, abdominal pain, stomatitis, nausea, fatigue, headache, arthralgia
- **Clinical Pearls:** LHRH agonist should be administered to pre-/perimenopausal women in combination with CDK inhibitors.

Futibatinib

- **Alias:** TAS-120
- **Type Mechanism:** An orally bioavailable inhibitor of the FGFR that selectively and irreversibly binds to and inhibits FGFR, which may result in the inhibition of both the FGFR-mediated signal transduction pathway and tumor cell proliferation and increased cell death in FGFR-overexpressing tumor cells. FGFR is an RTK essential to tumor cell proliferation, differentiation, and survival, and its expression is upregulated in many tumor cell types.
- **Drug Class:** FGFR inhibitor
- **Phase:** Phase 3
- **Indications:** Advanced cholangiocarcinoma harboring *FGFR2* gene rearrangements
- **Dose:** 20 mg PO daily
- **Half-life:** ~3 hours
- **Metabolism:** Major CYP3A4 substrate; P-glycoprotein/BCRP substrate
- **Side Effects:** Stomatitis, oral dysesthesia, transaminitis, diarrhea, hyperphosphatemia, constipation, hyperbilirubinemia, hyponatremia, increased lipase, increased CPK, dry mouth, decreased appetite

(Chatila et al., 2020)

Galunisertib

- **Alias:** LY2157299
- **Type Mechanism:** An orally available, small-molecule antagonist of the tyrosine kinase TGF-β receptor type 1 (TGFβR1) that specifically targets and binds to the kinase domain of TGFβR1, thereby preventing the activation of TGF-β–mediated signaling pathways. This may inhibit the proliferation of TGF-β–overexpressing tumor cells.
- **Phase:** Phase 1b/2
- **Indications:** Advanced HCC; unresectable, advanced pancreatic cancer
- **Dose:** 150 mg PO BID for 14 days on, 14 days off for a 28-day cycle
- **Half-life:** 8 hours
- **Side Effects:** Fatigue, thrombosis, dyspnea, thrombocytopenia, lymphopenia, anemia, neutropenia, increased bilirubin, hypoalbuminemia, peripheral edema

(Kelley et al., 2019)

Ganitumab

- **Alias:** AMG 479
- **Type Mechanism:** A recombinant fully human mAb that binds to membrane-bound IGF-1R, subsequently inhibiting cancer cell proliferation through disruption of the PI3K/AKT and MAPK pathways
- **Drug Class:** EGFR inhibitor
- **Phase:** Phase 2/3; granted orphan drug status for Ewing sarcoma in April 2017
- **Indications:** Metastatic Ewing sarcoma, mutant KRAS mCRC in combination with FOLFIRI, metastatic pancreatic cancer
- **Dose:** 12 mg/kg IV Q 2 weeks in combination with cytotoxic chemotherapy or targeted therapy
- **Half-life:** 7 days
- **Side Effects:** Hyperglycemia, fatigue, nausea/vomiting, anorexia, neutropenia, thrombocytopenia, increased AST

(Tap et al., 2012)

Gefitinib

- **Alias:** ZD1839
- **Brand Name:** Iressa
- **Type Mechanism:** A TKI that reversibly inhibits kinase activity of WT and select activation mutations of EGFR. It prevents autophosphorylation of tyrosine residues associated with the EGFR, which blocks downstream signaling and EGFR-dependent proliferation. Gefitinib has a

higher binding affinity for EGFR exon 19 deletion and exon 21 (L858R) substitution mutation than for WT EGFR.

- **Drug Class:** EGFR inhibitor
- **FDA Approval Date:** July 14, 2015
- **Indications:** First-line treatment for metastatic NSCLC with EGFR exon 19 deletions or exon 21 (L858R) substitution mutations
- **Dose:** 250 mg PO once daily with or without food
- **Half-life:** 48 hours
- **Metabolism:** Major CYP3A4 substrate; BCRP/ABCG2 substrate
- **Side Effects:** Skin rash (dry skin), nausea/vomiting, diarrhea, anorexia, pruritus, fatigue, acne vulgaris, stomatitis, ALT/AST elevation

Geldanamycin

- **Alias:** Tanespimycin (17AAG)
- **Type Mechanism:** Inhibits the ATPase activity of chaperone heat shock protein 90 (Hsp90), which maintains conformation, stability, and function of oncogenic protein kinases involved in signal transduction cascades, leading to proliferation and progression of cell cycle and apoptosis
- **Drug Class:** Benzoquinone ansamycin HSP90 inhibitors
- **Phase:** Phase 2
- **Indications:** Phase 2 in metastatic pancreatic cancer, metastatic melanoma, EGFR-mutated NSCLC, metastatic breast cancer
- **Dose:** RP2D: 220 mg/m^2 IV on days 1, 4, 8, and 11 of a 21-day cycle
- **Half-life:** 3.8 to 8.6 hours
- **Side Effects:** Diarrhea, transaminitis, hyperbilirubinemia, anorexia, fatigue, nausea, pleural effusion

(Gartner et al., 2012)

Gemtuzumab Ozogamicin

- **Alias:** CMA-676; CDP-771
- **Brand Name:** Mylotarg
- **Type Mechanism:** A humanized CD-33 directed monoclonal ADC, which is composed of the IgG4κ antibody gemtuzumab linked to a cytotoxic calicheamicin derivative. CD33 is expressed on leukemic cells in over 80% of patients with AML. It binds to the CD33 antigen, resulting in internalization of the antibody–antigen complex. Following internalization, the calicheamicin derivative is released inside the myeloid

cell. The calicheamicin derivative binds to DNA, resulting in double-strand breaks (DSB), inducing cell-cycle arrest and apoptosis.

- **FDA Approval Date:** September 1, 2017
- **Indications:** Relapsed/refractory CD33$^+$ AML; June 16,2020, FDA approved for CD33$^+$ pediatrics patients from 1 month old and beyond
- **Dose:** Induction: 3 mg/m^2 IV on days 1, 4, and 7; consolidation (2 cycles) 3 mg/m^2 IV on day 1 in combination with daunorubicin and cytarabine
- **Half-life:** Base on 9 mg/m^2 dose: Antibody portion is 62 hours after the first dose and 90 hours after the second dose.
- **Metabolism:** Calicheamicin is metabolized through nonenzymatic reduction of disulfide moiety.
- **Side Effects:** Hepatotoxicity (sinusoidal obstruction syndrome) (black box warning), severe infusion-related reactions (black box warning), skin rash, intracranial hemorrhage, increased ALT/AST, disseminated intravascular coagulopathy, HTN/hypotension, tachycardia, low-to-moderate emetogenicity, febrile neutropenia, fatigue, sepsis
- **Clinical Pearls:** Premedications recommended with methylprednisolone, diphenhydramine, and acetaminophen. May repeat steroid dose for any signs of infusion-related side effects. Prophylaxis to prevent TLS

Gilteritinib Fumarate

- **Alias:** ASP2215
- **Brand Name:** Xospata
- **Type Mechanism:** A TKI that inhibits multiple tyrosine kinases, such as FLT3. It inhibits FLT3 receptor signaling and proliferation in cells expressing FLT3 (including FLT3-ITD), tyrosine kinase domain (TKD) mutations FLT3-D835Y and FLT3-ITD-D835Y; it induces apoptosis in FLT3-ITD–expressing leukemia cells.
- **FDA Approval Date:** November 28, 2018
- **Indications:** Relapsed/refractory FLT3-mutated AML
- **Dose:** 120 mg PO daily
- **Half-life:** 113 hours
- **Metabolism:** Major CYP3A4 substrate
- **Side Effects:** Edema, hypotension, fatigue, malaise, headache, hyponatremia, stomatitis, nausea/vomiting, dysgeusia, febrile neutropenia, transaminitis, arthralgia, myalgia, renal insufficiency

Glasdegib Maleate

- **Alias:** PF-04449913
- **Brand Name:** Daurismo
- **Type Mechanism:** Binds to and inhibits Smoothened (SMO), which is a transmembrane protein involved in Hedgehog (Hh) signal transduction. Glasdegib blocks the translocation of SMO into cilia and prevents SMO-mediated activation of downstream Hh targets.
- **FDA Approval Date:** November 21, 2018
- **Indications:** AML for patients older than 75 years or have comorbidities
- **Dose:** 100 mg PO daily with or without food in combination with low-dose SC cytarabine
- **Half-life:** 17.4 hours
- **Metabolism:** Major CYP3A4 and UGT1A9 substrates
- **Side Effects:** Edema, arrhythmia, rash, chest pain, mucositis, anemia, neutropenia, myalgias, increased CK, transaminitis, QT prolongation, fatigue, decreased appetite, thrombocytopenia, fever, dyspnea
- **Clinical Pearls:** Avoid known cause of QTc prolongation medications.

Ibrutinib

- **Alias:** CRA-032765; PCI-32765
- **Brand Name:** Imbruvica
- **Type Mechanism:** A potent and irreversible inhibitor of BTK, an integral component of the BCR and cytokine receptor pathways. BTK inhibition results in decreased malignant B-cell proliferation and survival.
- **Drug Class:** BTK inhibitor
- **FDA Approval Date:** November 13, 2013
- **Indications:** Refractory, chronic graft-versus-host disease (GvHD), CLL/SLL, previously treated MCL, relapsed/refractory marginal zone lymphoma (MZL), and Waldenström macroglobulinemia
- **Dose:** 420 to 560 mg PO daily; in CLL and Waldenström, use in combination with rituximab at 420 mg dose.
- **Half-life:** 4 to 6 hours
- **Metabolism:** Major CYP3A4 substrate and minor CYP2D6 substrate
- **Side Effects:** HTN, peripheral edema, pruritus, skin rash, abdominal pain, decreased appetite, diarrhea, stomatitis, vomiting, gastric reflux, anemia, neutropenia, thrombocytopenia, lymphocytosis, infection

Icotinib

- **Alias:** BPI-2009H
- **Brand Name:** Conmana (China)

- **Type Mechanism:** A highly selective, first-generation EGFR-TKI that binds reversibly to the ATP-binding site of the EGFR protein, preventing completion of the signal transduction cascade. EGFR is an oncogenic receptor, and patients with activating somatic mutations, such as an exon 19 deletion or exon 21 L858R mutation, within the TKD display unchecked cell proliferation.
- **Drug Class:** EGFR inhibitor
- **Phase:** Phase 2/3
- **Indications:** Advanced NSCLC
- **Dose:** 125 mg PO TID
- **Half-life:** 5.5 hours
- **Side Effects:** Skin rash, diarrhea, ALT elevation, fatigue, loss of appetite, pruritus, leukopenia, dry skin, conjunctivitis, paronychia
- **Clinical Pearls:** Solely approved and marketed in China

(Shi et al., 2017)

Idecabtagene Vicleucel

- **Alias:** Ide-cel; BB2121; Ide-cel; Anti-BCMA
- **Brand Name:** Abecma
- **Type Mechanism:** A BCMA-directed genetically modified autologous T-cell immunotherapy in which a patient's T cells are reprogrammed via transduction with an anti-BCMA02 CAR lentiviral vector. The CAR construct includes an anti-BCMA scFv-targeting domain for antigen specificity, a transmembrane domain, a CD3-ζ T-cell activation domain, and a 4-1BB costimulatory domain. CD3-ζ signaling initiates activation and antitumor activity, whereas 4-1BB (CD137) signaling enhances T-cell expansion. Antigen-specific activation of idecabtagene vicleucel results in CAR-positive T-cell proliferation, cytokine secretion, and subsequent cytolytic killing of BCMA-expressing cells.
- **Drug Class:** CAR T-cell therapy
- **FDA Approval Date:** March 26, 2021
- **Indications:** Relapsed/refractory MM after four or more lines of prior therapies
- **Dose:** Target dose: 300 to 460 $\times$ 10^6 CAR-positive viable T cells. Administered 2 days after lymphodepleting chemotherapy completes
- **Half-life:** May persist in peripheral blood up to 1 year after infusion
- **Side Effects:** Edema, HTN or hypotension, skin rash, xeroderma, diarrhea, nausea, anemia, febrile neutropenia, lymphocytopenia, thrombocytopenia, CRS, antibody development, infections (viral, bacterial), encephalopathy, fatigue, elevated

ALT/AST, elevated activated partial thromboplastin time (aPTT)

- **Clinical Pearls:** Premedications with acetaminophen and diphenhydramine 30 minutes before cell infusion; administer prophylactic antibiotic, antiviral, and anti-PCP. Lymphodepleting chemotherapy will consist of 3 days of fludarabine and cyclophosphamide.

Idelalisib

- **Alias:** CAL-101; GS-1101
- **Brand Name:** Zydelig
- **Type Mechanism:** An orally bioavailable, small-molecule inhibitor of the δ isoform of the 110-kDa catalytic subunit of class I PI3K that inhibits the production of the second messenger PIP3, preventing the activation of the PI3K signaling pathway and inhibiting tumor cell proliferation, motility, and survival
- **FDA Approval Date:** July 23, 2014
- **Indications:** Relapsed CLL, follicular B-cell NHL, and relapsed SLL
- **Dose:** 150 mg BID regardless of food
- **Half-life:** 8.2 hours
- **Metabolism:** Major CYP3A4 substrate and UGT1A4 substrate; major CYP3A4 inhibitor

- **Side Effects:** Colitis, anemia, thrombocytopenia, neutropenia, fatigue, headache, skin rash, pneumonitis, elevated ALT/AST, infection, diarrhea, abdominal pain, nausea/vomiting, cough, pyrexia

---

Imatinib Mesylate

- **Alias:** STI-571; CGP-57148B; Glivec
- **Brand Name:** Gleevec
- **Type Mechanism:** An inhibitor of Bcr-Abl tyrosine kinase, the constitutive abnormal gene product of the Ph in CML. Inhibition of this enzyme blocks proliferation and induces apoptosis in Bcr-Abl–positive cell lines as well as in fresh leukemic cells in Ph+ CML. Also inhibits tyrosine kinase for PDGF, SCF, c-Kit, and cellular events mediated by PDGF and SCF.
- **Drug Class:** BCR-ABL TKI
- **FDA Approval Date:** May 10, 2001
- **Indications:** Ph+ ALL in adults and children; KIT (CD117)+ GISTs; Ph+ CML in adults and children in all phases; aggressive systemic mastocytosis, hypereosinophilic syndrome or chronic eosinophilic leukemia; myelodysplastic/myeloproliferative diseases with *PDGFR* gene rearrangement
- **Dose:** Dose range from 100 to 800 mg PO daily or in 2 divided doses depending on diagnosis

- **Half-life:** Parent drug = 18 hours; active metabolite *N*-desmethyl metabolite = ~40 hours
- **Metabolism:** Major CYP3A4 substrate; moderate CYP3A4 inhibitor
- **Side Effects:** Edema/fluid retention (periorbital edema), nausea/vomiting, diarrhea, abdominal pain, fever, myelosuppression, hemorrhage, musculoskeletal pain (arthralgia), fatigue, rash (pruritus), muscle cramps, liver dysfunction (transaminitis, increased bilirubin)
- **Clinical Pearls:** Tablets may be dispersed in water or apple juice (~50 mL for 100 mg tablets and ~200 mL for 400 mg tablets).

Imifoplatin

- **Alias:** PT-112
- **Type Mechanism:** Small molecule pyrophosphate conjugate that induces immunogenic cell death via the release of damage associated molecular patterns (DAMPs)
- **Phase:** Ongoing Phase 2 trials of PT-112 monotherapy in mCRPC, and in thymoma/thymic carcinoma, as well as the combination of PT-112 plus PD-L1 inhibition in NSCLC
- **Dose:** Recommended Phase 2 dose of 360 mg/m^2 IV on days 1, 8, and 15 of a 28-day cycle
- **Side Effects:** Fatigue, nausea, peripheral neuropathy and thrombocytopenia

Iniparib

- **Alias:** BSI-201
- **Type Mechanism:** A small-molecule iodobenzamide that has shown to have anticancer activity through a prodrug mechanism in which an active nitro radical ion is released through one- and two-electron cytosolic activation, rather than direct PARP inhibition
- **Phase:** Phase 2
- **Indications:** Malignant gliomas in combination with RT and temozolomide
- **Dose:** 3.6 mg/kg IV TIW for 6 cycles
- **Half-life:** Iniparib = 11 minutes; active metabolite IABM = 0.8 hours; and active metabolite IABA = 2.1 hours
- **Metabolism:** Nitro reduction pathway
- **Side Effects:** Fatigue, rash, thrombocytopenia, neutropenia, elevated ALT/AST, hyperbilirubinemia, abdominal pain, diarrhea, nausea, anorexia
- **Clinical Pearls:** Trials in phase 3 TNBC and squamous cell lung cancer and phase 2 in platinum-resistant ovarian cancer failed to show survival benefit. On June 2013, manufacture dropped the development of drug.

(Blakeley et al., 2019)

Inotuzumab Ozogamicin

- **Alias:** CMC-544; WAY-207294
- **Brand Name:** Besponsa
- **Type Mechanism:** A CD22-targeted cytotoxic immunoconjugate composed of a humanized IgG4 anti-CD22 antibody that is linked to a calicheamicin dimethyl hydrazide (CalichDMH), a potent cytotoxic antibiotic. After ADC binds to CD22, the CD22–conjugate complex is internalized and releases calicheamicin. Calicheamicin binds to the minor groove of DNA to induce double-strand cleavage and subsequent cell-cycle arrest and apoptosis.
- **Drug Class:** ADC
- **FDA Approval Date:** August 17, 2017
- **Indications:** Relapsed/refractory acute B-cell lymphoblastic leukemia
- **Dose:** Cycle 1: 0.8 mg/m² IV on day 1 and 0.5 mg/m² on days 8 and 15 of a 21-day cycle (may repeat twice if not in CR or CRi); subsequent cycles: 0.5 mg/m² IV on days 1, 8, and 15 of 21 days
- **Half-life:** 12.3 days
- **Side Effects:** Thrombocytopenia, asthenia, abdominal pain, transaminitis (increased AST/ALT and ALP), neutropenia, fever, fatigue, headache, elevated lipase/amylase, nausea, lymphocytopenia, hyperbilirubinemia, infection

Ipafricept

- **Alias:** OMP-54F28; Fzd8-Fc
- **Type Mechanism:** A proprietary fusion protein composed of the cysteine-rich domain of frizzled family receptor 8 (Fzd8) fused to the human Ig Fc domain that competes with the membrane-bound Fzd8 receptor for its ligand, Wnt proteins, thereby antagonizing Wnt signaling. This may result in the inhibition of Wnt-driven tumor growth. Fzd8, a member of the Frizzled family of G-protein–coupled receptors, is one of the components in the Wnt/β-catenin signaling pathway that plays key roles in embryogenesis and cancer growth.
- **Drug Class:** Wnt/β-catenin pathway inhibitor
- **Phase:** Phase 1b/2
- **Indications:** Untreated metastatic pancreatic adenocarcinoma (study terminated owing to bone-related toxicity in July 2020); platinum-sensitive ovarian cancer (study terminated after phase I owing to bone toxicity in August 2019)
- **Dose:** Pancreatic cancer dosing: 3.5 mg/kg IV days 1 and 15 of 28 days; ovarian cancer dosing: 6 mg/kg IV Q 3 weeks

- **Side Effects:** Elevated AST, fatigue, nausea, vomiting, anorexia, pyrexia, dysgeusia, rash

(Picozzi et al., 2019)

Ipatasertib

- **Alias:** GDC-0068; RG-7440
- **Type Mechanism:** An inhibitor of the serine/threonine protein kinase Akt (protein kinase B) that binds to and inhibits the activity of Akt in a non–ATP-competitive manner, which may result in the inhibition of the PI3K/Akt signaling pathway and tumor cell proliferation and the induction of tumor cell apoptosis
- **Drug Class:** AKT inhibitor
- **Phase:** Phase 2
- **Indications:** Metastatic prostate cancer with and without PTEN loss in combination with abiraterone
- **Dose:** 400 mg PO daily for 21 days on, 7 days off
- **Half-life:** 31.9 to 53 hours
- **Side Effects:** Diarrhea, nausea, vomiting, asthenia, rash, decreased appetite, hyperglycemia
- **Clinical Pearls:** Ipatunity-130 study failed both cohorts of TNBC and HR+ HER2− breast cancer.

(de Bono et al., 2019)

Ipilimumab

- **Alias:** MDX-010; MDX-CTLA-4
- **Brand Name:** Yervoy
- **Type Mechanism:** A recombinant human IgG1 mAb that binds to the CTLA-4. CTLA-4 is a downregulator of T-cell activation pathways. Blocking CTLA-4 allows for enhanced T-cell activation and proliferation.
- **Drug Class:** Anti-CTLA4 mAb
- **FDA Approval Date:** March 25, 2011
- **Indications:** Microsatellite instability high (MSI-H) or dMMR mCRC; HCC (in combination with nivolumab); unresectable, malignant pleural mesothelioma; unresectable or metastatic melanoma (in combination with nivolumab); metastatic/recurrent NSCLC with no EGFR or ALK; advanced RCC (in combination with nivolumab)
- **Dose:** Range of dose from 1 mg/kg IV Q 3 weeks, 3 mg/kg IV Q 3 weeks, or 10 mg/kg IV Q 3 weeks, up to 4 doses; NSCLC dose = 1 mg/kg IV Q 6 weeks until PD
- **Half-life:** 15.4 days
- **Side Effects:** Immune-mediated adverse effects (TEN, endocrine disorder, enterocolitis, hepatitis, neuropathy) (black box warning), fatigue, headache, rash/

pruritus, nausea/vomiting, diarrhea, abdominal pain, elevated amylase/lipase, elevated ALT/AST, hyperbilirubinemia

- **Clinical Pearls:** Some products contain polysorbate 80 that may require prophylaxis premedications with dexamethasone, H2 antagonist, acetaminophen, and diphenhydramine.

Isatuximab

- **Alias:** SAR650984; Isatuximab-irfc
- **Brand Name:** Sarclisa
- **Type Mechanism:** An IgG1-derived mAb directed against CD38 that is expressed on the surface of hematopoietic and tumor cells, including MM cells. Isatuximab has antitumor activity via antibody-dependent, cell-mediated cytotoxicity; complement-dependent cytotoxicity; and antibody-dependent cellular phagocytosis and directly inhibits the activity of CD38 ectoenzymes. Isatuximab can activate NK cells in the absence of CD38-positive target tumor cells and suppresses CD38-positive T-regulatory cells.
- **FDA Approval Date:** March 2, 2020
- **Indications:** Relapsed/refractory MM
- **Dose:** Cycle 1: 10 mg/kg IV on days 1, 8, 15, and 22 of 28 days; cycles 2+: 10 mg/kg IV on days 1 and 15 of 28 days
- **Side Effects:** Diarrhea, nausea, anemia, neutropenia, lymphocytopenia, thrombocytopenia, pneumonia, infusion-related side effects (chills, fevers, rigors)

Ivosidenib

- **Alias:** AG-120
- **Brand Name:** Tibsovo
- **Type Mechanism:** An inhibitor of isocitrate dehydrogenase type 1 (IDH1) that inhibits a mutated form of IDH1 in the cytoplasm, which inhibits the formation of the oncometabolite, 2HG. This may lead to both an induction of cellular differentiation and an inhibition of cellular proliferation in IDH1-expressing tumor cells. IDH1, an enzyme in the citric acid cycle, is mutated in a variety of cancers; it initiates and drives cancer growth by both blocking cell differentiation and catalyzing the formation of 2HG.
- **Drug Class:** IDH1 inhibitor
- **FDA Approval Date:** July 20, 2018
- **Indications:** Relapsed/refractory or newly diagnosed AML in adults older than ≥75 years with IDH1 mutation
- **Dose:** 500 mg PO daily. Do not take with high-fat meals due to 98% increase in C_{max}.
- **Half-life:** 93 hours

- **Metabolism:** Major CYP3A4 substrate
- **Side Effects:** Fatigue, diarrhea, nausea, decreased appetite, peripheral edema, prolonged QTc, dyspnea, anemia, HTN, transaminitis, leukocytosis due to differentiation syndrome, abdominal pain, skin rash, pruritus
- **Clinical Pearls:** ClarIDHy phase 3 trial demonstrated compelling results for treatment with previously treated, IDH1-mutant cholangiocarcinoma.

Lanreotide

- **Brand Name:** Somatuline Depot
- **Type Mechanism:** Octapeptide analog of somatostatin with affinity for somatostatin type 2 and 5 receptors (SSTR2 and SSTR5). It reduces growth hormone (GH) secretion and IGF-1 levels.
- **FDA Approval Date:** August 30, 2007
- **Indications:** Carcinoid syndrome and gastroenteropancreatic neuroendocrine tumor (GEP-NET)
- **Dose:** 120 mg SC Q 4 weeks
- **Half-life:** 23 to 30 days

Lapatinib Ditosylate

- **Alias:** GSK572016; GW2016; GW-572016

- **Brand Name:** Tykerb
- **Type Mechanism:** Reversibly blocks phosphorylation of the EGFR, HER2, and the ERK1, ERK2, and AKT kinases. Inhibits cyclin D protein levels in human tumor cell lines and xenografts
- **FDA Approval Date:** March 13, 2007
- **Indications:** Metastatic or advanced breast cancer with HER2 overexpression
- **Dose:** 1,250 mg once daily in combination with capecitabine 2,000 mg/m^2 daily, 1,500 mg once daily in combination with letrozole 2.5 mg once daily. Take 1 hour before or 1 hour after meals and avoid grapefruit juice.
- **Half-life:** 24 hours
- **Metabolism:** Major CYP3A4 and P-glycoprotein substrates
- **Side Effects:** Myelosuppression, hand-foot syndrome, liver dysfunction (increased bilirubin, transaminitis), fatigue, nausea/vomiting, diarrhea, rash, decreased LVEF
- **Clinical Pearls:** LVEF should be evaluated in patients before starting therapy, because a decreased EF can occur within the first 9 weeks of treatment. Oral steroids can decrease the levels of the drug and make it less effective. This drug can change the rhythm of the heart. Exercise caution with

patients who are already on medications to control irregular heart rhythm.

Larotrectinib

- **Alias:** LOXO-101; TRK inhibitor
- **Brand Name:** Vitrakvi
- **Type Mechanism:** An orally available TRK inhibitor that binds to TRK, thereby preventing neurotrophin–TRK interaction and TRK activation, which results in both the induction of cellular apoptosis and the inhibition of cell growth in tumors that overexpress TRK
- **Phase:** Phase 2
- **Indications:** Relapsed/refractory solid tumors, NHL, or histiocytic disorder with NTRK fusion
- **Dose:** 100 mg PO BID until PD
- **Half-life:** 3.5 hours
- **Side Effects:** Increased transaminases, fatigue, dizziness, anemia, dyspnea, neutropenia, constipation

(Hong et al., 2020; Laetsch et al., 2017)

Lenalidomide

- **Brand Name:** Revlimid
- **Type Mechanism:** A thalidomide analog that inhibits TNF-α production; stimulates T cells; reduces serum levels of the cytokines, VEGF, and bFGF; and inhibits angiogenesis. Also promotes G1 cell-cycle arrest and apoptosis of malignant cells
- **FDA Approval Date:** December 27, 2005
- **Indications:** MM, 5q-MDS, MCL, MZL, and FL with off-label use in relapsed/refractory CLL and DLBCL
- **Dose:** 25 mg once daily (MM and MCL); 10 mg PO daily (MDS); 20 mg once daily (FL and MZL); 10 mg once daily in combination with rituximab; 25 mg once daily
- **Half-life:** 3 to 5 hours
- **Metabolism:** P-glycoprotein substrate
- **Side Effects:** Bone marrow suppression (U.S. box warning), thromboembolic events (U.S. box warning), fatigue, weakness, constipation, nausea/vomiting, diarrhea, muscle cramp, pyrexia, rash (pruritus), URI
- **Clinical Pearls:** Lenalidomide may cause birth defects or miscarriage if taken during pregnancy. Women of childbearing age should practice effective birth control while on treatment. Routine scheduled pregnancy tests will be done before, during, and 4 weeks after discontinued.

Lenvatinib Mesylate

- **Alias:** E7080

- **Type Mechanism:** A multitargeted TKI of VEGF receptors VEGFR1 (FLT1), VEGFR2 (KDR), VEGFR3 (FLT4), FGFR1, FGFR2, FGFR3, FGFR4, PDGFRα, KIT, and RET
- **FDA Approval Date:** February 13, 2015
- **Indications:** Differentiated thyroid carcinoma, advanced RCC, or endometrial cancer or unresectable HCC
- **Dose:** 18 mg daily (in combination with everolimus in the RCC); 24 mg daily (thyroid cancer); 20 mg daily in combination with pembrolizumab (endometrial cancer and RCC); 12 mg daily (HCC)
- **Half-life:** 28 hours
- **Metabolism:** Major CYP3A4 substrate
- **Side Effects:** HTN, proteinuria, nausea/vomiting, diarrhea, stomatitis, anorexia, fatigue, QT prolongation, peripheral edema, arthralgia, cough

LGK974

- **Alias:** KB-145911
- **Type Mechanism:** Small-molecule inhibitor of porcupine (PORCN) protein, important for Wnt pathway signaling. No published clinical results
- **Phase:** Ongoing phase 1 trial as single agent and in combination with anti–PD-1 in solid tumors

- **Dose:** 10 mg once daily
- **Half-life:** 5 to 8 hours
- **Side Effect:** Dysgeusia

(Liu et al., 2013; Rodon et al., 2021)

Linifanib

- **Alias:** ABT 869
- **Type Mechanism:** VEGF and PDGF inhibitor. Exhibits potent antiproliferative and apoptotic effects on tumor cells whose proliferation is dependent on mutant kinases, such as FLT3
- **Phase:** Currently in phase 2 trials for breast cancer, NSCLC, RCC, and KRAS-positive CRC; phase 3 trial for HCC
- **Indications:** Breast cancer, NSCLC, RCC, and KRAS-positive CRC; HCC; potential for activity in AML patients
- **Dose:** 0.1 to 0.25 mg/kg PO daily
- **Half-life:** 15 to 19 hours

Linsitinib

- **Alias:** OSI-906; ASP7487
- **Type Mechanism:** An orally bioavailable small molecule that selectively inhibits IGF-1R
- **Phase:** Phase 3 trial in progress for adrenocortical carcinoma; phase 2 trials in

progress for liver, NSCLC, ovarian cancer, and MM
- **Dose:** 300 mg PO daily
- **Half-life:** 2 to 4 hours
- **Side Effects:** Hyperglycemia, nausea/vomiting, elevated lipase

(Lindsay et al., 2009)

Loncastuximab Tesirine

- **Alias:** ADCT-402
- **Brand Name:** Zynlonta
- **Type Mechanism:** An ADC that contains a humanized IgG1 mAb directed at CD19, conjugated to a pyrrolobenzodiazepine dimer cytotoxic alkylating agent (SG3199) via a protease-cleavable linker with SG3199 attached, which is the small-molecule cytotoxin, SG3249 (tesirine). The antibody component binds to CD19 (a transmembrane protein expressed on B-cell surfaces). After binding, loncastuximab tesirine is internalized and releases SG3199 via proteolytic cleavage. SG3199 then binds to the DNA minor groove and forms highly cytotoxic DNA interstrand cross-links and induces cell death.
- **Drug Class:** ADC
- **FDA Approval Date:** April 23, 2021
- **Indications:** Relapsed, refractory, large B-cell lymphoma
- **Dose:** 0.15 mg/kg IV on day 1 of 21 days for 2 cycles, then 0.075 mg/kg IV on day 1 Q 21 days until progression. NOTE: Administer premedications with dexamethasone 4 mg BID for 3 days beginning day before loncastuximab.
- **Half-life:** ~21 days
- **Metabolism:** Minor CYP3A4 and P-glycoprotein/ABCB1 substrates
- **Side Effects:** Edema, skin rash, pruritus, decreased albumin, GGT elevation, hyperglycemia, abdominal pain, loss of appetite, nausea, anemia, neutropenia, thrombocytopenia, transaminitis with ALT/AST elevations, fatigue, musculoskeletal pain
- **Clinical Pearls:** For patient with body mass index (BMI) $\geq$35 kg/m^2, use adjusted BW.

Lorlatinib

- **Alias:** Lorbrena
- **Type Mechanism:** Third-generation ALK inhibitor with increased potency and improved BBB penetration
- **FDA Approval Date:** November 2, 2018
- **Indications:** ALK-positive NSCLC
- **Dose:** 100 mg daily
- **Half-life:** 24 hours
- **Metabolism:** CY3A4 and UGT1A4
- **Side Effects:** HTN, edema, hyperlipidemia

(Shaw et al., 2017, 2019, 2020)

Lucitanib

- **Alias:** E-3810; AL3810
- **Type Mechanism:** Multikinase angiogenesis inhibitor of VEGFR1-3, PDGFRα/β, and FGFR1-3
- **Phase:** Phase 2/3 trial either alone and in combination with nivolumab for gynecologic cancers
- **Dose:** 6 mg PO once daily
- **Half-life:** 31 to 40 hours
- **Side Effects:** HTN, asthenia, proteinuria, rare thrombotic microangiopathy reported (two in phase 1 trial; one biopsy proven)

(Hui et al., 2020; Soria et al., 2015)

Lurbinectedin

- **Alias:** PM01183
- **Brand Name:** Zepzelca
- **Type Mechanism:** Alkylating agent that binds guanine residues in DNA, leading to cell-cycle disruption
- **FDA Approval Date:** June 15, 2020
- **Indications:** Metastatic SCLC
- **Dose:** 3.2 mg/m^2 IV Q 21 days
- **Half-life:** 51 hours
- **Metabolism:** Minor CYP3A4 substrate
- **Side Effects:** Cytopenias, hepatotoxicity, GI disorders

- **Clinical Pearls:** Body surface area (BSA) capped at 2 m^2 for dosing.

(Trigo et al., 2020)

Lutetium Lu 177 Dotatate

- **Brand Name:** Lutathera
- **Type Mechanism:** β- and γ-emitting radionuclide that binds to SSRT2. β Emission induces cellular damage by forming free radicals in somatostatin receptor–positive and surrounding cells.
- **Drug Class:** Radiopharmaceutical agent
- **FDA Approval Date:** January 26, 2018
- **Indications:** GEP-NETs
- **Dose:** 7.4 GBq (200 mCi) Q 7 weeks for 4 total doses
- **Half-life:** 71 ± 8 hours
- **Side Effects:** HTN, flushing, peripheral edema, alopecia, hyperglycemia, hyperkalemia, GGT elevation, nausea, vomiting, abdominal pain, anemia, diarrhea, loss of appetite, leukopenia, lymphocytopenia, neutropenia, ALT/AST elevations, hyperbilirubinemia, fatigue
- **Clinical Pearls:** 68Ga-DOTATATE PET may help identify lesions and evaluate response.

(Strosberg et al., 2017)

Margetuximab-cmkb

- **Alias:** MGAH22
- **Brand Name:** Margenza
- **Type Mechanism:** A chimeric IgG1κ mAb antagonist against HER2. It exerts its effect by inhibiting HER2 shedding and through antibody-dependent cellular toxicity.
- **Drug Class:** Anti-HER2 mAb
- **FDA Approval Date:** December 16, 2020
- **Indications:** HER2-positive metastatic breast cancer
- **Dose:** 15 mg/kg IV Q 3 weeks in combination with chemotherapy
- **Half-life:** 19.2 days
- **Side Effects:** Hand-foot syndrome, reduction in LVEF, cytopenias
- **Clinical Pearls:** Anthracyclines may enhance the adverse/toxic effects and should be avoided for up to 4 months after discontinuing margetuximab.

Matuzumab

- **Alias:** EMD 72000
- **Type Mechanism:** A humanized IgG1 EGFR mAb that binds to EGFR with high affinity
- **Phase:** Phase 2
- **Indications:** Platinum-resistant ovarian and primary peritoneal malignancies
- **Dose:** 800 mg weekly IV infusion
- **Half-life:** 4 to 7 days (at recommended dose)
- **Side Effects:** Acneiform skin effects, epidermolysis, nail bed infection, conjunctivitis, headache, diarrhea, fever, dry skin, fatigue

(Seiden et al., 2005)

Midostaurin

- **Alias:** PKC 412; CGP 41251
- **Brand Name:** Rydapt
- **Mechanism of Action:** A TKI that inhibits multiple receptors, such as WT FLT3, FLT3-mutant kinases ITD and TKD, KIT (WT and D816V mutant), PDGFRα/β, VEGFR2, and members of the serine/threonine PKC family. Midostaurin inhibits FLT3 receptor signaling and cell proliferation and induces apoptosis in ITD- and TKD-mutant–expressing leukemic cells, as well as in cells overexpressing WT FLT3 and PDGFR. It may also inhibit KIT signaling, cell proliferation, and histamine release (and induces apoptosis) in mast cells.
- **FDA Approval Date:** April 28, 2017
- **Indications:** FDA approved for mast cell leukemia, systemic mastocytosis, and FLT3-mutated AML

- **Dose:** 50 mg PO Q 12 hours on Days 8 to 21 of AML therapy after light meal; high-fat meal will increase the concentration of the drug; 100 mg Q 12 hours in mast cell leukemia and systemic mastocytosis
- **Half-life:** 19 hours (midostaurin); 32 hours (active metabolite CGP62221); 482 hours (active metabolite CGP52421)
- **Metabolism:** Major CYP3A4 substrate
- **Side Effects:** Nausea/vomiting/diarrhea, headache, fatigue, transient liver enzymes elevation, transient amylase elevation, QT prolongation, skin rash, hyperhidrosis, hyperglycemia, urinary tract infection, muscle pain, renal insufficiency

Milademetan

- **Alias:** RAIN-32
- **Type Mechanism:** A small-molecule inhibitor of MDM2 that disrupts the interactions between MDM2 and the tumor suppressor protein p53. This will result in sustained increase in p53 activity with resultant antitumor effect.
- **Phase:** Phase 2; phase 3 in liposarcoma
- **Indications:** Well-differentiated/dedifferentiated liposarcoma, intimal sarcoma, and advanced metastatic solid tumors with *MDM2* gene amplification
- **Dose:** RP2D: 260 mg PO daily on days 1 to 3 and days 15 to 17 of a 28-day cycle or 90 mg PO daily for 21 of 28 days
- **Metabolism:** Inhibitor of CYP3A4, P-glycoprotein, and BCRP
- **Side Effects:** Thrombocytopenia, neutropenia, anemia, nausea, decreased appetite, fatigue
- **Clinical Pearls:** Orphan drug designation for the treatment of liposarcoma.

(Takahashi et al., 2021)

Miransertib

- **Alias:** ARQ-092; MK-7075
- **Type Mechanism:** A small molecule that binds to and inhibits the activity of AKT1/2/3 isoforms in a non–ATP-competitive manner, which may result in the inhibition of the PI3K/AKT signaling pathway. This may lead to the reduction in tumor cell proliferation and the induction of tumor cell apoptosis.
- **Phase:** Phase 1b
- **Indications:** PIK3CA or AKT1-mutant ER+ endometrial or ovarian cancer
- **Dose:** 150 mg PO daily for 5 days on, 9 days off (in combination with anastrozole)

- **Side Effects:** ALT elevation, rash, hyperglycemia

(Hyman et al., 2018)

Mirvetuximab Soravtansine

- **Alias:** IMGN853
- **Type Mechanism:** An immunoconjugate consisting of the humanized mAb M9346A against FOLR1 conjugated, via the disulfide-containing cleavable linker sulfo-PDB, to the cytotoxic maytansinoid DM4. After antibody–antigen interaction and internalization, the immunoconjugate releases DM4, which binds to tubulin and disrupts microtubule assembly/disassembly dynamics, thereby inhibiting cell division and the growth of FOLR1-expressing tumor cells.
- **Phase:** Phase 3 studies of mirvetuximab versus standard of care in advanced, epithelial ovarian cancer, primary peritoneal cancer, and/or fallopian tube cancer; phase 1/2 studies ongoing in combinations with chemotherapy, antiangiogenesis agents, and checkpoint inhibitors
- **Dose:** 6 mg/kg IV Q 3 weeks. Dose is based on actual ideal BW. May need to use prophylactic steroid eye drops to reduce ocular toxicities
- **Half-life:** 79 to 121 hours (3–5 days)

- **Side Effects:** Hypophosphatemia, keratitis, fatigue, diarrhea, infusion-related reactions, peripheral neuropathy

(Moore et al., 2017; O'Malley et al., 2020)

MK-0752

- **Type Mechanism:** A synthetic small-molecule γ-secretase that inhibits the Notch signaling pathway
- **Phase:** Phase 1/2
- **Indications:** T-cell leukemia, breast cancer, brain tumors (gliomas), pancreatic cancer, colon cancer, cervical cancer, and salivary gland carcinoma
- **Dose:** 350 mg PO 3 days on, 4 days off Q week for 28 days; 1,500 to 1,800 mg PO once a week with or without food
- **Half-life:** 15 hours (terminal)
- **Side Effects:** Nausea/vomiting, diarrhea, fatigue, lymphopenia, hypokalemia, constipation

(Krop et al., 2012)

MK-2206

- **Type Mechanism:** An allosteric inhibitor of AKT (protein kinase B)
- **Phase:** Phase 2
- **Indications:** Solid tumors

- **Dose:** 60 mg PO QOD on empty stomach, 2 hours before meal or 2 hours after meal
- **Half-life:** 63 to 89 hours
- **Metabolism:** Major CYP3A4 substrate
- **Side Effects:** Skin rash, stomatitis, nausea, pruritus, hyperglycemia, diarrhea

(Yap et al., 2011)

MK-8242

- **Alias:** SCH 900242
- **Type Mechanism:** Inhibits MDM2, allowing TP53 to function and arrest cancer cell growth
  - For MK-8242 to work, TP53 itself has to be WT, because increasing the amount of abnormal TP53 would probably not stop cancer cells from growing.
- **Phase:** Phase 1
- **Indications:** Solid tumors and AML
- **Dose:** Oral dosing BID on fasting stomach 1 hour before dosing and remain in fasting for 1 hour after dosing
- **Half-life:** 6.5 to 8.9 hours
- **Metabolism:** CYP3A4 and possible major inhibitor of CYP3A4

(Wang et al., 2017)

MKC-1

- **Alias:** Ro-31-7453
- **Type Mechanism:** An orally bioavailable, small-molecule bisindolylmaleimide cell-cycle inhibitor that inhibits tubulin polymerization, blocking the formation of the mitotic spindle, which may result in cell-cycle arrest at the G2/M phase and apoptosis
  - Also shown to inhibit the activities of the oncogenic kinase AKT, the mTOR pathway, and importin-β, a protein essential to the transport of other proteins from the cytosol into the nucleus
- **Phase:** Phase 1b/2
- **Indications:** NSCLC, metastatic pancreatic cancer, metastatic ovarian cancer, and metastatic breast cancer
- **Dose:** Up to 1,000 mg PO daily for 4 days of each cycle
- **Half-life:** 9 hours
- **Side Effects:** Nausea/vomiting, diarrhea, fatigue, myelosuppression, mucositis, hyperbilirubinemia, transaminitis

(Tevaarwerk et al., 2012)

Mocetinostat

- **Alias:** MGCD0103
- **Type Mechanism:** Benzamide HDAC inhibitor of class I and IV HDACs (isoforms 1, 2, 3, and 11). It exhibits antiproliferative

activity through inducing cell-cycle arrest and apoptosis.

- **Phase:** Phase 1
- **Indications:** Promising activity in leukemias and lymphomas; currently in phase 1 clinical trial in combination with vinorelbine for rhabdomyosarcoma
- **Dose:** 45 mg PO TIW
- **Half-life:** 6.7 to 12.2 hours
- **Side Effects:** Fatigue, nausea/vomiting/diarrhea, anorexia, dehydration

(Batlevi et al., 2017; Siu et al., 2017)

Mogamulizumab-kpkc

- **Alias:** KW-0761; AMG-761
- **Brand Name:** Poteligeo
- **Type Mechanism:** A recombinant, humanized mAb of the IgG1κ isotype that targets CCR4-expressing cells; it may induce ADCC against CCR4-positive T cells.
- **FDA Approval Date:** August 8, 2018
- **Indications:** Relapsed/refractory mycosis fungoides; relapsed/refractory Sezary syndrome
- **Indications:** Approved in Japan for relapsed or refractory CCR4-positive PTCL and CTCL and chemotherapy-native CCR4-positive adult T-cell leukemia/lymphoma

- **Dose:** 1 mg/kg IV on days 1, 8, 15, and 22 of cycle 1, followed by 1 mg/kg on days 1 and 15 of subsequent 28-day cycle
- **Half-life:** 17.5 days
- **Side Effects:** Infusion-related side effects such as fevers, chills, rigors, neutropenia, transaminitis, thrombocytopenia, rash

(Kim et al., 2018; Makita & Tobinai, 2017)

Momelotinib

- **Alias:** GS-0387; CYT387
- **Type Mechanism:** An oral small-molecule inhibitor of JAK 1 and JAK 2. In preclinical models, it demonstrated increased iron availability for erythropoiesis via bone morphogenic protein receptor kinase activin A receptor type 1 (ActR1)
- **Phase:** Ongoing phase 3 trials in myelofibrosis
- **Dose:** 200 mg PO BID
- **Half-life:** 4 to 6 hours
- **Side Effects:** Diarrhea, peripheral neuropathy, thrombocytopenia, dizziness

(Gupta et al., 2017; Harrison et al., 2018; Mesa et al., 2017)

nab-Rapamycin

- **Alias:** ABI-009; nab-sirolimus

- **Type Mechanism:** The macrolide antibiotic rapamycin bound to nanoparticle albumin binds to the immunophilin FKBP-12 to generate a complex that binds to and inhibits the activation of the mTOR, a key regulatory kinase. In turn, inhibition of mTOR may result in the inhibition of the PI3K/Akt pathway and VEGF secretion, which may result in decreased tumor cell proliferation and tumor angiogenesis.
- **Drug Class:** mTOR inhibitor
- **Phase:** Phase 2
- **Indications:** Malignant PEComa, STS (in combination with pazopanib), advanced mCRC (in combination with FOLFOX and bevacizumab)
- **Dose:** 100 mg/m^2 IV Q week for 3 weeks of a 4-week cycle
- **Side Effects:** Mucositis, fatigue, nausea, weight loss, diarrhea, anemia, thrombocytopenia, pneumonitis, transaminitis, hypertriglyceridemia, neutropenia

(Gonzalez-Angulo et al., 2013)

Napabucasin

- **Alias:** BBI608
- **Type Mechanism:** An orally available cancer cell stemness inhibitor that targets and inhibits multiple pathways involved in cancer cell stemness. This may ultimately inhibit cancer stemness cell (CSC) growth as well as heterogeneous cancer cell growth. It is also a small-molecule inhibitor of STAT3.
- **Phase:** Phase 3
- **Indications:** Advanced CRC, pancreatic cancer, GEJ cancer, gastric cancer
- **Dose:** 240 mg PO Q 12 hours
- **Half-life:** 1.5 to 2.7 hours
- **Metabolism:** Inhibitor of CYP1A2, CYP2B6, CYP2C8, CYP2C9, CYP2D6, and CYP3A4
- **Side Effects:** Diarrhea, anorexia, nausea, abdominal pain, fatigue, weight loss, dehydration
- **Clinical Pearls:** Orphan drug designation for gastric, GEJ, and pancreatic cancers in June 2016

(Jonker et al., 2018)

Naquotinib Mesylate

- **Alias:** ASP8273
- **Type Mechanism:** An orally available, irreversible, mutant-selective, third-generation EGFR inhibitor that was found by mass spectrometry to covalently bind to a mutant EGFR (L858R/T790M) via cysteine residue 797 in the kinase domain of EGFR with long-lasting inhibition of EGFR phosphorylation

- **Drug Class:** EGFR inhibitor
- **Phase:** Phase 3
- **Indications:** EGFR-mutated NSCLC
- **Dose:** 300 mg PO daily
- **Side Effects:** Diarrhea, nausea, vomiting, thrombocytopenia, skin rash, mild interstitial lung disease–like events, anorexia, hyponatremia
- **Clinical Pearls:** Global phase 3 comparing naquotinib with gefitinib/erlotinib (SOLAR) was terminated on May 2017 because of poor performance. It was shown to perform worse than the first generation and had more side effects.

(Tan et al., 2016)

Navitoclax

- **Alias:** ABT-263
- **Type Mechanism:** An orally potent and highly selective inhibitor of antiapoptotic members of the BCL-2 family, with a nanomolar affinity for BCL-2, BCL-xL, and BCL-w
- **Phase:** Phase 3 studies in myelofibrosis; phase 1/2 studies in advanced solid tumors
- **Dose:** Up to 250 mg PO daily on a 21-day cycle
- **Half-life:** 15 hours

- **Side Effects:** Nausea/vomiting/diarrhea, fatigue/dizziness, thrombocytopenia, neutropenia, pyrexia, increased ALT

(Gandhi et al., 2011)

Nazartinib

- **Alias:** EGF816
- **Type Mechanism:** An orally available, irreversible, third-generation, mutant-selective EGFR inhibitor that covalently binds to and inhibits the activity of mutant forms of EGFR, including the T790M EGFR mutant, thereby preventing EGFR-mediated signaling. It will induce cell death and inhibit tumor growth in EGFR-overexpressing tumor cells.
- **Drug Class:** EGFR inhibitor
- **Phase:** Phase 2
- **Indication:** EGFR-mutant NSCLC
- **Dose:** 150 mg PO daily
- **Side Effects:** Diarrhea, maculopapular rash, pyrexia, cough, stomatitis, decreased appetite, pruritus, dermatitis acneiform, increased lipase

(Tan et al., 2020)

Necitumumab

- **Alias:** IMC-11F8

- **Type Mechanism:** A recombinant human IgG1 EGFR mAb that binds (with a high affinity) to the ligand-binding site of the EGFR to prevent receptor activation and downstream signaling
- **FDA Approval Date:** November 24, 2015
- **Indications:** FDA approved for metastatic SCC of the lungs (NSCLC)
- **Dose:** 800 mg IV over 60 minutes on days 1 and 8 of a 3-week cycle in combination with gemcitabine/cisplatin until PD
- **Half-life:** 14 days
- **Side Effects:** Headache, rash (acneiform eruption), electrolyte imbalance (potassium, phosphorus, calcium, magnesium), diarrhea, vomiting, stomatitis

Neratinib

- **Alias:** HKI-272; PB272
- **Type Mechanism:** Irreversible pan-EGFR inhibitor that can potentially overcome the acquired resistance of EGFR T790M mutation by targeting a cysteine residue in the ATP-binding pocket of the receptor
- **FDA Approval Date:** July 17, 2017
- **Indications:** FDA approved for extended adjuvant therapy in HER-2–positive breast cancer
- **Dose:** 240 mg PO daily with food

- **Half-life:** 14 hours (range 7–17 hours)
- **Side Effects:** Diarrhea, nausea/vomiting, fatigue, anorexia, skin rash, stomatitis
- **Clinical Pearls:** Recommend to use antidiarrheal prophylaxis with loperamide.

Nilotinib

- **Alias:** AMN107
- **Brand Name:** Tasigna
- **Type Mechanism:** Orally bioavailable BCR-ABL, KIT inhibitor
- **FDA Approval Date:** October 29, 2007
- **Indications:** FDA approved for (a) newly diagnosed Ph+ CML in chronic phase and (b) chronic- and accelerated-phase Ph+ CML in adult patients resistant to or intolerant to prior therapy that included imatinib
- **Dose:** (a) 300 mg PO BID; (b) 400 mg PO BID
- **Half-life:** 17 hours
- **Metabolism:** CYP2D6, CYP2C9, CYP2C19, CYP1A2, NAT2, and DPD substrates
- **Side Effects:** QT prolongation (U.S. box warning); nonhematologic: Rash, pruritus, headache, nausea, fatigue, myalgia, nasopharyngitis, constipation, diarrhea, abdominal pain, vomiting, arthralgia, pyrexia, upper respiratory tract infection,

back pain, cough, and asthenia; hematologic: myelosuppression (thrombocytopenia, neutropenia, anemia)

Nintedanib

- **Alias:** BIBF1120
- **Brand Name:** Ofev (the United States); Vargatef (European Union)
- **Type Mechanism:** A triple angiokinase inhibitor of VEGFR-1, VEGFR-2, VEGFR-3, PDGFRα, PDGFRβ, FGFR-1, FGFR-2, FGFR-3
- **FDA Approval Date:** October 15, 2014
- **Indications:** Approved in combination with docetaxel in EU for NSCLC after first-line therapy. FDA approved for chronic fibrosing interstitial lung disease and idiopathic pulmonary fibrosis
- **Dose:** 150 mg BID in lung diseases
- **Half-life:** 9.5 hours
- **Side Effects:** Diarrhea, nausea/vomiting, anorexia, liver dysfunction (hyperbilirubinemia, transaminitis), increased amylase/lipase, HTN

(Gandhi et al., 2011; Richeldi et al., 2014)

Niraparib

- **Alias:** MK-4827
- **Brand Name:** Zejula
- **Type Mechanism:** An inhibitor of PARP-1 and PARP-2
- **FDA Approval Date:** March 27, 2017
- **Indications:** FDA approved for recurrent epithelial ovarian cancer, fallopian tube or primary peritoneal cancer patients who are in CR or partial response (PR) to platinum-based chemotherapy
- **Dose:** 300 mg PO daily with or without food
- **Half-life:** 36 hours (range 33–46 hours)
- **Metabolism:** CYP1A2 and CYP3A4; P-glycoprotein
- **Side Effects:** Fatigue, insomnia, pneumonitis, anorexia, constipation, nausea/vomiting, neutropenia, thrombocytopenia

Nirogacestat

- **Alias:** PF-03084014
- **Type Mechanism:** An oral small-molecule γ-secretase inhibitor
- **Phase:** FDA granted orphan drug designation for desmoid tumors and European Commission for STSs
- **Dose:** 150 mg BID (changed from prior version)
- **Half-life:** 22 to 40 hours
- **Side Effects:** Diarrhea, nausea, fatigue, hypophosphatemia, vomiting

(Messersmith et al., 2015)

Nivolumab

- **Alias:** BMS-936558; MDX1106; ONO-4538
- **Brand Name:** Opdivo
- **Type Mechanism:** Fully human IgG4 mAb targeting PD-1 receptor on activated T cells
- **FDA Approval Date:** December 22, 2014
- **Indications:** FDA approved for recurrent or metastatic SCCHN, classic Hodgkin lymphoma, unresectable or metastatic melanoma or in adjuvant setting, metastatic NSCLC (nonsquamous), advanced RCC, RCC, HCC, MSI-H CRC, and locally advanced or metastatic urothelial carcinoma
- **Dose:** 3 mg/kg IV Q 2 weeks (H&N cancer, Hodgkin lymphoma, SCLC); 240 mg IV Q 2 weeks or 480 mg IV Q 4 weeks (melanoma, NSCLC, RCC, urothelial cancer, MSI-H CRC, esophageal cancer, HCC); mesothelioma 360 mg IV Q 3 weeks in combination with ipilimumab; combination and then increase it to 3 mg/kg or 240 mg when given alone (HCC, melanoma, RCC)
- **Half-life:** 25 days
- **Side Effects:** Fatigue, nausea, diarrhea, xerostomia, pruritus, immune-mediated colitis, pneumonitis, hyperglycemia, hypertriglyceridemia, hyponatremia, thyroid dysfunction

Obatoclax Mesylate

- **Alias:** GX15-070
- **Type Mechanism:** A small molecule and a pan inhibitor of Bcl-2 family proteins, with proapoptotic activity. GX015-070 is a selective antagonist of the BH3-binding groove of the Bcl-2 family proteins, which are frequently overexpressed in cancers, including CLL. This agent induces/restores apoptosis in cancer cells by inhibiting apoptosis suppressors in multiple members of the Bcl-2 family simultaneously.
- **Drug Class:** Pan-bcl2 inhibitor
- **Phase:** Phase 2
- **Indications:** SCLC, MDSs, relapsed/refractory MCL
- **Dose:** 60 mg IV over 24 hours Q 2 weeks
- **Side Effects:** Euphoria, nausea, diarrhea, anemia, ataxia, thrombocytopenia, pneumonia
- **Clinical Pearls:** Phase 2 with topotecan for relapsed SCLC did not show superiority over historic response rate with topotecan alone.

(Paik et al., 2011)

Obinutuzumab

- **Alias:** GA101; R05072759; R7159
- **Brand Name:** Gazyva

- **Type Mechanism:** A glycoengineered type 2 anti-CD20 mAb that is expressed on the surface of pre-B and mature B lymphocytes; upon binding to CD20, obinutuzumab activates complement-dependent cytotoxicity, ADCC, and antibody-dependent cellular phagocytosis, resulting in cell death
- **FDA Approval Date:** November 1, 2013
- **Indications:** FDA approved for CLL and FL
- **Dose:** (1) For CLL—cycle 1: 100 mg IV on day 1, followed by 900 mg on day 2, followed by 1,000 mg weekly for 2 doses. For cycles 2 to 6: 1,000 mg IV on day 1 of each 28-day cycle. (2) FL—cycle 1 (in combination with bendamustine): 1,000 mg IV weekly for 3 doses. For cycles 2 to 6: 1,000 mg IV on day 1 of each 28-day cycle. If used as monotherapy, 1,000 mg IV Q 2 months for 2 years
- **Half-life:** 26.4 to 36.8 days
- **Side Effects:** Hypophosphatemia, hypocalcemia, myelosuppression, transaminitis, infection, muscle and back pain, weakness, increased SCr, cough, URI

(Marcus et al., 2017)

Ofatumumab

- **Alias:** HuMax-CD20
- **Brand Name:** Arzerra
- **Type Mechanism:** A fully human, high-affinity IgG1 mAb directed against the B-cell CD20 cell-surface antigen
- **Phase:** Currently in clinical trials for other hematologic malignancies
- **FDA Approval Date:** October 26, 2009
- **Indications:** FDA approved for the treatment of CLL refractory to fludarabine and alemtuzumab
- **Dose:** 300 mg IV initial dose, followed 1 week later by 2,000 mg weekly for 7 doses, followed 4 weeks later by 2,000 mg Q 4 weeks for 4 doses for total of 12 doses
- **Half-life:** 4 days (between doses 4 and 12)
- **Side Effects:** U.S. box warning: Hepatitis B virus reactivation, progressive multifocal leukoencephalopathy, fatigue, skin rash, neutropenia/anemia, diarrhea, infection, infusion-related reactions (50% in the first dose)

Olaparib

- **Alias:** AZD2281; KU-0059436
- **Brand Name:** Lynparza
- **Type Mechanism:** A small-molecule inhibitor of the nuclear enzyme PARP with potential chemosensitizing and radiosensitizing properties
- **FDA Approval Date:** December 19, 2014

- **Indications:** Advanced ovarian cancer, HER2-negative and BRCA mutation breast cancer, MCRPC with HRD, and pancreatic cancer as maintenance therapy after first-line chemotherapy
- **Dose:** 400 mg Q 12 hours. No grapefruit or Seville oranges
- **Half-life:** 11.9 ± 4.8 hours
- **Side Effects:** Nausea/vomiting, leukopenia/lymphopenia, increased creatinine, fatigue, abdominal pain, diarrhea, anemia, thrombocytopenia, muscle pain, infection

Olaratumab

- **Alias:** Antibody IMC-3G3, IMC-3G3; LY3012207
- **Brand Name:** Lartruvo
- **Type Mechanism:** A fully human IgG1 mAb that selectively binds to PDGFRα, blocking the binding of its ligand, PDGF; signal transduction downstream of PDGFR through the MAPK and PI3K pathways is inhibited, which may result in the inhibition of angiogenesis and tumor cell proliferation
- **Drug Class:** PDGFRα blocker
- **FDA Approval Date:** October 19, 2016
- **Indications:** A confirmatory phase 3 randomized, blinded trial in patients with unresectable locally advanced or metastatic STS comparing olaratumab plus doxorubicin to placebo plus doxorubicin found no significant difference in overall survival because of the addition of olaratumab to doxorubicin (Tap, 2020). Owing to the trial results, the manufacturer has withdrawn olaratumab from the market.

- **Dose:** 15 mg/kg IV on days 1 and 8 Q 3 weeks (in combination with doxorubicin) for 8 cycles; after 8 cycles are completed, continue olaratumab as a single agent. Premedicate with diphenhydramine IV and dexamethasone 10 mg IV on cycle 1 day 1 of olaratumab.
- **Half-life:** 11 days (range 6–24 days)
- **Side Effects:** Fatigue, neuropathy, headache, alopecia, hyperglycemia, electrolyte depletion (potassium, phosphorus, and magnesium), mucositis, nausea/vomiting, diarrhea, loss of appetite, myelosuppression, musculoskeletal pain, dry eyes, infusion-related reactions

Olmutinib

- **Alias:** BI 1482694
- **Type Mechanism:** Third-generation EGFR-TKIs with covalent binding to the receptors demonstrating irreversible enzymatic

inhibition of activating EGFR mutations and T790M mutation (a common reason for acquired EGFR-TKI resistance), while sparing WT EGFR
- **Phase:** Phase 2
- **Indications:** NSCLC harboring T790 resistance mutation
- **Dose:** RP2D: 800 mg PO daily
- **Half-life:** 4.8 to 7.4 hours
- **Side Effects:** Diarrhea, pruritus, rash, palmar–plantar erythrodysesthesia, ALT elevation, hyperkeratosis, pyrexia, nausea
- **Clinical Pearls:** Granted breakthrough therapy designation in NSCLC by FDA in December 2015. First global approval in South Korea in May 2016 for locally advanced or metastatic EGFR T790M mutation–positive NSCLC. However, study stopped owing to inferior response compared to other EGFR.

(Park et al., 2019, 2021)

Onartuzumab

- **Alias:** MetMAb; RO5490258
- **Type Mechanism:** An IgG1 humanized monovalent mAb that is directed against MET by binding to the extracellular domain, preventing the binding of its ligand, HGF
- **Phase:** Phase 3
- **Indications:** NSCLC and MET+ GE cancer
- **Dose:** 15 mg/kg IV Q 3 weeks
- **Half-life:** 8 to 12 days
- **Side Effects:** Fatigue, peripheral edema, nausea, hypoalbuminemia

(Salgia et al., 2014)

Onatasertib

- **Alias:** CC-223
- **Type Mechanism:** A potent, selective, and orally bioavailable inhibitor of mTOR kinase, demonstrating inhibition of mTORC1 (pS6RP and p4EBP1) and mTORC2 [pAKT(S473)] in cellular systems. mTOR kinase inhibition in cells, by CC-223, resulted in more complete inhibition of the mTOR pathway biomarkers and improved antiproliferative activity as compared with rapamycin.
- **Drug Class:** mTOR inhibitor
- **Phase:** Phase 2
- **Indications:** Non-pNETs, MM, and NHL
- **Dose:** 30 mg PO daily for 28 days
- **Half-life:** 4.86 to 5.64 hours
- **Side Effects:** Diarrhea, fatigue, stomatitis, hyperglycemia, rash, thrombocytopenia, decreased appetite, transaminitis

(Mortensen et al., 2015)

Osimertinib

- **Alias:** AZD9291
- **Brand Name:** Tagrisso
- **Type Mechanism:** An orally available, irreversible, third-generation, mutant-selective EGFR inhibitor that selectively and covalently binds to and inhibits the activity of the mutant forms of EGFR, including the T790M EGFR mutant form, thereby preventing EGFR-mediated signaling. This may both induce cell death and inhibit tumor growth in EGFR-overexpressing tumor cells.
- **FDA Approval Date:** November 13, 2015
- **Indications:** Metastatic NSCLC with exon 19 del, exon 21 L858R mutation–positive, or EGFR T790 mutation–positive patients who have progressed on or after EGFR-TKI therapy
- **Dose:** 80 mg daily with or without food. May be dissolved in water if needed. (Off label 160 mg daily with brain or leptomeningeal metastases)
- **Half-life:** 48 hours
- **Metabolism:** CYP3A4 substrate
- **Side Effects:** Fatigue, skin rash, diarrhea, decreased appetite, nausea, stomatitis, thrombocytopenia, neutropenia, cough

Pacritinib

- **Alias:** SB1518
- **Type Mechanism:** A JAK2/tyrosine kinase 3 inhibitor with minimal activity against JAK1 that also inhibits IRAK1 (IL-1 receptor–associated kinase 1)
- **Phase:** Phase 3
- **Indications:** Myelofibrosis
- **Dose:** 200 to 400 mg PO daily or in split doses
- **Half-life:** 2 to 3 days
- **Side Effects:** Diarrhea, nausea, thrombocytopenia

(Gerds et al., 2020)

Palbociclib

- **Alias:** PD0332991
- **Brand Name:** Ibrance
- **Type Mechanism:** A reversible small-molecule CDK inhibitor that is selective for CDK 4 and CDK 6. CDKs have a role in regulating progression through the cell cycle at the G1/S phase by blocking Rb hyperphosphorylation. It reduces the proliferation of breast cancer cell lines by preventing progression from the G1 to the S cell-cycle phase.
- **FDA Approval Date:** February 3, 2015

- **Indications:** FDA approved with hormone therapy for HR-positive, HER2-negative breast cancer or advanced breast cancer as initial endocrine-based therapy or upon PD with endocrine therapy
- **Dose:** 125 mg PO daily for 21 days of the 28-day cycle. No grapefruit juice
- **Half-life:** 29 ± 5 hours
- **Metabolism:** Major CYP3A4 substrate
- **Side Effects:** Fatigue, nausea/vomiting, diarrhea, constipation, rash, peripheral edema, dyspnea, myelosuppression, stomatitis

(Finn et al., 2016)

Panitumumab

- **Alias:** ABX-EGF; mAb ABX-EGF; rHuMAb-EGFr
- **Brand Name:** Vectibix
- **Type Mechanism:** A fully human mAb that binds specifically to EGFR on both normal and tumor cells and competitively inhibits the binding of ligands for EGFR
  - First antibody to demonstrate the use of KRAS as a predictive biomarker
- **FDA Approval Date:** September 27, 2006
- **Indications:** FDA approved for RAS WT mCRC
- **Dose:** 6 mg/kg IV infusion (over 60 or 90 minutes) Q 14 days

- **Half-life:** 7.5 days (range 4–11 days)
- **Side Effects:** Dermatologic toxicity (rash, dermatitis acneiform, pruritus) (U.S. box warning), infusion reactions (fevers, chills, bronchospasms) (U.S. box warning), hypomagnesemia, paronychia, fatigue, nausea/vomiting, diarrhea
- **Clinical Pearls:** Severity of acne-form rash can be minimized with the use of topical steroid cream, topical antibiotic gel, and doxycycline. Presence and severity of rash may correlate improved response and survival.

(Peeters et al., 2009)

Panobinostat

- **Alias:** LBH-589
- **Brand Name:** Farydak
- **Type Mechanism:** Hydroxamic acid that acts as a nonselective HDAC inhibitor
- **FDA Approval Date:** February 23, 2015
- **Indications:** FDA approved in MM after two prior standard therapies
- **Dose:** 20 mg/m^2 IV weekly in combination with dexamethasone and bortezomib
- **Half-life:** 16 hours
- **Side Effects:** Nausea, fatigue, diarrhea, thrombocytopenia

(Prince & Bishton, 2009; San-Miguel et al., 2017)

Parsaclisib

- **Alias:** INCB050465
- **Type Mechanism:** An inhibitor of the δ isoform of PI3K that inhibits the δ isoform of PI3K and prevents the activation of the PI3K/AKT signaling pathway. This both decreases proliferation and induces cell death in PI3K-δ–overexpressing tumor cells. Unlike other isoforms of PI3K, PI3K-δ is expressed primarily in hematopoietic disease and cell lineages.
- **Drug Class:** PI3K-δ inhibitor
- **Phase:** Phase 2
- **Indications:** Relapsed/refractory B-cell malignancies (NHL, FL, DLBCL, MZL, and MCL)
- **Dose:** 20 mg PO daily for 9 weeks, followed by 20 mg PO Q weekly
- **Half-life:** 8.6 to 11.5 hours
- **Side Effects:** Neutropenia, lymphopenia, thrombocytopenia, pneumonitis, anemia, diarrhea/colitis, nausea, fatigue, rash, pyrexia, hypotension, abdominal pain, decreased appetite, pruritus
- **Clinical Pearls:** Advantage over first-generation PI3K-δ inhibitor in terms of hepatotoxicity or hyperglycemia

(Forero-Torres et al., 2019)

Pazopanib Hydrochloride

- **Alias:** GW786034
- **Brand Name:** Votrient
- **Type Mechanism:** Selectively inhibits VEGFR-1, VEGFR-2, VEGFR-3, FGFR-1, FGFR-3, KIT, and PDGFR, preventing angiogenesis
- **FDA Approval Date:** October 19, 2009
- **Indications:** FDA approved for RCC and STS
- **Dose:** 800 mg daily on fasting stomach, at least 1 hour before or 2 hours after a meal; avoid grapefruit juice
- **Half-life:** 31 hours
- **Metabolism:** Major CYP3A4 substrate
- **Side Effects:** Diarrhea, nausea/vomiting, anorexia, HTN, hair color changes (lightening)
- **Clinical Pearls:** Avoid concurrent medications, which can prolong the QTc interval. Because VEGFR is inhibited, surgical intervention should be avoided.

Pelareorep

- **Alias:** DS-1062
- **Brand Name:** Reolysin®
- **Type Mechanism:** Reovirus serotype 3-dearing strain, a double-stranded

replication-competent RNA nonenveloped icosahedral virus
- **Phase:** Phase 2
- **FDA Approval Date:** July 7, 1905
- **Indications:** Orphan drug designation in ovarian cancer, malignant glioma, and pancreatic cancer
- **Dose:** 3×10^{10} tissue culture effective dose ($TCID_{50}$) well tolerated
- **Side Effects:** Fever, chills, myalgias, cold-like symptoms, GI upset, fatigue

(Gollamudi et al., 2017; Mahalingam et al., 2020)

Pembrolizumab

- **Alias:** MK-3475; SCH 900475
- **Brand Name:** Keytruda
- **Type Mechanism:** A humanized IgG4 mAb directed against human cell-surface receptor PD-1, an inhibitory signaling receptor expressed on the surface of activated T cells. This results in the activation of T-cell–mediated immune responses against tumor cells.
- **FDA Approval Date:** September 4, 2014
- **Indications:** FDA approved for recurrent or metastatic SCCHN, adult and pediatric patients with relapsed or refractory Hodgkin lymphoma, unresectable or metastatic melanoma, adjuvant therapy for melanoma, unresectable or metastatic MSI-H cancers, metastatic NSCLC with PD-L1 expression, or locally advanced or metastatic urothelial carcinoma
- **Dose:** 200 mg IV Q 3 weeks or 400 mg IV Q 6 weeks
- **Side Effects:** Fatigue, rash, hyperglycemia, hypertriglyceridemia, hyponatremia, diarrhea, decreased appetite, anemia, muscle pain, increased SCr, infection, thyroid disorder, immune-mediated pneumonitis

Pemetrexed

- **Alias:** LY231514; MTA
- **Brand Name:** Alimta
- **Type Mechanism:** An inhibitor of TS, DHFR, GARFT, and AICARFT, the enzymes involved in folate metabolism and DNA synthesis, resulting in the inhibition of purine and thymidine nucleotide and protein synthesis
- **FDA Approval Date:** February 4, 2004
- **Indications:** FDA approved for unresectable, malignant mesothelioma in combination with cisplatin and metastatic or locally advanced, nonsquamous NSCLC; off-label use for metastatic bladder cancer, recurrent cervical cancer, platinum-resistant ovarian cancer, and metastatic thymoma
- **Dose:** 500 mg/m^2 IV over 10 minutes Q 21 days. NOTE: Start vitamin supplements with folic acid and vitamin B_{12} 7 days before

pemetrexed dose. Give dexamethasone 4 mg PO BID for 3 days, starting 24 hours before pemetrexed dose.

- **Half-life:** 3.5 hours
- **Side Effects:** Fatigue, desquamation, skin rash, nausea, anorexia, vomiting, stomatitis, anemia, neutropenia, edema, transaminitis

Pemigatinib

- **Brand Name:** Pemazyre
- **Type Mechanism:** Oral competitive inhibitor of FGFR1-3 inhibiting FGFR phosphorylation
- **FDA Approval Date:** April 17, 2020
- **Indications:** FDA approved for locally advanced, unresectable, or metastatic cholangiocarcinoma with FGFR2 alteration
- **Dose:** 13.5 mg once daily on days 1 to 14 of a 21-day cycle
- **Half-life:** 15.4 hours
- **Metabolism:** Primarily hepatic through CYP3A4
- **Side Effects:** Edema, hyperphosphatemia, ocular toxicity (retinal pigment epithelial detachment)

(Abou-Alfa et al., 2020)

Peposertib

- **Alias:** Nedisertib; MSC2490484A; M3814

423

- **Type Mechanism:** A small-molecule, selective DNA-PK inhibitor that blocks DNA-PK activity inhibiting its ability to function in the DNA repair process. This leads to DNA DSB persistence and subsequent cellular death.
- **Phase:** Phase 1 in combination with RT and/or chemotherapy
- **Dose:** 400 mg BID
- **Half-life:** ~5.5 hours
- **Side Effects:** Nausea/vomiting, fatigue, rash, pyrexia

(van Bussel et al., 2021)

Perifosine

- **Alias:** KRX-0401; D-21266
- **Type Mechanism:** Inhibits AKT and MAPK pathways and modulates the balance between the MAPK and proapoptotic SAPK/JNK pathways, thereby inducing apoptosis
- **Phase:** Phase 2/3
- **Indications:** MM, advanced RCC, prostate cancer, and NSCLC
- **Dose:** 200 mg PO daily
- **Half-life:** 4 to 5 days
- **Metabolism:** Potential substrate for CYP450, subfamilies unknown

- **Side Effects:** Nausea/vomiting, diarrhea, musculoskeletal pain, fatigue, anorexia

Pertuzumab

- **Alias:** 2C4; rhuMAb-2C4
- **Type Mechanism:** A humanized recombinant mAb directed against the extracellular dimerization domain of the HER2
- **FDA Approval Date:** June 8, 2012
- **Indications:** FDA approved for HER2-positive breast cancer
- **Dose:** A loading dose of 840 mg IV infusion (over 60 minutes); a maintenance dose of 420 mg IV infusion (over 30–60 minutes) Q 3 weeks; approved to be given in combination with trastuzumab and docetaxel
- **Half-life:** 18 days
- **Side Effects:** Diarrhea, fatigue, neutropenia, rash, nausea/vomiting, stomatitis, embryo–fetal toxicity/cardiotoxicity (U.S. box warning)

Pexidartinib

- **Type Mechanism:** A small-molecule TKI with strong activity against CSF1 receptor; also with inhibition of KIT and FLT3-ITD
- **FDA Approval Date:** August 2, 2019
- **Indications:** FDA approved for giant-cell tumor of the tendon sheath

- **Dose:** 400 mg BID
- **Half-life:** 26.6 hours
- **Metabolism:** Oxidation via CYP3A4 and glucuronidation via UGT1A4
- **Side Effects:** Diarrhea, vomiting, abdominal pain, fatigue, transaminase elevation, rash, dizziness

(Tap et al., 2018)

Pilaralisib

- **Alias:** SAR245408; XL-147
- **Type Mechanism:** An orally bioavailable small molecule targeting the class I PI3K family
- **Phase:** No ongoing trials registered
- **Indications:** Currently in phase 2 trial for endometrial cancers, phase 1b/2 trial for HR-positive breast cancer
- **Dose:** 600 mg PO daily as continuous dosing
- **Half-life:** 70 to 88 hours
- **Side Effects:** Maculopapular rash, nausea, diarrhea, decreased appetite

(Matulonis et al., 2015)

Pimasertib

- **Alias:** MSC1936369B; AS703026
- **Type Mechanism:** Selective noncompetitive ATP inhibitor of MEK1/2
- **Phase:** Phase 1/2
- **Dose:** 60 mg PO daily

- **Side Effects:** Diarrhea, CPK increase
- **Clinical Pearls:** Crosses BBB

(Awada et al., 2012; Lebbé et al., 2020)

Pomalidomide

- **Alias:** CC-4047; 3-amino-thalidomide
- **Brand Name:** Pomalyst
- **Type Mechanism:** Derivative of thalidomide that acts as an antiangiogenic agent and immunomodulator
- **FDA Approval Date:** February 8, 2013
- **Indications:** FDA approved for the treatment of relapsed or refractory MM and accelerated approval for Kaposi sarcoma after failure of highly active antiretroviral therapy (HAART) or when negative for HIV
- **Dose:** 4 mg PO daily on days 1 to 21 of the 28-day cycle
- **Half-life:** 9.5 hours in healthy patients, 7.5 hours in patients with MM
- **Metabolism:** Primarily metabolized by CYP1A2 and CYP3A, but is also a substrate of P-glycoprotein. Inhibitors of these enzymes should be avoided.
- **Side Effects:** Fatigue, asthenia, neutropenia, anemia, constipation, diarrhea, nausea, back pain, dyspnea
- **Clinical Pearls:** Given high risk of clotting events, thromboprophylaxis is recommended.

(Polizzotto et al., 2018)

Ponatinib Hydrochloride

- **Alias:** AP24534
- **Brand Name:** Iclusig
- **Type Mechanism:** A multitargeted RTK inhibitor of WT and all mutated forms of BCR-ABL, including T315I, the highly drug therapy–resistant missense mutation of BCR-ABL
  - Also inhibits VEGFR, FGFR, TIE2, and FLT3
- **FDA Approval Date:** December 14, 2012
- **Indications:** Chronic myeloid leukemia with T315I-positive mutation in chronic, accelerated, or blastic phase or have resistance or intolerance to at least two prior kinase inhibitors. Also indicated for acute lymphoblastic leukemia with Philadelphia chromosome-positive (Ph+) for which no other kinase inhibitors are indicated or ALL Ph+ with T315I mutation positive.
- **Dose:** 45 mg PO with or without food
- **Half-life:** 24 hours
- **Metabolism:** Moderate CYP3A4 substrate
- **Side Effects:** HTN, peripheral edema, rash, nausea/vomiting, abdominal pain, myelosuppression, fatigue/weakness, diarrhea or constipation, increased lipase, hyperglycemia, arterial thrombosis/hepatotoxicity (U.S. box warning)

Poziotinib

- **Alias:** HM781-36B; NOV120101; pan-HER kinase inhibitor HM781-36B
- **Type Mechanism:** A quinazoline-based, small molecular and irreversible inhibitor of EGFR (HER1 or ErbB1), ceritinib HER2, HER4, and EGFR mutants with exon 20 insertion
- **Phase:** Phase 2
- **Indications:** EGFR-mutated advanced NSCLC with exon 20 insertion mutations, HER2-positive metastatic breast cancer patients who have received two prior lines of HER2 therapies, and in HER2-positive gastric cancer patients
- **Dose:** 12 to 16 mg PO daily for 14 days on, 7 days off in a fasted state
- **Half-life:** 5.1 to 9.9 hours on day 1 and similar on day 14
- **Side Effects:** Diarrhea, rash, fatigue, pruritus, stomatitis, anorexia

(Kim et al., 2018; Park et al., 2018)

Pralatrexate

- **Alias:** PDX
- **Brand Name:** Folotyn
- **Type Mechanism:** An antifolate analog that inhibits DNA, RNA, and protein synthesis by selectively entering cells expressing RFC-1, gets polyglutamylated by FPGS, and then competes for the DHFR folate-binding site to inhibit DHFR
- **FDA Approval Date:** September 24, 2009
- **Indications:** FDA approved for relapsed or refractory PTCL
- **Dose:** 30 mg/m^2 IV Q week for 6 weeks with 1 week off for a 7-week treatment cycle. NOTE: Initiate vitamin supplements with folic acid and vitamin B_{12} IM 2 weeks before pralatrexate dose.
- **Half-life:** 12 to 18 hours
- **Side Effects:** Edema, fatigue, rash, pruritus, mucositis, nausea, constipation, diarrhea, thrombocytopenia, anemia, neutropenia, transaminitis, fever, pain

Pralsetinib

- **Alias:** BLU-667
- **Brand Name:** Gavreto
- **Type Mechanism:** A next-generation small-molecule RET inhibitor designed to target oncogenic RET fusions and mutations
- **Phase:** Phase 3
- **FDA Approval Date:** September 4, 2020
- **Indications:** Accelerated FDA approval for RET fusion–positive NSCLC and RET fusion or mutation-positive thyroid cancer

- **Dose:** 400 mg PO once daily
- **Half-life:** 16 hours after single dose, 20 hours after multiple doses
- **Metabolism:** Major CYP3A4 substrate
- **Side Effects:** Increased AST/ALT, cytopenias, fatigue, HTN, hypophosphatemia

(Subbiah et al., 2020)

Prexasertib

- **Alias:** LY2606368
- **Type Mechanism:** An ATP-competitive inhibitor of CHK1 and CHK2 that selectively binds CHK1 to prevent DNA damage repair
- **Phase:** Phase 1/2 trials
- **Dose:** 105 mg/m^2 IV Q 14 days in a 28-day cycle
- **Half-life:** 13 to 27 hours
- **Side Effects:** Cytopenias with risk for febrile neutropenia

(Hong et al., 2019; Lee et al., 2018)

Pyrotinib

- **Type Mechanism:** An orally irreversible pan-ErbB receptor tyrosine kinase inhibitor that targets HER1, HER2, and HER4
- **Indications:** Approved in China and used in combination with capecitabine for HER2-positive, advanced metastatic breast cancer following anthracycline or taxane
- **Dose:** 400 mg PO once daily
- **Half-life:** 11.4 to 15.9 hours
- **Metabolism:** CYP3A4 most active enzyme, primarily excreted through feces
- **Side Effects:** Diarrhea, hand-foot syndrome, vomiting

(Ma et al., 2019; Xu et al., 2021)

Quizartinib

- **Alias:** AC220
- **Brand Name:** Vanflyta
- **Type Mechanism:** An orally available small molecule that selectively inhibits class 3 RTKs, including FLT3/STK1, CSF1R/FMS, SCFR/KIT, and PDGFR
- **Phase:** Phase 2/3
- **Indications:** Approved in Japan for FLT3-ITD–positive AML
- **Dose:** 30 to 60 mg PO daily (continuous dosing)
- **Half-life:** 1.5 days
- **Side Effects:** Nausea/vomiting/diarrhea, prolonged QTc, anorexia/dysgeusia, fatigue, hypocalcemia

(Cortes et al., 2013, 2019)

Ramucirumab

- **Alias:** IMC-1121B
- **Brand Name:** Cyramza
- **Type Mechanism:** A recombinant, fully human mAb directed against VEGFR-2. Has a high affinity for VEGFR2, binding to it and blocking the binding of VEGFR ligands VEGF-A, VEGF-C, and VEGF-D to inhibit the activation of VEGFR2, thereby inhibiting ligand-induced proliferation and migration of endothelial cells. VEGFR2 inhibition results in reduced tumor vascularity and growth.
- **FDA Approval Date:** April 21, 2014
- **Indications:** FDA approved for mCRC, advanced or metastatic gastric cancer, metastatic NSCLC, HCC
- **Dose:** 8 mg/kg IV Q 2 weeks (CRC and gastric cancer); 10 mg/kg IV Q 21 days (NSCLC)
- **Half-life:** 14 days
- **Side Effects:** Nausea/vomiting, headache, fatigue, proteinuria, HTN, abdominal pain, DVT

(Tabernero et al., 2015; Wilke et al., 2014)

Razuprotafib

- **Alias:** AKB-9778
- **Type Mechanism:** A small-molecule inhibitor of VE-PTP, the most critical negative regulator of Tie-2 in diseased blood vessels. It binds to and inhibits the intracellular catalytic domain of VE-PTP that inactivates Tie-2. Inhibition of VE-PTP has shown the ability to activate the Tie-2 receptor irrespective of extracellular levels of its binding ligands, ANG-1 (agonist) or ANG-2 (antagonist).
- **Drug Class:** Tie-2 activator and antiangiogenesis
- **Mechanism of Action:** Vascular endothelial protein tyrosine phosphatase inhibitor
- **Phase:** Phase 1
- **Indications:** Undergoing trials in metastatic breast cancer and RCC
- **Dose:** SC dosing in diabetic retinopathy

(Goel et al., 2013)

RC48-ADC

- **Type Mechanism:** A novel humanized anti-HER2 antibody conjugated with a cleavable linker to MMAE
- **Phase:** Phase 1/2
- **Dose:** 2.0 mg/kg IV over 30 to 90 minutes Q 2 weeks
- **Half-life:** 1 to 1.5 days
- **Side Effects:** AST/ALT increase, hypoesthesia, cytopenias

(Sheng et al., 2021)

Rebastinib

- **Alias:** DCC-2036
- **Type Mechanism:** Switch-control inhibitor targeting tunica interna endothelial cell kinase (Tie-2)
- **Phase:** Phase 1/2
- **Dose:** 50 mg BID PO in combination with paclitaxel
- **Half-life:** 12 to 15 hours
- **Side Effects:** Constipation, fatigue, alopecia, peripheral edema, dysgeusia, peripheral neuropathy, diarrhea, arthralgia

(Janku et al., 2020)

Refametinib

- **Alias:** BAY 86-9766; RDEA119
- **Type Mechanism:** Highly selective, orally bioavailable inhibitor of MEK 1/2
- **Phase:** Phase 1/2
- **Indications:** Highly selective, orally bioavailable inhibitor of MEK 1/2
- **Dose:** 100 mg PO daily
- **Half-life:** 12 hours
- **Metabolism:** Substrates of CYP3A4 and CYP2C19; concomitant use of inhibitors or inducers of these enzymes should be avoided.

- **Side Effects:** Acneiform dermatitis, diarrhea, nausea/vomiting, lymphedema, fatigue, rash

(Weekes et al., 2013)

Regorafenib

- **Alias:** BAY 73-4506
- **Type Mechanism:** Orally bioavailable VEGFR, TIE2, KIT, RAF, RET, PDGFR, FGFR inhibitor
- **FDA Approval Date:** September 27, 2012
- **Indications:** FDA approved for mCRC and unresectable or metastatic GISTs and HCC
- **Dose:** 160 mg PO with food, once daily for the first 21 days of each 28-day cycle
- **Half-life:** 28 hours (range 14–58 hours)
- **Metabolism:** Major CYP3A4 substrate
- **Side Effects:** Hepatotoxicity (U.S. box warning), asthenia/fatigue, diarrhea, anorexia, HTN, mucositis, dysphonia
- **Clinical Pearls:** Assure liver function tests before initiation; monitor blood pressure closely; for diarrhea, prescribe imodium— up to 8 tabs/day. If resistant, first add budesonide 3-mg tab TID, and possibly

also add third drug, lomotil, 2 tab four times daily (QID). For mucositis, avoid sodas, acidic fruits, tomatoes, and spicy food. Gargle with baking soda/water mixture am/pm and after each meal. Swish with carafate after baking soda to coat the mouth and protect. May also add viscous lidocaine to assist with diminishing painful eating. For anorexia, add supplemental nutrition to each meal: ensure/boost TID if feasible.

Ridaforolimus

- **Alias:** AP23573; MK-8669; deforolimus
- **Type Mechanism:** Orally bioavailable mTOR inhibitor
- **Phase:** Phase 2
- **Indications:** Soft-tissue and bone sarcoma (SUCCEED) improved PFS, but did not result in FDA approval.
- **Dose:** 40 mg QID $\times$ 5 days/week for 28 days
- **Half-life:** 42 hours
- **Side Effects:** Stomatitis, fatigue, mucosal inflammation, rash, mouth ulceration, anemia, diarrhea, thrombocytopenia

(Mita et al., 2013)

Rigosertib

- **Alias:** ON-01910 sodium salt
- **Type Mechanism:** A benzyl styryl sulfone compound developed as a non–ATP-competitive, multikinase inhibitor. The precise mechanism of action is unclear, with early report describing it as PLK1 inhibitor and recent reports of it exerting effects through RAS pathway.
- **Phase:** Phase 2/3
- **Indications:** MDS and pancreatic cancer
- **Dose:** Varying doses; MDS 1,800 mg Q 24 hours $\times$ 3 days Q 2 weeks
- **Half-life:** 27 hours
- **Side Effects:** Skeletal, abdominal, and tumor pain, nausea, diarrhea

(Jimeno et al., 2008; Kowalczyk et al., 2021)

Rilotumumab

- **Alias:** AMG 102
- **Type Mechanism:** A fully human IgG2 mAb that binds to and neutralizes the human HGF, preventing the binding to its receptor, MET
- **Phase:** Phase 2
- **Indications:** NSCLC and GI cancers
- **Dose:** 10 to 20 mg/kg IV Q 21 days with chemotherapy

- **Half-life:** 14 to 22 days
- **Side Effects:** Fatigue, constipation, nausea/vomiting, anorexia, myalgia, hypotension, hypoxia, dyspnea, GI hemorrhage, colonic fistula

(Gordon et al., 2010)

Ripretinib

- **Brand Name:** Qinlock
- **Type Mechanism:** A switch-control TKI active against a broad spectrum of KIT and PDGFRα mutations through binding to WT and mutant forms, preventing switch from inactive to active conformations
- **Phase:** Phase 3
- **Indications:** FDA approved the fourth-line treatment of GIST
- **Dose:** 150 mg daily
- **Half-life:** 14.8 hours
- **Side Effects:** Increased lipase, HTN, hypophosphatemia, diarrhea, anemia

(Blay et al., 2020)

Rituximab

- **Alias:** IDEC-C2B8; anti-CD20 mAb
- **Brand Name:** Rituxan
- **Type Mechanism:** A recombinant chimeric murine/human antibody directed against the CD20 antigen, a hydrophobic transmembrane protein located on normal pre-B and mature B lymphocytes
- **Phase:** Currently in clinical trials for other hematologic malignancies
- **FDA Approval Date:** September 26, 1997
- **Indications:** FDA approved for the treatment of B-cell NHL and CLL
- **Dose:** IV infusion. 375 mg/m^2 on day 1 of each cycle, used in combination with chemotherapy for NHL; 375 mg/m^2 on day before FL in cycle 1, then 500 mg/m^2 on day 1 for cycles 2 to 6 in CLL
- **Half-life:** 22 days (range 6–52 days) in NHL; 32 days (range 14–62 days) in CLL
- **Side Effects:** U.S. box warning: Infusion reactions, severe mucocutaneous reactions, hepatitis B virus reactivation, progressive multifocal leukoencephalopathy, fever, lymphopenia, chills, infection, asthenia, neutropenia

Romidepsin

- **Alias:** FK228; FR901228; NSC 630176
- **Brand Name:** Istodax
- **Type Mechanism:** A bicyclic depsipeptide antibiotic isolated from the bacterium *Chromobacterium violaceum* that binds to

and inhibits HDAC, resulting in alterations in gene expression and the induction of cell differentiation, cell-cycle arrest, and apoptosis. It also inhibits hypoxia-induced angiogenesis and depletes several Hsp90-dependent oncoproteins.

- **FDA Approval Date:** November 5, 2009
- **Indications:** FDA approved for cutaneous T cell and PTCL patients who have had one prior systemic chemotherapy
- **Dose:** 14 mg/m^2 IV over 4 hours on days 1, 8, and 15 of a 28-day cycle
- **Half-life:** 3 hours
- **Metabolism:** Major CYP3A4 substrate. Avoid grapefruit juice.
- **Side Effects:** EKG changes, hypotension, fatigue, headache, chills, pruritus, dermatitis, hyperglycemia, hypocalcemia, dysgeusia, anorexia, nausea, diarrhea or constipation, thrombocytopenia, anemia, leukopenia, neutropenia, transaminitis, weakness, fever

Rovalpituzumab Tesirine

- **Alias:** Rova-T; ADC SC16LD6.5
- **Type Mechanism:** An ADC containing an antibody (SC16) directed against an as-of-yet undisclosed protein and conjugated to the cytotoxic agent D6.5 that will selectively bind to the target on tumor cell surfaces and cause DNA damage
- **Indications:** Phase 3 metastatic NSCLC; phase 1b/2 MTC, melanoma, neuroendocrine carcinoma, and neuroendocrine prostate cancer
- **Dose:** 0.3 mg/kg IV Q 42-day cycle
- **Half-life:** 10 to 14 days
- **Side Effects:** Thrombocytopenia, fatigue, rash, serosal effusions, capillary leak syndrome, peripheral edema

(Kavalerchik et al., 2018)

Rucaparib Camsylate

- **Alias:** AG014699; CO-338; PF-01367338
- **Brand Name:** Rubraca
- **Type Mechanism:** The camsylate salt form of rucaparib, an inhibitor of the nuclear enzyme polyadenosine 5′-diphosphoribose PARP, with chemosensitizing, radiosensitizing, and antineoplastic activities. Rucaparib selectively binds to PARP-1, PARP-2, and PARP-3 and inhibits PARP1-mediated repair of single-strand DNA (ssDNA) breaks via the base-excision repair pathway. This enhances the accumulation of DNA strand breaks and promotes genomic instability and apoptosis. Rucaparib may potentiate the cytotoxicity of DNA-damaging agents and reverse tumor cell resistance to chemotherapy and RT.

- **FDA Approval Date:** December 19, 2016
- **Indications:** FDA approved as monotherapy for the treatment of patients with deleterious BRCA mutation (germline or somatic) associated with advanced ovarian cancer in advanced or recurrent setting (as maintenance) and approved for BRCA-mutated MCRPC
- **Dose:** 600 mg BID
- **Half-life:** 17 to 19 hours
- **Side Effects:** Fatigue, increased cholesterol, nausea/vomiting, constipation, decreased appetite, dysgeusia, abdominal pain, thrombocytopenia, anemia, transaminitis, weakness, increased SCr, photosensitivity

(Abida et al., 2020; Jenner et al., 2016)

Ruxolitinib Phosphate

- **Alias:** INCB18424; Jakavi (Canada)
- **Brand Name:** Jakafi
- **Type Mechanism:** An oral kinase inhibitor that inhibits JAK1 and JAK2
- **FDA Approval Date:** November 16, 2011
- **Indications:** FDA approved for intermediate- or high-risk myelofibrosis, GvHD, and polycythemia vera (PV)
- **Dose:** Platelets $\geq$200,000/mm^3, start 20 mg PO BID; platelets $\geq$100,000/mm^3, start 15 mg PO BID; platelets $\geq$50,000/mm^3, start 5 mg PO BID; may titrate all doses in increments of 5 mg PO BID Q 2 weeks to maximum dose of 25 mg PO BID with or without food (myelofibrosis); 10 mg PO BID (GvHD and PV)
- **Half-life:** 5.8 hours
- **Metabolism:** Potent CYP3A4 substrate
- **Side Effects:** Diarrhea, peripheral edema, dizziness/headache, increased ALT/AST, myelosuppression (thrombocytopenia, neutropenia, anemia), ecchymosis

Sacituzumab Govitecan

- **Brand Name:** Trodelvy
- **Type Mechanism:** An ADC with a humanized TROP2 antibody with a topoisomerase inhibitor SN-38 payload via a cleavable linker
- **FDA Approval Date:** April 22, 2020
- **Indications:** Approved for advanced, refractory, or metastatic TNBC after two or more treatments and locally advanced or metastatic urothelial cancer after platinum and checkpoint inhibitor
- **Dose:** 10 mg/kg IV on days 1 and 8 of a 21-day cycle
- **Half-life:** 15.3 hours
- **Metabolism:** SN38 primarily metabolized via UGT1A1

- **Side Effects:** Cytopenias including neutropenia, diarrhea, hypersensitivity, neuropathy

(Bardia et al., 2019; Tagawa et al., 2021)

Sapanisertib

- **Alias:** TAK228; MLN0128; INK128
- **Type Mechanism:** An orally bioavailable mTOR1/2 inhibitor
- **Phase:** Ongoing phase 1 trials either alone and in combination
- **Dose:** 5 mg daily or 30 mg weekly
- **Half-life:** 5.9 to 9.4 hours
- **Side Effects:** Hyperglycemia, rash, stomatitis, asthenia

(Voss et al., 2020)

Saracatinib

- **Alias:** AZD0530
- **Type Mechanism:** An orally available 5-, 7-substituted anilinoquinazoline that is a dual-specific inhibitor of SRC and ABL
  - Specifically inhibits SRC kinase–mediated osteoclast bone resorption
- **Phase:** Phase 2
- **Indications:** HR-positive breast cancer, NSCLC, and osteosarcoma in the lung; phase 3 for ovarian cancer
- **Indications:** Phase 1 studies suggest saracatinib may have therapeutic benefit in metastatic bone disease.
- **Dose:** 175 mg/day
- **Half-life:** 40 hours
- **Side Effects:** Anemia, diarrhea, asthenia

(Baselga et al., 2010; Hannon et al., 2012)

Selinexor

- **Alias:** KPT-330
- **Type Mechanism:** A small-molecule inhibitor of CRM1 (chromosome region maintenance 1 protein, exportin 1 or XPO1), with potential antineoplastic activity
  - Modifies the essential CRM1 cargo–binding residue cysteine-528, thereby irreversibly inactivating CRM1-mediated nuclear export of cargo proteins such as tumor suppressor proteins, including p53, p21, BRCA1/2, pRB, FOXO, and other growth regulatory proteins
  - Restores endogenous tumor suppressing processes to selectively eliminate tumor cells, while sparing normal cells
- **FDA Approval Date:** July 3, 2019
- **Indications:** Approved in relapsed or refractory DLBCL and MM
- **Dose:** DLBCL: 60 mg/dose on days 1 and 3 each week; MM Sd regimen: 80 mg/dose on

days 1 and 3 each week; MM SVd regimen: 100 mg once weekly on day 1

- **Half-life:** 6 to 7 hours
- **Side Effects:** Anorexia, asthenia, cytopenias, edema, fatigue, hyponatremia, liver function elevations

(Abdul Razak et al., 2016)

Selitrectinib

- **Alias:** LOXO-195
- **Type Mechanism:** Selective second-generation TRK inhibitor to maintain potency against multiple TRK domain mutations
- **Phase:** Phase 1/2
- **Half-life:** 3 hours
- **Side Effects:** Dizziness/ataxia, gait disturbance, nausea/vomiting, anemia, thrombocytopenia, myalgia, abdominal pain

(Hyman et al., 2019)

Selpercatinib

- **Alias:** LOXO-292
- **Brand Name:** Retevmo
- **Type Mechanism:** An ATP-competitive selective small-molecule RET kinase inhibitor
- **Drug Class:** RET inhibitor

- **FDA Approval Date:** May 8, 2020
- **Indications:** RET fusion–positive NSCLC or thyroid cancer or RET-mutant MTC
- **Dose:** >50 kg: 160 mg BID; <50 kg: 120 mg BID
- **Half-life:** 32 hours
- **Metabolism:** Predominantly CYP3A4
- **Side Effects:** Dry mouth, fatigue, HTN

(Wirth et al., 2020)

Selumetinib

- **Alias:** AZD6244; ARRY-142886
- **Brand Name:** Koselugo
- **Type Mechanism:** An orally bioavailable small molecule that inhibits MEK or MAPK/ERKs 1 and 2
- **Phase:** Phase 3
- **Indications:** FDA approved for neurofibromatosis type 1 with symptomatic, inoperable plexiform neurofibromas
- **Dose:** 50 to 75 mg PO BID
- **Half-life:** 8.3 hours
- **Side Effects:** Nausea/vomiting, weight gain, acneiform dermatitis, diarrhea, peripheral edema

(Gross et al., 2020)

Serabelisib

- **Alias:** TAK-117; INK-1117; MLN-1117
- **Type Mechanism:** A selective oral PI3Kα isoform inhibitor demonstrating greater selectivity than other class I PI3K family members and mTOR, and a high degree of selectivity against many other kinases
- **Phase:** Ongoing phase 1–2 studies
- **Dose:** TIW of 900 mg daily oral (e.g., MWF/MTuW) or 150 mg PO oral daily
- **Half-life:** ~11 hours
- **Side Effects:** Nausea, hyperglycemia, hyperglycemia, elevated liver transaminases

(Juric et al., 2017)

Sintilimab

- **Brand Name:** Tyvyt
- **Type Mechanism:** Fully human IgG4 mAb that targets checkpoint inhibitor PD-1 and blocks its interaction with PD-L1 and PD-L2; this results in releasing the PD-1 pathway–mediated inhibition of the immune response, including antitumor immune response, thereby decreasing tumor growth
- **Phase:** Phase 3 pending FDA approval
- **Indications:** FDA accepted for review the Biologics License Application (BLA) for sintilimab in combination with pemetrexed and platinum chemotherapy for the first-line treatment of nonsquamous NSCLC chemotherapy
- **Dose:** 200 mg IV Q 3 weeks
- **Half-life:** 35.6 hours
- **Side Effects:** Hypothyroidism, rash, diarrhea, increased liver function tests, pruritis

(Yang et al., 2020)

Sipuleucel-T

- **Alias:** APC8015
- **Brand Name:** Provenge
- **Type Mechanism:** A cell-based vaccine composed of autologous antigen-presenting peripheral blood mononuclear cells that have been exposed to a recombinant protein consisting of GM-CSF fused to PAP, a protein expressed by prostate cancer cells resulting in antitumor T-cell response against tumor cells
- **FDA Approval Date:** April 29, 2010
- **Indications:** FDA approved for the treatment of asymptomatic or minimally symptomatic MCRPC (hormone-refractory)
- **Dose:** Each dose contains >50 million autologous CD54$^+$ cells (leukapheresis) activated with PAP-GM-CSF; dose given at ~2-week intervals for a total of 3 doses.

Premedications with acetaminophen PO and diphenhydramine are needed.

- **Side Effects:** Chills, fatigue, headache, dizziness, pain, nausea/vomiting, anemia, severe infusion-related side effects, back pain, myalgias, weakness, HTN, hematuria, flulike symptoms

---

Sirolimus

- **Alias:** Rapamycin
- **Brand Name:** Rapamune
- **Type Mechanism:** A natural macrocyclic lactone produced by the bacterium *Streptomyces hygroscopicus* that binds to the immunophilin FKBP-12 to generate an immunosuppressive complex that binds to and inhibits the activation of mTOR
- **Indications:** Currently under investigation in phase 1/2 clinical single-agent and combination trials in different cancer types
- **Dose:** 2 mg PO daily maintenance dose following loading; lymphangioleiomyomatosis 2 mg PO daily starting dose (dose titrated per trough concentration)
- **Half-life:** 57 to 63 hours
- **Metabolism:** Major CYP3A4 substrate
- **Side Effects:** Peripheral edema, hypertriglyceridemia, HTN, hypercholesterolemia, creatinine increase, abdominal pain, diarrhea
- **Clinical Pearls:** Monitor fasting triglycerides and cholesterol because levels may increase while on treatment; may consider rapamune-level monitoring.

(Martin Liberal et al., 2012)

Sitravatinib

- **Alias:** MGCD-516
- **Type Mechanism:** An oral spectrum-selective TKI that targets TAM (TYRO3/AXL/MERTK) and split (VEGFR2/KIT) family RTKs as well as MET. Inhibition of TAM may promote depletion of myeloid-derived suppressor cells, causing repolarization of macrophages in tumor, allowing reversal of checkpoint inhibitor resistance.
- **Phase:** Phase 3 study in combination with chemoimmunotherapy in NSCLC
- **Dose:** 120 mg once daily
- **Half-life:** 40 to 53 hours
- **Side Effects:** Fatigue, diarrhea, HTN, nausea, vomiting

(Bauer et al., 2016; Percent et al., 2020)

Sonidegib

- **Alias:** Erismodegib; LDE225
- **Brand Name:** Odomzo
- **Type Mechanism:** An orally bioavailable SMO antagonist that selectively binds to the Hh-ligand cell-surface receptor SMO, which may result in the suppression of the Hh signaling pathway
- **FDA Approval Date:** July 24, 2015
- **Indications:** FDA approved for locally advanced basal cell carcinoma
- **Dose:** 200 mg daily
- **Half-life:** 28 days (<10% is orally absorbed)
- **Metabolism:** Major CYP3A4 substrate
- **Side Effects:** Fatigue, alopecia, hyperglycemia, weight loss, transaminitis, increased amylase/lipase, anemia, increased CPK, muscle spasms, increased SCr, myalgias

(Dummer et al., 2019; Migden et al., 2015)

Sonolisib

- **Alias:** PX-866; CHEBI:65345; DJM-166
- **Type Mechanism:** An irreversible, small-molecule wortmannin analog inhibitor of the α, γ, and δ isoforms of PI3K
- **Phase:** Phase 1/2
- **Indications:** CRC, melanoma, glioblastoma multiforme, SCCHN, and prostate cancer

- **Dose:** 8 mg PO daily on fasting stomach 2 hours before meals and fast for 1 hour after dosing
- **Half-life:** 4 hours
- **Side Effects:** Nausea/vomiting, diarrhea, fatigue, thrombocytopenia, increased AST

(Hong et al., 2012)

Sorafenib

- **Alias:** BAY 43-9006
- **Brand Name:** Nexavar
- **Type Mechanism:** Orally bioavailable inhibitor of RAF, VEGFR, PDGFRβ, and RET
- **FDA Approval Date:** December 20, 2005
- **Indications:** FDA approved for RCC, HCC, and differentiated thyroid carcinoma
- **Dose:** 400 mg PO BID without food (at least 1 hour before or 2 hours after a meal)
- **Half-life:** 25 to 48 hours
- **Metabolism:** UGT1A1 inhibitor; a weak substrate of CYP3A4
- **Side Effects:** Rash, redness, itching, or peeling of skin; alopecia; diarrhea; nausea/vomiting; anorexia; abdominal pain; fatigue
- **Clinical Pearls:** Avoid direct sunlight, use moisturizers after bathing, use mild soap for bathing, and antihistamine for itching. Monitor the patient's blood pressure while on therapy. Instruct the patient on home monitoring. Monitor PTT/INR (International

normalized ratio) closely for patients taking Coumadin.

Sotatercept

- **Alias:** ACE-011
- **Type Mechanism:** A soluble fusion protein composed of the extracellular domain of the ActR2A linked to the Fc portion of human IgG1 with anabolic bone activity. Sotatercept selectively binds to activin, inhibiting its binding to ActR2A and ActR2A signaling, resulting in the stimulation of osteoblast activity and the inhibition of osteoclast activity and also normal bone formation and increased bone mineral density and strength.
- **Phase:** Phase 2
- **Indications:** Myeloproliferative disorder associated with myelofibrosis; MDS; PV; essential thrombocytopenia
- **Dose:** 0.75 m/kg or 1 mg/kg SC Q 3 weeks
- **Half-life:** 23 days
- **Side Effects:** Myalgias, bone pain, injection site reaction, HTN

(Bose et al., 2016)

Sotorasib

- **Alias:** AMG510
- **Brand Name:** Lumakras
- **Type Mechanism:** A small molecule that specifically and irreversibly inhibits KRAS G12C through interaction at the P2 pocket, trapping it in the inactive GDP-bound state
- **Phase:** Ongoing phase 3 studies
- **Indications:** Approved in locally advanced or metastatic KRAS G12C-mutated NSCLC
- **Dose:** 960 mg PO once daily
- **Half-life:** 5 hours
- **Metabolism:** CYP3A4 substrate and moderate inducer of CYP3A4
- **Side Effects:** Diarrhea, cytopenias, hepatotoxicity, fatigue, edema, hyponatremia, rash

(Hong et al., 2020; Skoulidis et al., 2021)

Spartalizumab

- **Alias:** PDR001
- **Type Mechanism:** A humanized checkpoint inhibitors mAb directed toward PD-1.
- **Phase:** Ongoing phase 1–3 studies
- **Dose:** 400 mg Q 4 weeks or 300 mg Q 3 weeks
- **Half-life:** 11 to 41 days
- **Side Effects:** Fatigue, diarrhea, hypothyroidism, hyponatremia, transaminase elevation

(Naing et al., 2020)

Sunitinib

- **Alias:** SU11248

- **Type Mechanism:** Antiangiogenesis inhibitor of PDGFR and VEGFR, as well as KIT and RET
- **FDA Approval Date:** January 26, 2006
- **Indications:** FDA approved in GIST, pNET, and RCC
- **Dose:** 50 mg daily, 4 weeks on treatment followed by 2 weeks off. pNET dose: 37.5 mg daily, continuously without a scheduled off-treatment period
- **Half-life:** 40 to 60 hours
- **Side Effects:** Hepatotoxicity (U.S. box warning), yellowing of skin, fatigue, pyrexia, diarrhea, nausea/vomiting, rash
- **Clinical Pearls:** Swelling of the face, upper, and lower extremities is a possible side effect. Higher risk of complications such as osteonecrosis when taking bisphosphonates with this drug is also possible.

TAK580

- **Alias:** MLN2480
- **Type Mechanism:** A novel pan-RAF inhibitor that disrupts RAF homodimerization or heterodimerization, leading to MEK inhibition
- **Phase:** Phase 1

(Suzuki et al., 2020)

Taladegib

- **Alias:** LY2940680
- **Type Mechanism:** An orally bioavailable potent inhibitor of human Smoothened (hSmo) receptor, a key Hh pathway component, that inhibits binding of an ShSmo agonist
- **Phase:** Phase 1/2 studies
- **Dose:** 400 mg
- **Half-life:** 19 hours
- **Side Effects:** Fatigue, nausea, muscle spasms

(Bendell et al., 2018)

Talazoparib Tosylate

- **Alias:** BMN-673
- **Type Mechanism:** A potent PARP1/2 inhibitor, with both strong catalytic inhibition and a PARP-trapping potential that is significantly greater than other PARP inhibitors. Catalytic inhibition causes cell death due to accumulation of irreparable DNA damage; talazoparib also traps PARP–DNA complexes, which may be more effective in cell death than enzymatic inhibition alone.
- **FDA Approval Date:** October 16, 2018
- **Indications:** Breast cancer, locally advanced or metastatic, BRCA mutated, HER2 negative

- **Dose:** 1 mg PO daily regardless of meals
- **Half-life:** 90 ± 58 hours
- **Metabolism:** Major P-glycoprotein/ABCB1 substrate; BCRP/ABCG2 substrate
- **Side Effects:** Fatigue, headache, alopecia, mild nausea/vomiting, diarrhea, anemia, neutropenia, thrombocytopenia, transaminitis, lymphopenia
- **Clinical Pearls:** Dose adjustment needed for creatinine clearance (CrCl) <60 mL/hr.

Taletrectinib

- **Alias:** DS-6051b; AB-106
- **Type Mechanism:** A selective ROS1/NTRK inhibitor that induces dramatic growth inhibition of both WT and G2032R-mutant ROS1-rearranged cancers or NTRK-rearranged cancers
- **Drug Class:** NTRK inhibitor
- **Phase:** Phase 1/2
- **Indications:** Neuroendocrine tumors or tumors harboring ROS1/NTRK rearrangements or patients with crizotinib-refractory ROS1+ NSCLC; phase 2 for NTRK fusion–driven solid tumors
- **Dose:** RP2D: 800 mg PO daily
- **Side Effects:** Nausea/vomiting, diarrhea

(Papadopoulos et al., 2020)

Talimogene Laherparepvec

- **Alias:** T-VEC; GM-CSF–encoding oncolytic HSV
- **Brand Name:** Istodax
- **Type Mechanism:** A genetically modified attenuated HSV oncolytic virus that selectively replicates in and lyses tumor cells. It is modified through the deletion of two viral genes, *ICP24.5* and *ICP47*. Virally derived GM-CSF recruits and activates APCs, leading to antitumor immune response.
- **FDA Approval Date:** October 27, 2015
- **Indications:** FDA approved for unresectable cutaneous, SC, and nodal lesions in patients with melanoma recurrent after initial surgery.
- **Dose:** Intralesional injection into cutaneous, SC, and/or nodal lesions that are visible, palpable, or detectable. Inject up to 4 mL at a concentration of 1 million PFU/mL into largest lesions first and then in the remaining lesions until maximum injectable volume is reached. May give second injection 3 weeks after initial treatment at 4 mL at a concentration of 100 million PFU/mL. May give subsequent injections 2 weeks after previous treatment.

- **Side Effects:** Fatigue, chills, headache, nausea/vomiting, diarrhea, myalgia, arthralgia, flulike symptoms, fevers, dizziness

---

Talquetamab

- **Alias:** JNJ 64407564
- **Type Mechanism:** A bispecific humanized mAb against human CD3, a T-cell surface antigen, and human G-protein–coupled receptor family C group 5 member D (GPRC5D), a TAA that binds to both CD3 on T cells and GPRC5D expressed on certain tumor cells. This results in the cross-linking of T cells and tumor cells and induces a potent CTL response against GPRC5D-expressing tumor cells. GPRC5D is overexpressed on certain tumors, such as MM.
- **Phase:** Phase 2
- **Indications:** Relapsed/refractory MM
- **Dose:** RP2D: 405 mcg/kg SC Q week (step-up doses of 10 mcg/kg and then 60 mcg/kg are recommended to decrease the severity of neutropenia)
- **Side Effects:** Neutropenia, maculopapular rash, CRS, anemia, dysgeusia delirium, confusion, decreased level of consciousness, lipase elevation

(Berdeja et al., 2021)

Tazemetostat Hydrobromide

- **Alias:** EPZ6438; E7438
- **Brand Name:** Tazverik
- **Type Mechanism:** A potent and selective inhibitor of histone methyltransferase EZH2 (enhancer of zeste homolog 2) that inhibits some EZH2 gain-of-function mutations (including Y646X and A687V), as well as EZH1. EZH2 is overexpressed or mutated in many cancer types and plays a role in tumor proliferation.
- **Drug Class:** EZH2 inhibitor
- **FDA Approval Date:** January 23, 2020
- **Indications:** Metastatic or locally advanced epithelioid sarcoma; relapsed/refractory FL who are EZH2 mutation positive; salvage relapsed/refractory FL
- **Dose:** 800 mg PO BID with or without food
- **Half-life:** 3.1 hours
- **Metabolism:** Major CYP3A4 substrate; weak CYP3A4 inducer
- **Side Effects:** Alopecia, skin rash, hypoalbuminemia, increased triglycerides, abdominal pain, decreased appetite, diarrhea, musculoskeletal pain, anemia, neutropenia, thrombocytopenia, prolonged PTT, fatigue, headache, increased SCr

Teclistamab

- **Alias:** JNJ 64007957
- **Type Mechanism:** A bispecific humanized mAb against human CD3, a T-cell surface antigen, and human BCMA (TNFRSF17), a TAA expressed on plasma cells that binds to both CD3 on T cells and BCMA expressed on malignant plasma cells. This results in the cross-linking of T cells and tumor cells and induces a potent CTL response against BCMA-expressing plasma cells.
- **Phase:** Phase 2
- **Indications:** Relapsed/refractory MM
- **Dose:** RP2D: 1,500 mcg/kg SC once a week with step-up doses of 60 mcg/kg and 300 mcg/kg used to mitigate risk for severe CRS
- **Side Effects:** Neurotoxicity, neutropenia, thrombocytopenia, anemia, leukopenia, diarrhea, fatigue, injection site reactions

(Krishnan et al., 2021)

Telaglenastat

- **Alias:** CB839
- **Type Mechanism:** An orally bioavailable inhibitor of glutaminase that selectively and irreversibly inhibits glutaminase, a mitochondrial enzyme that is essential for the conversion of the amino acid glutamine into glutamate. By blocking glutamine utilization, proliferation in rapidly growing cells is impaired. Glutamine-dependent tumors rely on the conversion of exogenous glutamine into glutamate and glutamate metabolites to both provide energy and generate building blocks.
- **Drug Class:** Glutaminase inhibitor
- **Indications:** NRF2-mutated, nonsquamous NSCLC; metastatic/refractory RAS WT CRC; advanced MDS; phase 2 in combination with cabozantinib and telaglenastat failed to meet primary end point in RCC
- **Dose:** 800 mg PO BID
- **Half-life:** 2 to 4 hours
- **Side Effects:** Fatigue, nausea, ALT/AST increase, photophobia, vomiting, ALP increase, decreased appetite

(Harding et al., 2021)

Telatinib

- **Alias:** BAY 57-9352
- **Type Mechanism:** An orally bioavailable mesylate salt of the 17-AAG small-molecule inhibitor of several receptor protein tyrosine kinases
  - Binds to and inhibits VEGFR-1 and VEGFR-2, PDGFRβ, and KIT, which

may result in the inhibition of angiogenesis and cellular proliferation in tumors in which these receptors are upregulated

- **Phase:** Phase 2
- **Indications:** Advanced gastric carcinoma or GEJ carcinoma
- **Dose:** 900 mg PO BID
- **Half-life:** 5 to 10 hours
- **Side Effects:** HTN, diarrhea, anorexia, fatigue, pulmonary embolism, hand-foot reaction, neutropenia

(Ko et al., 2010)

Temsirolimus

- **Alias:** CCI-779
- **Brand Name:** Torisel
- **Type Mechanism:** An ester analog of rapamycin that binds to and inhibits mTOR, resulting in a reduced expression of mRNAs necessary for cell-cycle progression and arresting cells in the G1 phase of the cell cycle
- **FDA Approval Date:** May 30, 2007
- **Indications:** RCC
- **Dose:** 25 mg infusion over 30 to 60 minutes once a week. Pretreatment with antihistamine recommended.
- **Half-life:** 17.3 hours
- **Metabolism:** Major CYP3A4 substrate

- **Side Effects:** Rash, asthenia, mucositis, nausea, edema, anorexia, anemia, hyperglycemia, hyperlipidemia
- **Clinical Pearls:** For management of fatigue: Encourage exercise and good sleep hygiene, initiate oral care early on (soft toothbrush, salt, and soda swish), avoid direct sunlight, use moisturizers after bathing, use mild soap for bathing, antihistamines for itching, be aware of possibility of lung toxicity, monitor fasting triglycerides and cholesterol. Levels may increase while on treatment.

Tepotinib

- **Alias:** MSC2156119J; EMD1214063
- **Brand Name:** Tepmetko
- **Type Mechanism:** An oral highly selective MET inhibitor that inhibits MET phosphorylation and downstream signaling
- **FDA Approval Date:** February 3, 2021
- **Indications:** FDA approved for metastatic NSCLC with MET alterations
- **Dose:** 500 mg PO daily 30 minutes after breakfast
- **Half-life:** 46 hours
- **Side Effects:** Peripheral edema, increased lipase/amylase, nausea, diarrhea, blood creatinine increased

(Falchook et al., 2020; Paik et al., 2020)

Thalidomide

- **Brand Name:** Thalomid
- **Type Mechanism:** Exhibits immunomodulatory and antiangiogenic characteristics through suppression of angiogenesis, prevention of free-radical–mediated DNA damage, increased cell-mediated cytotoxic effects, and altered expression of cellular adhesion molecules
- **FDA Approval Date:** July 16, 1998
- **Indications:** MM; erythema nodosum leprosum
- **Dose:** 200 mg PO at bedtime (in combination with dexamethasone in MM)
- **Half-life:** 5.5 to 7.3 hours
- **Side Effects:** DVT, edema, ischemic heart disease, hyperglycemia, constipation, fatigue, dizziness, peripheral neuropathy, asthenia, tremor, nausea

Tipifarnib

- **Alias:** R115777
- **Brand Name:** Zarnestra
- **Type Mechanism:** An orally bioavailable, nonpeptidomimetic quinolinone that binds to and inhibits the enzyme farnesyl protein transferase, an enzyme involved in protein processing (farnesylation) for signal transduction, resulting in the prevention of the activation of RAS oncogenes
- **Indications:** Although theoretically promising as a new agent, the development of this drug has not proceeded successfully to date.
- **Dose:** 300 mg PO BID
- **Half-life:** 16 hours
- **Side Effects:** Nausea/vomiting, headache, fatigue, anemia, hypotension, liver enzyme elevation, neutropenia, thrombocytopenia

(Zujewski et al., 2000)

Tirabrutinib

- **Alias:** ONO-GS-4059
- **Type Mechanism:** A selective, irreversible, second-generation, small-molecule BTK inhibitor. Tirabrutinib irreversibly binds to C481 of BTK with greater target selectivity.
- **Drug Class:** BTK inhibitor
- **Phase:** Phase 2
- **Indications:** Relapsed/refractory Waldenström macroglobulinemia; relapsed/refractory B-cell NHL and CLL; FL
- **Dose:** 480 mg PO daily or 300 mg PO BID
- **Side Effects:** Diarrhea, neutropenia, rash, leukopenia, vomiting, anemia

- **Clinical Pearls:** Approved in Japan in March 2020 for the treatment of recurrent or refractory primary CNS lymphoma

(Munakata et al., 2019)

Tisagenlecleucel

- **Alias:** Autologous CART-19 TCR:4-1BB cells
- **Brand Name:** Kymriah
- **Type Mechanism:** Autologous T lymphocytes transduced with a modified lentiviral vector expressing a CAR consisting of an anti-CD19 scFv and the ζ chain of the TCR/CD3 complex (CD3-ζ), coupled to the signaling domain of 4-1BB (CD137) resulting in immune-modulating effects by inducing a selective toxicity in CD19-expressing tumor cells. After binding to CD19-expressing cells, the CAR transmits a signal to promote T-cell expansion, activation, target cell elimination, and persistence of the tisagenlecleucel cells. Tisagenlecleucel is prepared from the patient's peripheral blood cells obtained via leukapheresis.
- **FDA Approval Date:** August 30, 2017
- **Indications:** Relapsed/refractory ALL; relapsed/refractory DLBCL
- **Dose:** A treatment course consists of lymphodepleting chemotherapy with fludarabine and cyclophosphamide followed by tisagenlecleucel 2 to 14 days following completion of the fludarabine/cyclophosphamide regimen. Premedicate with acetaminophen and diphenhydramine (or another H1-antihistamine) ~30 to 60 minutes before tisagenlecleucel infusion. Do not use corticosteroids at any time (except for life-threatening situations).
  - <25 years and >50 kg: IV: 0.1 to 2.5×10^8 CAR-positive viable T cells
  - <25 years and ≤50 kg: IV: 0.2 to 5×10^6 CAR-positive viable T cells per kg BW
- **Half-life:** Tisagenlecleucel is present in blood and bone marrow and is measurable beyond 2 years; T1/2 ~16.2 days in responding patients
- **Side Effects:** CRS, tachycardia, infection, hypotension, transaminitis, headaches, pancytopenia, acute renal failure, fatigue

---

Tisotumab Vedotin-tftv

- **Alias:** HuMax-TF-ADC
- **Brand Name:** Tivdak
- **Type Mechanism:** An ADC composed of tisotumab, a mAb against human tissue factor (TF) covalently coupled, via

a protease-cleavable peptide linker, to MMAE, an auristatin derivative and potent microtubule-disrupting agent. It binds to cell-surface TF and is internalized. Later, the MMAE moiety is released by proteolytic cleavage. It then binds to tubulin and inhibits its polymerization, which results in G2/M phase arrest and apoptosis.

- **Drug Class:** ADC
- **FDA Approval Date:** September 20, 2021
- **Indications:** Recurrent or metastatic cervical cancer
- **Dose:** 2 mg/kg (for patients ≥100 kg, cap dose at 200 mg) IV Q 3 weeks
- **Half-life:** Tisotumab vedotin = ~4 days
  ○ MMAE = ~2.5 days
- **Metabolism:** Major CYP3A4 substrate
- **Side Effects:** Conjunctival eye dryness, corneal toxicity, blepharitis, severe ulcerative keratitis, CK elevation, abdominal pain, pruritus, skin rash, alopecia, anemia, neutropenia, hemorrhage, leukopenia, lymphocytopenia, diarrhea, fever, nausea, vomiting
- **Clinical Pearls:** Need ophthalmic care and premedications with topical corticosteroid ophthalmic eye drops, topical vasoconstrictor eye drops, cooling packs for eyes during infusion, topical lubricating eye drops.

Tivantinib

- **Alias:** ARQ 197
- **Type Mechanism:** An orally bioavailable small molecule that binds to the MET protein and disrupts MET signal transduction pathways
- **Phase:** Phase 2/3
- **Indications:** HCC and in phase 2 clinical trials with many cancer types, including NSCLC, prostate, breast, and H&N
- **Dose:** 240 to 360 mg PO BID
- **Half-life:** 2 hours
- **Side Effects:** Fatigue, nausea, neutropenia, anemia, asthenia

(Rosen et al., 2011; Yap et al., 2011)

Toripalimab

- **Alias:** TAB001
- **Type Mechanism:** A humanized IgG4 mAb directed against the negative immunoregulatory human cell-surface receptor PD-1. It binds to PD-1 and inhibits the binding of PD-1 to its ligands, PD-L1 and PD-L2. This prevents the activation of PD-1 and its downstream signaling pathways. This may restore immune function through the activation of both T cells and T-cell–mediated immune responses against tumor cells.

- **Drug Class:** Anti–PD-1 mAb
- **Phase:** Phase 2/3
- **Indications:** Neoadjuvant treatment in resectable stage 3 NSCLC, advanced melanoma
- **Dose:** 3 or 10 mg/kg IV days 1 and 15 of 28 days or flat dose of 240 or 360 mg IV day 1 of a 21-day cycle
- **Half-life:** 7.7 to 14 days
- **Side Effects:** Peripheral neuropathy, leukopenia, anemia, neutropenia, ALT/AST elevations, nausea, decreased appetite, thrombocytopenia, asthenia, maculopapular rash, pneumonitis

(Tang et al., 2020)

Trabectedin

- **Alias:** ET 743; ecteinascidin
- **Brand Name:** Yondelis
- **Type Mechanism:** A tetrahydroisoquinoline alkaloid isolated from the marine tunicate *Ecteinascidia turbinata* that binds to the minor groove of DNA and interferes with the transcription-coupled nucleotide excision repair machinery to induce lethal DNA strand breaks and blocks the cell cycle in the G2 phase
- **FDA Approval Date:** October 23, 2016
- **Indications:** FDA approved in the treatment of unresectable or metastatic STS (liposarcoma or leiomyosarcoma) in patients who have received a prior anthracycline-containing regimen.
- **Dose:** 1.5 mg/m^2 continuous infusion over 24 hours once Q 3 weeks. Premedications with dexamethasone 10 to 20 mg IV + ondansetron 8 to 16 mg IV 30 minutes before infusion
- **Half-life:** ~175 hours
- **Metabolism:** Potent CYP3A4 substrate
- **Side Effects:** Peripheral edema, diarrhea, nausea, vomiting neutropenia, anemia, thrombocytopenia, hyperbilirubinemia, transaminitis, fatigue, increase serum creatinine, dyspnea, and arthralgias

---

Trabedersen

- **Alias:** AP 12009
- **Type Mechanism:** An antisense oligonucleotides that binds to TGF-β2 mRNA causing the inhibition of protein translation, thereby decreasing TGF-β2 protein levels
- **Phase:** Phase 1/2
- **Indications:** Pancreatic cancer, malignant melanoma, and CRC
- **Dose:** 140 mg/m^2/day IV 4 days on, 10 days off; 10 to 80 μM
- **Half-life:** 1.12 to 2.08 hours
- **Side Effect:** Thrombocytopenia

(Bogdahn et al., 2011; Oettel et al., 2021)

Trametinib

- **Alias:** GSK1120212; JTP-74057
- **Brand Name:** Mekinist
- **Type Mechanism:** An orally bioavailable molecule that specifically binds to and inhibits MEK1/2
- **FDA Approval Date:** May 29, 2013
- **Indications:**
  - FDA approved for (1) BRAF V600E– or V600K-mutated metastatic melanoma, and (2) in combination with dabrafenib for BRAF V600E–mutated metastatic NSCLC
  - First FDA-approved MEK inhibitor
- **Dose:** 2 mg PO daily
- **Half-life:** 4 to 5 days
- **Metabolism:** Weak CYP2C8 inhibitor and weak/moderate CYP3A4 inducer
- **Side Effects:** Rash or dermatitis acneiform, diarrhea, peripheral edema, fatigue, HTN, transaminitis
- **Clinical Pearls:** To prevent rash, avoid sun exposure and harsh soaps. Encourage patients to avoid spicy and acidic foods. Remain hydrated. Encourage antidiarrheal and antacid medication. Instruct patients to report visual changes immediately. Obtain baseline retinal and retinal vein examination.

Trastuzumab

- **Alias:** Biosimilar ABP 980; biosimilar PF-05280014
- **Brand Name:** Herceptin
- **Type Mechanism:** A recombinant humanized mAb directed against the HER2, inducing an ADCC against tumor cells that overexpress HER2
- **FDA Approval Date:** September 25, 1998
- **Indications:** FDA approved for the treatment of HER2-overexpressing breast cancer in adjuvant or metastatic setting and HER2-overexpressing gastric cancer
- **Dose:** Adjuvant or metastatic breast: Initial dose of 4 mg/kg over 90-minute IV infusion followed by subsequent weekly doses of 2 mg/kg as 30-minute IV infusion. Metastatic gastric: Initial dose of 8 mg/kg over 90-minute IV infusion followed by 6 mg/kg over 30- to 90-minute IV infusion Q 3 weeks
- **Half-life:** 2 days (for doses <10 mg)
- **Metabolism:** Cardiomyopathy, infusion reactions, embryo–fetal toxicity, and pulmonary toxicity (U.S. box warning); headache; diarrhea; nausea; chills; neutropenia

- **Side Effects:** Infusion reaction common—observe closely during loading dose; LVEF should be evaluated in patients before starting therapy and monitored Q 2 months.

Trebananib

- **Alias:** AMG 386
- **Type Mechanism:** ANG-1 and ANG-2 neutralizing peptibody (ligands of TIE-2 receptor), with potential antiangiogenic activity
- **Phase:** Phase 2/3
- **Indications:** Ovarian, glioblastoma, brain, colorectal prostate, and kidney cancers
- **Dose:** 175 mg/m^2 (10 mg/kg) Q 3 hours IV Q 3 weeks (with chemotherapy)
- **Half-life:** 3 to 6 hours
- **Side Effects:** Fatigue, peripheral edema, insomnia, upper abdominal pain, back pain, nausea/vomiting

(Herbst et al., 2011)

Tremelimumab

- **Alias:** CP-675,206; CP-675; anti-CTLA4 human mAb CP-675,206
- **Type Mechanism:** A human IgG2 mAb directed against the human TCR protein CTLA4 that binds to CTLA4 on activated T lymphocytes and blocks the binding of the APC ligands B7-1 (CD80) and B7-2 (CD86) to CTLA4, resulting in the inhibition of CTLA4-mediated downregulation of T-cell activation
- **Phase:** Phase 2
- **Indications:** Advanced HCC or biliary tract cancer, TNBC, germ cell tumor, esophageal cancer, urothelial carcinoma (phase 3 global study), high-risk STS, and NSCLC
- **Dose:** 1 mg/kg IV Q 4 weeks for 6 doses, then Q 12 weeks for 3 doses
- **Half-life:** 22 days
- **Side Effects:** Diarrhea, colitis, fatigue, nausea, skin rash, hypophysitis, pruritus

(Comin-Anduix et al., 2016)

Tucatinib

- **Alias:** ARRY380; irbinitinib; ONT-380
- **Brand Name:** Tukysa
- **Type Mechanism:** A TKI that is highly selective for the HER2 kinase domain, with minimal inhibition of EGFR. It inhibits HER2 and HER3 phosphorylation, resulting in downstream inhibition of MAPK and AKT signaling and cell proliferation; tucatinib demonstrated antitumor activity in HER2-expressing tumor cells and inhibited the growth of HER2-expressing tumors.

- **Drug Class:** HER2 TKI
- **FDA Approval Date:** April 17, 2020
- **Indications:** Advanced, unresectable, or metastatic HER2-positive breast cancer
- **Dose:** 300 mg PO BID (in combination with trastuzumab and capecitabine)
- **Half-life:** ~8.5 hours
- **Metabolism:** Major CYP2C8; minor CYP3A4; major CYP3A4; P-glycoprotein/ABCB1 inhibitors
- **Side Effects:** Palmar–plantar erythrodysesthesia, skin rash, hypomagnesemia, hypophosphatemia, weight loss, loss of appetite, diarrhea, nausea, stomatitis, vomiting, anemia, ALT/AST elevations, hyperbilirubinemia, peripheral neuropathy, headache, fatigue

Ulixertinib

- **Alias:** BVD-523
- **Type Mechanism:** An inhibitor of ERK1 and ERK2 that inhibits both ERK1 and ERK2, thereby preventing the activation of ERK-mediated signal transduction pathways. This results in the inhibition of ERK-dependent tumor cell proliferation and survival.
- **Drug Class:** ERK1/2/3 inhibitor
- **Mechanism of Action:** Inhibitor of ERK1, ERK2, and MAPK

- **Phase:** Phase 2 MATCH
- **Indications:** Patients with specific genetic alterations and tumor histologies that result in aberrant MAPK pathway signaling (e.g., GI cancers); relapsed/refractory NHL or histiocytic disorders in pediatric patients
- **Dose:** RP2D: 600 mg PO BID
- **Half-life:** 1 to 2.5 hours
- **Side Effects:** Diarrhea, fatigue, nausea, dermatitis acneiform
- **Clinical Pearls:** FDA granted immediate Expanded Access Program for patients with MAPK pathway aberrant cancer.

(Sullivan et al., 2018)

Uprosertib

- **Alias:** GSK2141795
- **Type Mechanism:** Akt inhibitor GSK2141795 binds to and inhibits the activity of Akt, which may result in inhibition of the PI3K/Akt signaling pathway and tumor cell proliferation and the induction of tumor cell apoptosis. Activation of the PI3K/Akt signaling pathway is frequently associated with tumorigenesis, and dysregulated PI3K/Akt signaling may contribute to tumor resistance to a variety of antineoplastic agents.
- **Drug Class:** AKT inhibitor

- **Phase:** Phase 1
- **Indications:** TNBC or BRAF WT advanced melanoma (phase 1 study terminated); relapsed/refractory cervical cancer (phase 2 trial terminated); MUM
- **Dose:** 25 to 50 mg PO daily (in combination with trametinib)
- **Side Effects:** Diarrhea, rash, mucositis, colitis
- **Clinical Pearls:** Phase 1 study terminated early owing to futility in continuous dosing and intermittent dosing.

(Tolcher et al., 2020)

Urelumab

- **Alias:** BMS-663513; anti-4-1BB mAb
- **Type Mechanism:** A humanized agonistic mAb targeting the CD137 receptor with potential immunostimulatory and antineoplastic activities. Urelumab specifically binds to and activates CD137-expressing immune cells, stimulating an immune response, in particular a cytotoxic T-cell response, against tumor cells.
- **Drug Class:** Anti-4-1BB/CD137 mAb
- **Phase:** Phase 1/2
- **Indications:** Stages I to 2B pancreatic cancer before and after surgery; PD-L1–negative melanoma; NSCLC after failing PD-1/PD-L1 therapy

- **Dose:** 0.1 mg/kg IV Q 3 weeks
- **Half-life:** ~18 days
- **Side Effects:** Nausea, fatigue, ALT/AST elevations, rash, pruritus, decreased appetite, pyrexia, diarrhea, leukopenia, thrombocytopenia, asthenia

(Segal et al., 2017)

Vadastuximab Talirine

- **Alias:** SGN-CD33A
- **Type Mechanism:** An immunoconjugate consisting of a humanized mAb that is engineered to contain cysteine residues that are conjugated to the synthetic, DNA cross-linking, pyrrolobenzodiazepine dimer SGD-1882, via the protease-cleavable linker maleimidocaproyl-valine-alanine dipeptide. It binds to the cell-surface antigen CD33 and gets internalized, then releases the cytotoxic moiety SGD-1882.
- **Drug Class:** ADC
- **Clinical Pearls:** Phase 3 CASCADE trial in frontline treatment of AML has been terminated because of patients' death.

Valproic Acid

- **Brand Name:** Depakote; Depakene
- **Type Mechanism:** An HDAC inhibitor that inhibits NKG2D expression in NK cells as well as STAT3

- **Drug Class:** HDAC inhibitor
- **FDA Approval Date:** February 28, 1978
- **Indications:** Solid tumors or hematologic cancers
- **Dose:** 5 mg/kg/day in 2 divided doses use in combination with chemotherapy due to synergy
- **Half-life:** 9 to 19 hours
- **Metabolism:** Minor substrate of CYP2C9, CYP2B6, and CYP2C19
- **Side Effects:** Diarrhea, nausea, vomiting, dizziness, drowsiness, insomnia, diplopia, edema
- **Clinical Pearls:** Only check levels if suspect toxicity due to high serum levels.

(Roccaet al., 2009)

Vandetanib

- **Alias:** AZD6474; ZD6474; Zactima; Zictifa
- **Brand Name:** Caprelsa
- **Type Mechanism:** A multikinase inhibitor including EGFR, VEGF, RET, protein tyrosine kinase 6, TIE-2, EPH kinase receptors, and SRC kinase receptors, selectively blocking intracellular signaling, angiogenesis, and cellular proliferation
- **Drug Class:** Multikinase inhibitor
- **FDA Approval Date:** April 6, 2011
- **Indications:** Locally advanced or metastatic MTC

- **Dose:** 300 mg PO daily
- **Metabolism:** Major CYP3A4 substrate
- **Side Effects:** QT prolongation, HTN, acneiform rash, pruritus, skin rash, xeroderma, hypocalcemia, abdominal pain, diarrhea, colitis, headache, fatigue, ALT elevation

Vanucizumab

- **Alias:** RG7221; RO5520985
- **Type Mechanism:** An antiangiogenic, first-in-class, bispecific mAb targeting VEGF-A and ANG-2
- **Phase:** Phase 2
- **Indications:** With FOLFOX versus FOLFOX + bevacizumab in untreated, mCRC
- **Dose:** 2,000 mg IV Q 2 weeks in combination with chemotherapy
- **Half-life:** 6 to 9 days
- **Side Effects:** HTN, asthenia, headache, hemorrhage, thrombosis

(Hidalgo et al., 2018)

Vatalanib

- **Alias:** PTK787; ZK222584; CGP-79787
- **Type Mechanism:** A small-molecule TKI of VEGFR1/2/3 preventing VEGF-mediated angiogenesis

- **Drug Class:** VEGF inhibitor
- **Phase:** Phase 2
- **Indications:** Metastatic or advanced pancreatic adenocarcinoma; phase 3 in CRC did not meet primary objectives.
- **Dose:** MTD: 1,250 mg PO daily
- **Half-life:** 4 to 6 hours
- **Side Effects:** HTN, neutropenia, fatigue, abdominal pain, elevated ALP, pulmonary embolism

(Dragovich et al., 2014)

Veliparib

- **Alias:** ABT-888
- **Type Mechanism:** A PARP-1 and PARP-2 inhibitor with chemosensitizing and antitumor activities. With no antiproliferative effects as a single agent at therapeutic concentrations, ABT-888 inhibits PARPs, thereby inhibiting DNA repair and potentiating the cytotoxicity of DNA-damaging agents.
- **Drug Class:** PARP inhibitor
- **Phase:** Phase 3
- **Indications:** Advanced squamous cell lung cancer; locally, advanced unresectable BRCA-associated breast cancer; high-grade serous epithelial ovarian, fallopian, or primary peritoneal carcinoma with BRCA mutation

- **Dose:** 120 to 150 mg PO BID for 7 days or 5 days on, 2 days off, or continuously (in combination with paclitaxel and carboplatin), then continue as maintenance at dose of 300 to 400 mg PO BID (without chemotherapy)
- **Half-life:** 5.18 hours
- **Side Effects:** Nausea, vomiting, fatigue, anemia, thrombocytopenia, neutropenia, diarrhea, leukopenia, loss of appetite

(Gojo et al., 2017; Isakoff et al., 2016)

Vemurafenib

- **Alias:** RO5185426; PLX4032; RG7204
- **Brand Name:** Zelboraf
- **Type Mechanism:** A PARP-1 and PARP-2 inhibitor with chemosensitizing and antitumor activities. With no antiproliferative effects as a single agent at therapeutic concentrations, ABT-888 inhibits PARPs, thereby inhibiting DNA repair and potentiating the cytotoxicity of DNA-damaging agents.
- **Drug Class:** BRAF kinase inhibitor
- **FDA Approval Date:** August 17, 2011
- **Indications:** Unresectable, metastatic melanoma; Erdheim–Chester disease with BRAF V600 mutation
- **Dose:** 960 mg PO Q 12 hours
- **Half-life:** 57 hours

- **Metabolism:** Major CYP3A4 substrate
- **Side Effects:** Prolonged QT, HTN, peripheral edema, headache, skin rash, neuropathy, fatigue, palmar–plantar erythrodysesthesia, nausea, vomiting, decreased appetite, diarrhea, cutaneous papilloma, SCC of skin, myalgia/arthralgia, increased GGT

Venetoclax

- **Alias:** ABT 199; GDC-0199; RG7601; SureCN523816; UN2-N54AIC43PW
- **Type Mechanism:** An orally bioavailable, selective small-molecule inhibitor of the antiapoptotic protein BCL-2
- **FDA Approval Date:** April 11, 2016
- **Indications:** FDA approved in April 2016 for patients with CLL who have 17p deletion chromosome
- **Dose:** Escalation weekly up to 400 mg PO daily. Give on a fasting stomach (food will increase bioavailability of drug). Dose escalation to gradually debulk and reduce the risk of TLS. Consider antihyperuricemic therapy and hydration based on tumor lysis risk.
- **Half-life:** 26 hours
- **Side Effects:** Peripheral edema, nausea/ diarrhea, fatigue, upper respiratory tract infection, cough, TLS, neutropenia, thrombocytopenia

Vevorisertib

- **Alias:** ARQ 751
- **Type Mechanism:** A pan inhibitor of the serine/threonine protein kinase AKT (protein kinase B) enzyme family that selectively binds to and inhibits the activity of the AKT isoforms 1, 2, and 3, which may result in the inhibition of the PI3K/ AKT signaling pathway. This may lead to a reduction in tumor cell proliferation and the induction of tumor cell apoptosis.
- **Drug Class:** Pan-AKT inhibitor
- **Phase:** Phase 1b
- **Indications:** Hormone-positive/HER− metastatic breast cancer; solid tumors harboring mutations in the AKT/PI3K/PTEN pathways
- **Dose:** RP2D: 75 mg PO daily

(**EORTC/AACR**/NCI Symposium, 2018)

Vismodegib

- **Alias:** GDC-0449
- **Type Mechanism:** An orally bioavailable small molecule that targets the Hh signaling pathway, blocking the activities of the Hh-ligand cell-surface receptors patched and/or SMO and suppressing Hh signaling

- **FDA Approval Date:** January 30, 2012
- **Indications:**
  - FDA approved for metastatic and locally advanced basal cell carcinoma
  - First FDA-approved Hh signaling agent
- **Dose:** 150 mg PO once daily
- **Half-life:** 12 days after single dose, 4 days after continuous once-daily dosing
- **Metabolism:** Weak CYP2C9 and CYP3A4 substrates
- **Side Effects:** Embryo–fetal death and severe birth defects (U.S. box warning), muscle spasms, alopecia, dysgeusia, weight loss, fatigue, nausea, diarrhea
- **Clinical Pearls:** For the management of alopecia, encourage to cut long hair short. Use mild shampoo. Avoid dyes and blow drying. For dysgeusia, consider zinc supplementation.

Vistusertib

- **Alias:** AZD2014
- **Type Mechanism:** An inhibitor of the mTOR that inhibits the activity of mTOR, which may result in the induction of tumor cell apoptosis and a decrease in tumor cell proliferation
- **Drug Class:** mTOR kinase inhibitor
- **Phase:** Phase 2
- **Indications:** Phase 2 in metastatic ovarian cancer and NSCLC shows promise. November 2018, Astra Zeneca drops vistusertib owing to the lack of efficacy and toxicity. December 2019, Vistusertib was shown to be less effective in combination with fulvestrant than everolimus and fulvestrant.

Vocimagene Amiretrorepvec

- **Alias:** TOCA 511
- **Type Mechanism:** A replication-competent retroviral vector, derived from the Moloney murine leukemia virus, encoding a modified form of the yeast suicide gene *CD* (Toca 511) that will enter and transfect tumor cells and express CT, an enzyme that catalyzes the intracellular conversion of the prodrug flucytosine (5-FC) into the antineoplastic agent 5FU
- **Phase:** Phase 2/3
- **Indications:** Phase 2/3 in combination with lomustine, temozolomide, or bevacizumab in recurrent high-grade glioma; phase 1/2

combination with Toca FC as intralesional, intratumoral, or IV infusion in solid tumor or lymphoma patients

- **Dose:** Toca 511 dose ranged from 1.4×10^7 to 4.8×10^9 transducing units with Toca FC from 130 to 220 mg/kg/day taken PO.
- **Side Effects:** Very minimal side effects; associated with injections

(Cloughesy et al., 2020)

Vopratelimab

- **Alias:** JTX-2011
- **Type Mechanism:** An agonist mAb that specifically binds to the inducible CO-stimulator of T cells (ICOS) to generate an antitumor immune response. ICOS, a T-cell–specific, CD28 superfamily costimulatory molecule and immune checkpoint protein, is normally expressed on certain activated T cells and plays a key role in the proliferation and activation of T cells.
- **Drug Class:** ICOS mAb
- **Phase:** Phase 2
- **Indications:** NSCLC with TISvopra predictive biomarker; urothelial cancer
- **Dose:** 0.03 to 0.1 mg/kg IV Q 3 weeks (usually in combination with ipilimumab 3 mg/kg IV for 4 doses or nivolumab 240 mg IV Q 3 weeks)

- **Side Effects:** Anemia, hypoxia, diarrhea, infusion reactions with chills, pyrexia, neck pain, dizziness, nausea (can be delayed up to 6 hours post infusion)

(Martinez-Cannon et al., 2017)

Vorinostat

- **Alias:** MK 0683; SAHA
- **Brand Name:** Zolinza
- **Type Mechanism:** An orally available, synthetic hydroxamic acid derivative that binds to the catalytic domain of the HDACs, allowing the hydroxamic moiety to chelate zinc ion, thereby inhibiting deacetylation and leading to an accumulation of both hyperacetylated histones and transcription factors
- **FDA Approval Date:** October 6, 2006
- **Indications:** CTCL that is progressive, persistent, or recurrent after two lines of treatment
- **Dose:** 400 mg PO daily with food. Take with plenty of water and keep hydrated.
- **Half-life:** 2 hours
- **Side Effects:** Fatigue, peripheral edema, alopecia, nausea/diarrhea, pruritus, hyperglycemia, proteinuria

Xentuzumab

- **Alias:** BI 836845
- **Type Mechanism:** Binds to both IGF-1 and IGF-2 and inhibits the binding of these ligands to their receptor, IGF-1R. This blocks the IGF signaling pathway, which is upregulated in a number of cancer cell types and plays a key role in cancer cell proliferation and chemoresistance. It also prevents the binding of IGF-2 to insulin receptor variant A (IR-A), preventing its activation.
- **Drug Class:** A humanized IgG1 IGF mAb
- **Indications:** Metastatic ER/PR-positive, HER2-negative breast cancer; NSCLC
- **Dose:** RP2D: 1,000 mg IV Q week for 28-day cycle (for breast cancer: combine with everolimus and exemestane)
- **Side Effects:** Stomatitis, decreased appetite, hyperglycemia, mucosal inflammation

(Cortes et al., 2016)

Zalutumumab

- **Alias:** HuMax-EGFR
- **Type Mechanism:** A fully human IgG1 mAb that selectively binds to the EGFR and blocks the receptor binding of EGF and TGF-α
- **Phase:** Phase 3
- **Indications:** Designed for the treatment of SCCHN
- **Dose:** A loading dose of 8 mg/kg followed by 2 weekly doses of 4 mg/kg by IV infusion over 60 minutes
- **Half-life:** Increased with dose from 5 hours for 0.15 mg/kg to 66 hours for 8.0 mg/kg dose
- **Side Effects:** Rash, anemia, pyrexia, headache, skin and nail disorder

(Bastholt et al., 2007; Machiels et al., 2011)

Zanidatamab

- **Alias:** ZW25
- **Type Mechanism:** An engineered IgG1 bispecific mAb that targets two different nonoverlapping epitopes of the human TAA HER2, ECD2 and ECD4 resulting in dual HER2 signal blockade, HER2 clustering, and receptor internalization and downregulation. This also induces a CTL response and ADCC against tumor cells that overexpress HER2.
- **Drug Class:** Bispecific mAb
- **Phase:** Phase 3
- **Indications:** HER2-positive, metastatic breast cancer; first-line HER2-positive GE adenocarcinoma, HER2-amplified advanced, metastatic biliary tract cancer including cholangiocarcinoma and gallbladder cancer

- **Dose:** Three dosing schema are being studied: (1) 30 mg/kg IV Q 3 weeks, (2) 20 mg/kg IV Q 2 weeks, and (3) 1,200/1,600 mg IV Q 2 weeks.
- **Side Effects:** Diarrhea, infusion-related side effects (chills, fevers), fatigue, nausea/vomiting, dysgeusia, loss of appetite, peripheral neuropathy
- **Clinical Pearls:** Infusions should be premedicated with acetaminophen and diphenhydramine and given over 2 hours.

(Ku et al., 2021)

Zanubrutinib

- **Alias:** BGB-3111
- **Brand Name:** Brukinsa
- **Type Mechanism:** A highly selective BTK inhibitor that forms a covalent bond with a cysteine residue in the BTK active site to inhibit BTK activity. BTK is a signaling molecule of the BCR and cytokine receptor pathways. BTK signals activation of pathways necessary for B-cell proliferation, trafficking, chemotaxis, and adhesion. It inhibits malignant B-cell proliferation and reduces tumor growth.
- **Drug Class:** BTK inhibitor
- **Mechanism of Action:** BTK inhibitor
- **FDA Approval Date:** November 14, 2019

- **Indications:** Relapsed or refractory MCL and MZL; Waldenström macroglobulinemia
- **Half-life:** ~2 to 4 hours
- **Metabolism:** Major CYP3A4 substrate; weak CYP3A4 inducer
- **Side Effects:** HTN, fatigue, skin rash, hyperuricemia, hypokalemia, diarrhea, lymphocytosis, neutropenia, thrombocytopenia, bruising, petechiae, hyperbilirubinemia, ALT increase, second primary malignant neoplasm
- **Clinical Pearls:** Consider initiating prophylactic antiviral to prevent HSV infection or other bacteria.

Ziv-Aflibercept

- **Brand Name:** Zaltrap
- **Type Mechanism:** Fusion protein inhibitor of VEGF
- **FDA Approval Date:** August 3, 2012
- **Indications:** FDA approved for mCRC that is resistant to or has progressed following an oxaliplatin-containing regimen
- **Dose:** 4 mg/kg IV infusion over 1 hour Q 2 weeks in combination with FOLFIRI
- **Half-life:** 6 days
- **Side Effects:** Diarrhea, proteinuria, increased AST and ALT, stomatitis, fatigue,

HTN, weight reduced, decreased appetite, epistaxis, abdominal pain, dysphonia, increased SCr, headache; hematologic: leukopenia, neutropenia, thrombocytopenia

Zotatifin

- **Alias:** eFT226
- **Brand Name:** Zotatifin
- **Type Mechanism:** A selective inhibitor of the eukaryotic translation initiation factor 4A (eIF4A) by targeting and binding to eIF4A, and promotes eIF4A binding to mRNA with specific polypurine motifs within their 5′-untranslated region (5′-UTR), leading to the formation of a stable sequence-specific ternary complex with eIF4A and mRNA (eIF4A-zotatifin-mRNA). This results in the translational repression of key oncogenes and antiapoptotic proteins involved in tumor cell proliferation, survival, and metastasis, such as KRAS, Myc, myeloid cell leukemia-1 (Mcl-1), B-cell lymphoma 2 (Bcl-2), CDK4 and CDK6, cyclin D, FGFR-1 and FGFR-2, HER2 (ERBB2), and β-catenin.
- **Drug Class:** eIF4A inhibitor
- **Phase:** Phase 2
- **Indications:** KRAS-mutant NSCLC and breast cancer
- **Dose:** 0.07 mg/kg IV on days 1 and 8 of a 21-day cycle

Index